AF882509

Atlas of Ocular Inflammatory Diseases

C. Stephen Foster, MD, FACR, FACS
Pooja Bhat, MD
Tyagan Yilmaz, BS
Rene Cervantes, MD
John Mauro, DO

Atlas of Ocular Inflammatory Diseases

ISBN-13: 978-1-7332376-4-2

C. Stephen Foster, MD, FACR, FACS
Pooja Bhat, MD
Tyagan Yilmaz, BS
Rene Cervantes, MD
John Mauro, DO

Executive Editor: John Mauro, DO
Associate Editors:
C. Stephen. Foster, MD
Fouad R. Zakka, MD
Pooja V Bhat MD
Pranjal Thakuria, MD

Contributors:
Sarah Acevedo-Roman, MD
Peter Chang, MD
Miguel Cordero-Coma, MD
Michael J Gallagher, MD,
Ioannis P. Glavas, MD
David Hinkle, MD
Karina Quinones, MD

(also available in eBook format)

OIUF
Ocular Immunology and Uveitis Foundation
www.uveitis.org

To all of the Fellows — past, present and future, who have trained in Ocular Immunology with me over the past 30 years.

— C. Stephen Foster, M.D.

The idea of an atlas devoted to ocular inflammatory disease seen at the Massachusetts Eye Research and Surgery Institution (MERSI) was conceived by Mr. Taygan Yilmaz, an ophthalmic photographer at MERSI. The Ocular Immunology Fellows at MERSI eagerly took up and championed the idea, convincing me that there was a need for such a resource, and that they could easily do it all, with minimal involvement on my part.

For my part, I saw an educational opportunity, a chance for young doctors to learn by experience just how difficult constructing a textbook, even an atlas, is and at the same time to produce a product of which they could collectively be very proud. The project has taken nearly 4 years. Fellows have come and gone, each benefiting from the experience of contributing to the team and from the education gained regarding manuscript preparation and the various stages which follow.

I am very pleased with the result of this group effort, and I suspect that you will be too. Although the text may be uneven as a consequence of the many authors, it is the photography which is the centerpiece of the Work, and it is those pictures I believe, which will be of most value to you.

— C. Stephen Foster, M.D. Cambridge, Massachusetts

The caring for the patient with ocular inflammation has gained more import over the past few years and at the same time it has become more intricate. Indeed it has become an area of intense interest because of the fact that it touches so many aspects of medicine. Inflammatory diseases of the eye often have an important systemic component, and the Eye MD plays an integral part in the care of the patient. Research studies have shown that ocular mechanisms as they become delineated reflect patterns of responses that are shared by many organ specific disorders. And within Ophthalmology itself, the inflammatory aspects of disease have reached new import as we discover that diseases such as age related macular degeneration and diabetes may have significant immune mechanisms.

Dr. C. Stephen Foster has been a pioneer and continued leader in the development of ocular inflammation as a subspecialty in Ophthalmology. His broad medical training provided him with a solid foundation upon which to work and help push forward his chosen area of ophthalmic interest. This book represents a wonderful visual compendium of the vast array of ocular inflammatory disorders with which the clinician needs to be concerned. The photos presented to the reader will encompass both intraocular and extraocular disease, reflecting Dr. Foster's and his team's great expertise. It will help the reader recognize the important complications of the myriad disorders that the eye care physician must contend with. It is an important addition to the ophthalmic literature.

— Robert B. Nussenblatt, MD

Table of Contents

Part One:

The Basic Principles of Ocular Inflammatory Disease

Clinical Diagnosis of Uveitis

Uveitis is defined as inflammation of the uveal tract, which is the vascular layer of the eye composed of the iris, ciliary body, and choroid. Since it usually involves surrounding structures, uveitis commonly refers to inflammation in any intraocular structure. Diagnosis is based on an extensive review of the patient's personal and family history, review of symptoms, systemic and ocular examinations, and a targeted laboratory workup.

Indeed, the diagnosis of uveitis has evolved considerably over the past 200 years. It was believed to be exclusively infectious in nature. Specific testing and associations with systemic disease led to the important realization that there may be other causes of intraocular inflammation. This has led physicians to recognize the importance of searching for the underlying etiology of the patient's uveitis. This not only helps guide treatment options, but may be life-saving in some cases.

Uveitis may be the first manifestation of a systemic disease, or it may help confirm a suspected diagnosis. It is clearly important to continue diagnostic investigations in patients who have continuing inflammation. An extensive analysis reviewing all the records of patients evaluated by Foster between 1982 and 1992, disclosed that 35% of patients were labeled with "idiopathic uveitis." An underlying cause or diagnosis could not be pinpointed in these cases. Even so, additional, longitudinal laboratory testing may reveal abnormalities in these patients. A careful and unwearied follow-up may indeed disclose a definitive diagnosis.

I. Classification of Uveitis

In 2005, the First International Workshop on Standardization of Uveitis Nomenclature (SUN) established a standardized set of criteria to classify, grade, and describe all aspects of intraocular inflammation.

a. Anatomic Location

The SUN group established that an anatomic classification of uveitis should be used and should serve as a framework for subsequent work on diagnostic criteria for specific uveitic diagnoses. It was agreed that the classification of the anatomic location of the uveitis should be on the basis of the site(s) of inflammation and not on the presence of structural complications. Table 1 lists the most current classification scheme.

Anterior uveitis is the most common type of uveitis, most typically noninfectious. Infectious anterior uveitis is most commonly due to herpes virus. Further classification into granulomatous or nongranulomatous inflammation helps refine the diagnosis.

Intermediate uveitis (IU) includes a subset of uveitis where the vitreous is the major site of the inflammation. The diagnostic term pars planitis should be used only for that subset of intermediate uveitis where there is "snowbanks" or "snowball" formation occurring in the absence of an associated infection or systemic disease (that is, "idiopathic"). IU is usually idiopathic and noninfectious in etiology. Definable causes of IU include: Sarcoidosis, borreliosis, bartonellosis, multiple sclerosis, toxocariasis, and masquerades (lymphoma, amyloid, foreign body, ophthalmia nodosa). Patients who present with intermediate uveitis should undergo evaluation for these possibilities.

Posterior uveitis is more commonly infectious. The prevalence of specific causative organisms depends on the patient's demographic characteristics as well as exposure history. Toxoplasmosis is a common cause of posterior uveitis. When history, exam, and laboratory findings do not suggest an infectious origin, rigorous investigations should be pursued to rule out a more serious systemic disease. This is especially important in patients presenting with retinal vasculitis, as retinal vessel inflammation may presage vasculitis elsewhere. Sarcoidosis, systemic lupus erythematosus (SLE), polyarteritis nodosa, Adamantiades-Behcet's disease, granulomatosis with polyangiitis, and multiple sclerosis are just some of the systemic conditions which may present with retinal vasculitis.

Table 1: The SUN* Working Group Anatomic Classification of Uveitis

Type	Primary site of inflammation**	Includes
Anterior uveitis	Anterior chamber	Iritis Iridocyclitis Anterior cyclitis
Intermediate uveitis	Vitreous	Pars planitis Posterior cyclitis Hyalitis
Posterior uveitis	Retina or choroid	Focal, multifocal, or diffuse choroiditis Chorioretinitis Retinochoroiditis Retinitis Neuroretinitis
Panuveitis	Anterior chamber, vitreous, and retina or choroid	

*SUN Standardization of Uveitis Nomenclature. Adapted from Reference 1.
**As determined clinically

Panuveitis encompasses inflammation in all of the above mentioned locations. The term panuveitis should be reserved for those situations in which there is no predominant site of inflammation, but inflammation is observed in the anterior chamber, vitreous, and retina and/or choroid. It occurs in 15 to 25 % of patients with uveitis.

b. Course and Onset of Inflammation

Table 2 outlines the terms to be used when describing the clinical course, onset, and/or duration of the uveitis. These were obtained from the Standardized Uveitis Nomenclature group.

Table 2: The SUN Working Group Descriptors of Uveitis

Category	Descriptor	Comment
Onset	Sudden Insidious	
Duration	Limited Persistent	≤ 3 months duration > 3 months duration
Course	Acute	Episode characterized by sudden onset and limited duration
	Recurrent	Repeated episodes separated by periods of inactivity without treatment ≥ 3 months in duration
	Chronic	Persistent uveitis with relapse in < 3 months after stopping treatment

*SUN Standardization of Uveitis Nomenclature. Adapted from Reference 1.

c. Patient Age

Even though uveitis may occur at any age, some inflammatory conditions are more prevalent in certain age groups. For example, juvenile idiopathic arthritis associated uveitis is common in patients younger than 16 years of age. Older adults are more likely to suffer from a systemic illness such as SLE or late latent syphilis.

d. Social and Geographic Characteristics

Social and geographic factors are helpful in guiding our diagnostic evaluation. Demographic characteristics, lifestyle, place of residency, and recent or distant travel should always be documented.

e. Source of Ocular Inflammation

Determining whether intraocular inflammation results from exogenous or endogenous stimuli is important when considering an infectious source of inflammation. History of previous ocular surgery, trauma, or recent systemic illness may help establish the offending agent.

f. Associated Involvement of the Cornea and Sclera

Corneal involvement is frequently observed in patient with anterior uveitis. We believe that many cases of uveitis with an associated corneal pathology are most commonly due to herpetic infection. Corneal hypoesthesia, unexplained corneal scars and history of cold sores are additional clues to the diagnosis of herpetic ocular disease. Scleral inflammation is divided into anterior/posterior and sectoral/diffuse. Necrotizing scleritis is typically offensive in nature and is characteristically associated with potentially lethal systemic conditions.

II. History

Ocular inflammatory disease is frequently one manifestation of an occult systemic disease. This makes history-taking invaluable when further investigating the underlying diagnosis. A comprehensive diagnostic survey should scrutinize information regarding the patient's family and personal medical history, including demographic information, geographic history, habits, occupational exposures, and detailed review of medical systems. The physician will then dwell upon any pertinent positives or negatives, depending on the presenting signs and symptoms. (Appendix 1)

III. Clinical Examination

a. Ocular examination and findings

i. Visual acuity, pupils and extraocular motility

Best-corrected visual acuity is commonly assessed with a Snellen acuity chart. Other methods are available for preverbal children and for patients with media opacities, to judge their visual potential. When evaluating pupillary response, both direct and consensual responses should be present. Light-near dissociation occurs in neurosyphilis, multiple sclerosis, and in sarcoidosis. Relative afferent pupillary defects (RAPD) are seen with asymmetric optic nerve involvement. Ocular motility testing may be abnormal (i.e. painful, limited movements) in orbital inflammatory processes, including posterior scleritis and granulomatosis with polyangiitis.

ii. Conjunctiva, episclera, and sclera

Variations in conjunctival / episcleral color may help distinguish inflammation in these layers from scleritis, which appears violaceous, or bluish-gray in color. Tenderness upon palpation further suggests scleritis versus painless episcleral inflammation.

iii. Cornea

Characterization of keratic precipitates (KPs) usually reveals nongranulomatous KPs (small, round, white) or granulomatous KPs (large, yellow). They are commonly distributed along the inferior corneal endothelium. Patterns different from the above mentioned should alert the physician to some specific syndrome. For example, stellate KPs are pathognomonic of Fuchs' heterochromic iridocyclitis, especially if the KP are distributed widely across the entire geographic extent of the endothelium. Interstitial keratitis may accompany uveitis secondary to viruses, syphilis, leprosy, sarcoidosis, Lyme disease, tuberculosis, psoriasis, and inflammatory bowel disease. Congenital syphilis, Cogan's syndrome, mumps, collagen vascular disorders present with bilateral keratitis. Advanced band keratopathy, calcium deposits in Bowman's membrane, causes significant visual loss in patients with chronic juvenile idiopathic arthritis.

iv. Anterior chamber

In anterior uveitis, breakdown of the blood-ocular barrier results in accumulation of inflammatory cells and protein in the anterior chamber. These are graded by the clinician in order to follow the course of the patient's intraocular inflammation and to adjust the treatment plan. In chronic uveitis, persistent flare (protein in the anterior chamber) is unresponsive to treatment because of permanent breakdown of the barrier. Tables 3 and 4 outline the current grading scheme of anterior chamber cells and flare.

Table 3: The SUN* Working Group Grading Scheme for Anterior Chamber Cells

Grade	Cells in Field'
0	<1
0.5+	1-5
1+	6-15
2+	16-25
3+	26-50
4+	> 50

*SUN Standardization of Uveitis Nomenclature. Adapted from Reference 1
**Field size is a 1 mm by 1 mm slit beam.

Table 4: The SUN' Working Group Grading Scheme for Anterior Chamber Flare

Grade	Description
0	None
1 +	Faint
2 +	Moderate (iris and lens details clear)
3 +	Marked (iris and lens details hazy)
4 ±	Intense (fibrin or plastic aqueous)

*SUN Standardization of uveitis nomenclature. Adapted from Reference 1.

v. Iri

Iris apposition to the anterior lens capsule (posterior synechiae) is a sign of chronic anterior chamber inflammation. Iris atrophy, seen with retro illumination, should alert the physician of herpetic uveitis.

vi. Lens

Cataract formation can be secondary to chronic inflammation or chronic corticosteroid therapy. The degree of lenticular opacification provides insight into the duration of the uveitis. Posterior subcapsular cataracts are the most common in uveitic patients.

vii. Intraocular pressure.

Intraocular pressure can be altered from obstruction to aqueous outflow resulting from the accumulation of inflammatory cells and debris. Infectious uveitis, particularly herpetic, is associated with elevated IOP. Corticosteroid therapy may help resolve or may aggravate the problem. Hypotony can be a result of decreased aqueous production or cyclitic membranes.

viii. Vitreous

Inflammation involving the ciliary body, retina, and choroid may result in accumulation of inflammatory cells in the vitreous body. The grading of vitreous haziness provides a measure of the optical effects of protein leakage and cellular infiltration. Anterior vitreous cells are evaluated in terms of their form, color, and apposition to the vitreous fibrils. Active vitritis presents with white, evenly distributed cells between the liquid and formed vitreous, whereas inactive, old cells appear small, pigmented and fixed to fibrils. Focal accumulation of these cells may form clumps known as snowballs, which typically precipitate onto the peripheral retina in intermediate uveitis. Tables 5 and 6 list the grading system used at our institute.

ix. Retina and choroid

Maintenance of the blood-retinal barrier is essential for adequate retinal function. In uveitis, this structure is altered leading to increased permeability and subsequent accumulation of inflammatory cells. Retinitis imparts the retina yellowish-white appearance. Retinal vasculitis may affect arteries or veins, or both. Accumulation of fluid in the retina can result in cystoid macular edema, one of the most common vision-robbing elements in uveitis. Choroidal inflammation may not involve the vitreous because the retinal pigmented epithelium is not affected, preventing the migration of inflammatory cells. Choroiditis can appear as a thickened choroid with prominent infiltrates and/or granulomas.

Table 5: Grading Scheme for Vitreous Chamber Cells

Grade	Cells in Field*
0	< 1
0.5+	1-10
1 +	11-20
2 +	20-30
3 +	30-100
4+	>100

*Field size is a 1 mm by 1 mm slit beam

Table 6: Grading Scheme for Vitreous Chamber

Grade	Description
0	None
1+	Clear optic disc and vessels; hazy nerve fiber layer
2+	Hazy optic disc and vessels
3+	Only optic disc visible
4+	Optic disc not visible

x. Pars plana

Scleral depression permits an adequate view of the peripheral retina and pars plana. It may be affected with exudate deposition, snowbanking, and neovascularization. These are more prominent inferiorly.

xi. Optic disc

Inflammation of the optic nerve can occur with or without other signs of uveitis. Papillitis, neovascularization, infiltration, and cupping are pathologic inflammatory changes involving this area.

b. Extraocular examination

Extraocular manifestations may help support the diagnostic considerations that were obtained as a result of the history and ocular examination. Altered mental status may point towards a systemic vasculitis or infectious condition. Epidermal changes occur in many conditions associated with uveitis. Poliosis, or whitening of the eyelashes or eyebrows, are common findings in Vogt-Koyanagi-Harada syndrome. Additional skin changes include hypopigmentation, loss of hair, and scaling of the skin. Vesicular lesions appearing in a dermatomal fashion are characteristic of herpetic disease. Nail abnormalities are observed in psoriatic arthritis, reactive arthritis syndrome, and vasculitis. Mucosal ulcerations of both oral and genital mucosa are typical in Adamantiades-Behcet's disease (ABD) and reactive arthritis syndrome. Articular abnormalities, arthralgias, and arthritis are components of the seronegative spondyloarthropathies, juvenile idiopathic arthritis, ABD, sarcoidosis, relapsing polychondritis, and Lyme disease, among others.

Nasal cartilage loss should make one suspicious of granulomatosis with polyangiitis, relapsing polychondritis, and syphilis. Regional lymphadenopathy, neuropathy, and hearing loss should promote further investigations. The information provided in this section will help the physician in making a more informed, accurate diagnosis. It will also provide the groundwork towards obtaining targeted laboratory and ancillary tests.

Appendix 1: Massachusetts Eye Research and Surgery Institution Ocular Inflammatory Disease Review of Systems Questionnaire

References:

1) The Standardization of Uveitis Nomenclature (SUN) Working Group. Standardization of Uveitis Nomenclature for Reporting Clinical Data. Results of the First International Workshop. *Am J Ophthalmol* 2005;140:509 16.
2) McCannel CA, Holland GN, Helm CJ, et al: Causes of uveitis in the general practice of ophthalmology. *Am J Ophthalmol* 1996; 121:35.
3) Harper SL, Chorich LI, Foster CS. Diagnosis of Uveitis. In: Foster CS, Vitale A, ed. *Diagnosis and treatment of uveitis.* Philadelphia, PA: WB Saunders Co.;2001:79-97.

Diagnostic Imaging Studies

Ancillary testing is crucial for accurate diagnosis and proper treatment of ocular inflammatory disease. Objective, reproducible examination methods eliminate inter-observer variability and facilitate outcomes analysis.

Fluorescein angiography (FA) was developed by Novotony and Alvis in 1959. FA delineates inflammatory involvement of the scleral, iris, retinal and choroidal circulations. Cystoid macular edema and retinal vasculitis are frequent occult findings.

Indocyanine green angiography (ICG) was described by Flower and Hocheimer in the 1970s. Unlike FA, ICG fluorescence is not blocked by blood because the fluorescent wavelengths are poorly absorbed by hemoglobin. ICG more selectively images choroidal circulation abnormalities in conditions such as lupus, and the white dot syndromes.

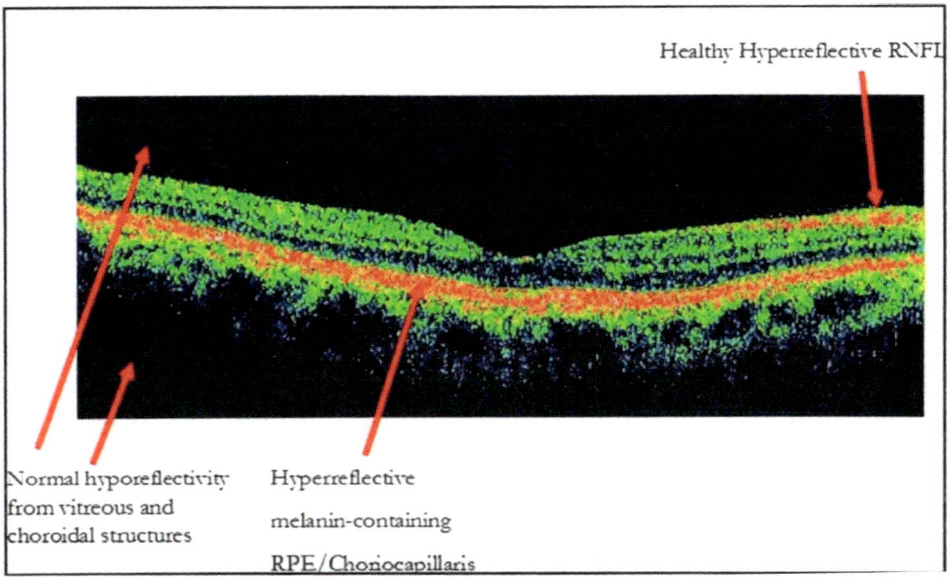

Figure 1: Normal Optical Coherence Tomography

Optical coherence tomography is useful for monitoring macular edema, vitreoretinal interface interactions, in addition to the important role of retinal nerve fiber layer analysis in glaucoma, a common co-morbid condition. Subjects with poor cooperation frequently tolerate OCT better than longer, more invasive angiographic and electrophysiologic studies. OCT should never be relied upon as a diagnostic tool.

Automated visual field testing remains the standard of care in glaucoma management. Characteristic visual field changes occur in white dot syndromes including multiple evanescent white dot syndrome and acute zonal occult outer retinopathy. Full field electroretinography is useful in monitoring retinal toxicity and diseases with diffuse involvement such as birdshot retinochoroidopathy. Multifocal electroretinography is more sensitive for early, focal, and macular pathology. Electrooculography is a useful adjunct to automated visual field testing in infiltrative and inflammatory optic pathway diseases.

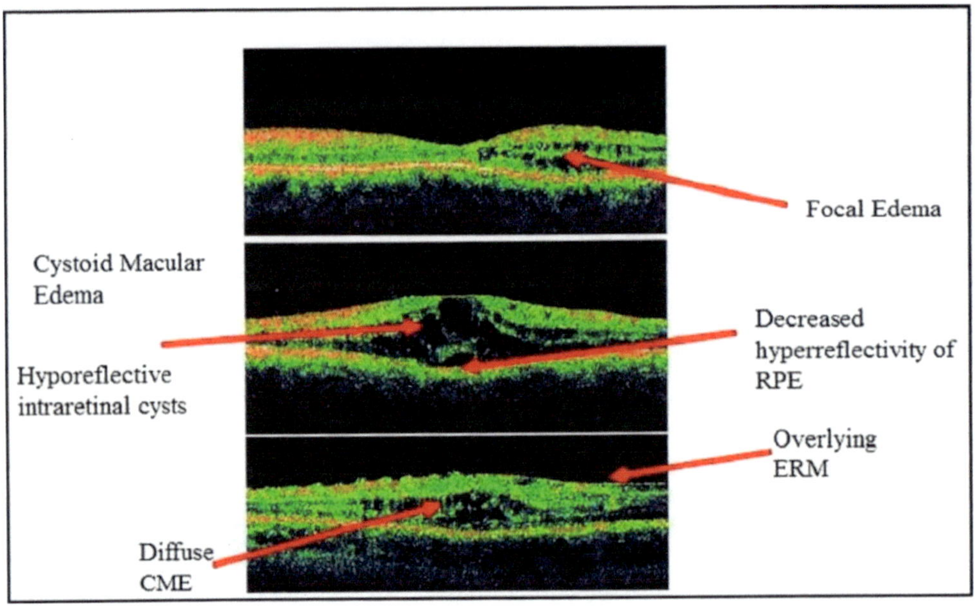

Figure 2: Patterns of Uveitic Macular Edema

Chest roentgenogram and lumbosacral spine films have a low yield in the diagnostic work-up of uveitis unless ordered in the context of pertinent clinical signs, symptoms, and review of systems.

High resolution computed tomography improves the ability to diagnose sarcoidosis, granulomatosis with polyangiitis, idiopathic orbital inflammation, and orbital masquerade syndromes. Magnetic resonance imaging has important prognostic significance in cases of optic neuritis and intraocular lymphoma. Gallium scanning is an underutilized technique in evaluation of sarcoidosis and tubulointerstitial nephritis and uveitis syndrome.

Reference:

1) Chan R, Tawansy KA, El-Helw T, Foster CS, Carter BL. Diagnostic Imaging Studies for Inflammatory Systemic Diseases with Eye Manifestations; in: Foster CS, Vitale AT. *Diagnosis and treatment of uveitis.* Saunders. Philadelphia 2002:104-39.

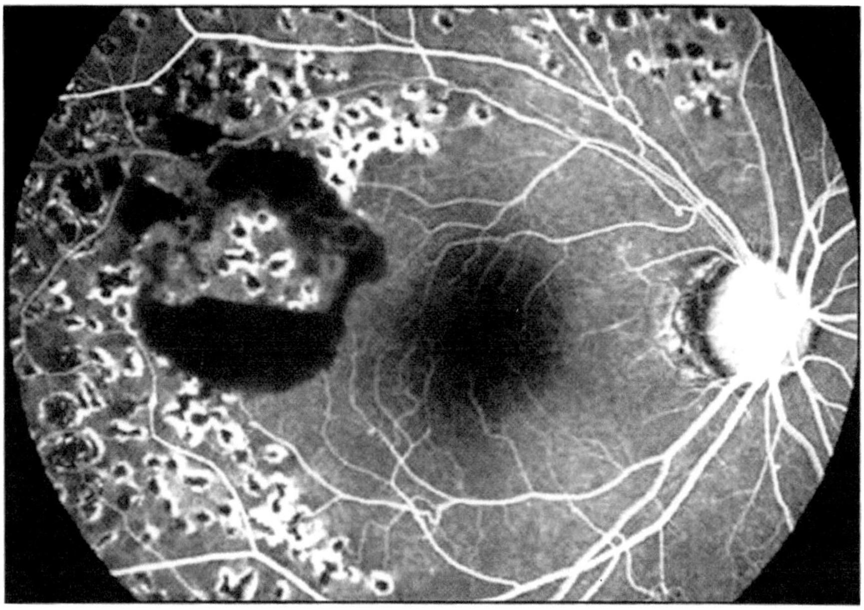

<u>Figure 3:</u> Persistent neovascularization elsewhere despite aggressive panretinal photocoagulation secondary to lupus-related vasculitis as seen on fluorescein angiogram.

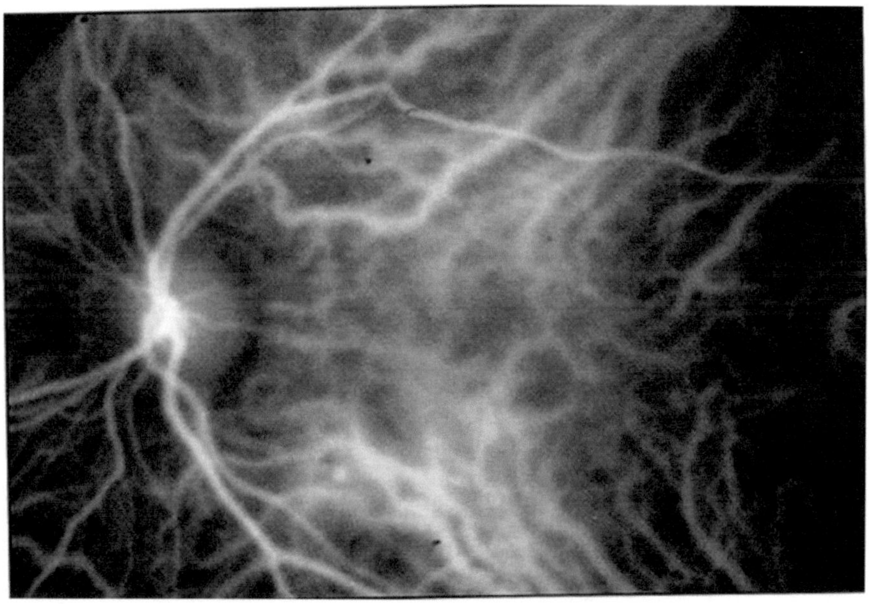

<u>Figure 4:</u> Early phase indocyanine green angiogram showing filling of the medium and large choroidal vessels.

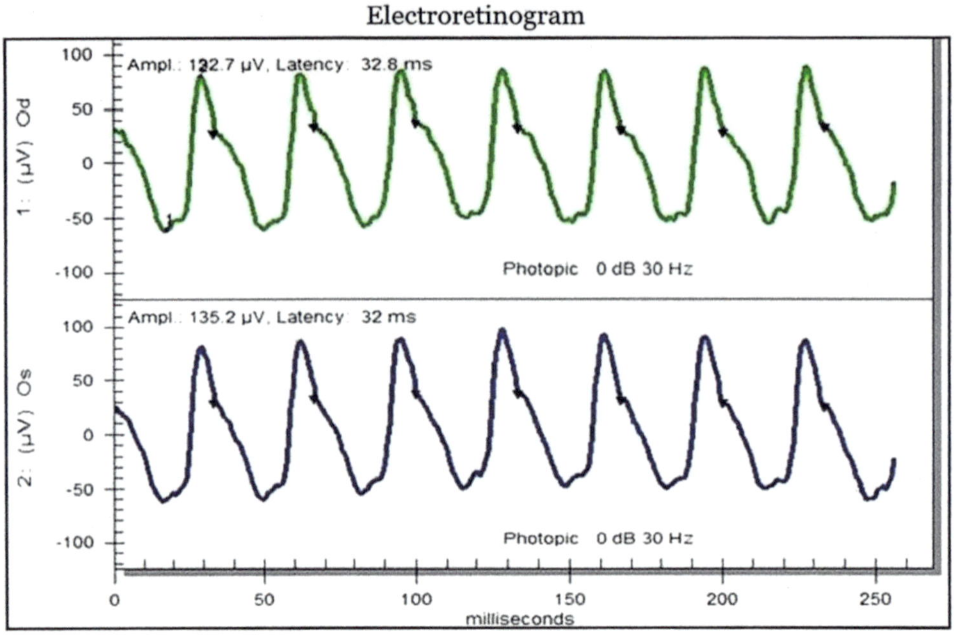

Figure 5: Normal electroretinogram (30 Hz implicit time) in a patient with bird-shot retinochoroidopathy.

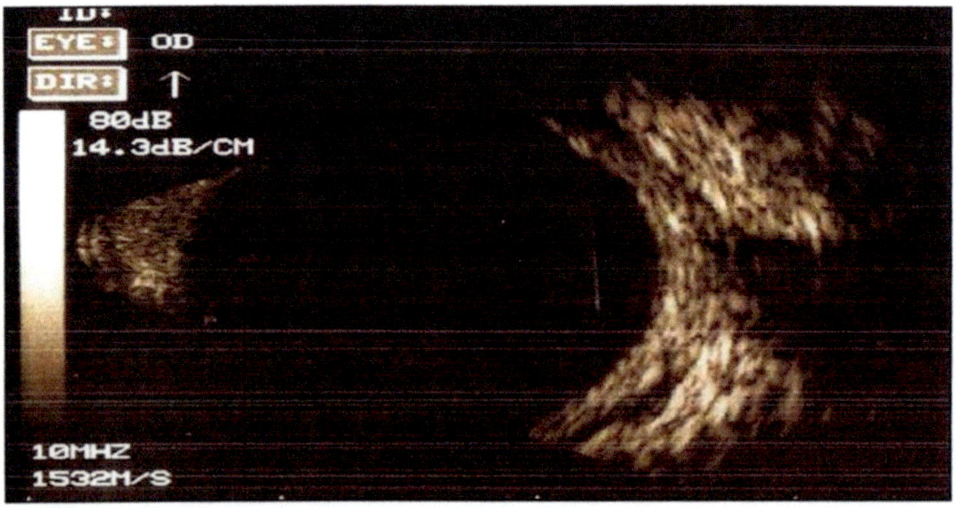

Figure 6: B-Scan ultrasonography demonstating choridal thickening in orbital pseudotumor.

Laboratory Testing

Once a thorough medical history, review of systems, ocular and physical exam are completed, a preliminary differential diagnosis is formulated. Laboratory testing targeting the contenders on the differential diagnosis list is then appropriate. There are a large number of laboratory tests that can aid in the diagnosis of the 85 possible causes of ocular inflammation. Appropriate antigen markers and antibody titering must be included in the lab work-up to rule out the possible causes (e.g. FTA-ABS for syphilis, Borrelia antibodies in the presence of intermediate uveitis, herpes virus infection in all forms of uveitis, Toxoplasma gondii IgG and IgM, etc). Other specific immunological markers are antinuclear antibodies (ANA), which can help in the diagnosis of several diseases, such as juvenile idiopathic arthritis (ANA Hep-2), systemic lupus erythematosus (double- stranded DNA, mouse kidney), polyarteritis nodosa, rheumatoid arthritis, and others. Although the level of ANA may not correlate with the clinical course of a particular autoimmune disease state, the various patterns of nuclear staining may be associated with specific disease states. It should be noted that the incidence of positive ANA increases in apparently normal individuals, particularly in the 5th to 7th decade of life, so this test can have low sensitivity.

Recently, determination of the titers of several interleukins has shown to help in the diagnosis of ocular inflammatory diseases. They can act as predictors of disease activity and severity. Interleukin-1 (IL-1) is well known as an endogenous pyrogen because of its ability to increase body temperature. It is secreted by macrophages in response to infection, but can also be elevated in chronic inflammatory diseases such as rheumatoid arthritis and ankylosing spondylitis. Interleukin-2 (IL-2) is produced by T lymphocytes in response to IL-1. IL-2 plays an important role in the presentation of foreign antigens to CD4+ T cells as well as playing a key role in T cell immunologic memory. IL-2 levels can be elevated in inflammatory bowel disease and other autoimmune diseases. Interleukin-6 (IL-6) is secreted by both macrophages and T cells in response to trauma and, especially, during burn injuries. It also has some effect on osteoclast and bone resorption. It is an unspecific inflammatory agent for inflammatory diseases and cancer, which can be found elevated in rheumatic diseases like psoriatic and rheumatoid arthritis. Interleukin-10 (IL-10), otherwise known as human cytokine synthesis inhibitory factor (CSIF), is an anti-inflammatory cytokine, capable of inhibiting synthesis of pro-inflammatory cytokines like interferon-gamma, IL-2, IL-3, TNF and GM-CSF by cells, such as macrophages and Type 2 T-helper (TH2) cells. It is mainly expressed in monocytes, TH2, mast cells and a certain subset of activated T cells and B cells. Low levels of IL-10 can prognosticate failure in the intrinsic mechanism of the immune response regulation. Interleukin-12 (IL-12) is involved in the differentiation of T cells into Th1 cells, which is important in resistance against pathogens. It stimulates the production of interferon gamma and tumor necrosis factor alpha from T and natural killer (NK) cells, and reduces IL-4 mediated suppression of interferon gamma. IL-12 is linked with autoimmunity, so in patients with elevated levels of IL-12 we can predict a more severe level of activity in the disease.

Other useful immunological testing comprises of complement elements like C3, C4, CH50 total complement and Raji cell analysis (indirect ANA test) to assess vasculitic processes. Tumor necrosis factor alpha (TNF-a) can be measured in serum and promotes an inflammatory response, which in turn causes many of the clinical problems associated with autoimmune disorders such as rheumatoid arthritis, ankylosing spondylitis, Crohn's disease, and psoriasis. In Sjogren disease's it is useful to determine the presence of SSA and SSB antibodies, SSA being more specific. These antibodies are part of the diagnostic criteria for Sjogren's syndrome. When screening for sarcoidosis, one should test levels of serum calcium, serum lysozyme levels and angiotensin converting enzyme (ACE). These markers are elevated during active sarcoidosis inflammation. ACE testing can be controversial in children and can be elevated in normal children. Anti-neutrophil cytoplasmic antibodies (ANCA) are subdivided in two groups: pANCA (perinuclear staining) and cANCA (cytoplasmic staining). The pANCA pattern occurs because during ethanol fixation some antigen targets artifactually localize around the nucleus. Antibody staining therefore results in flourescence of the region around the nucleus (i.e. perinuclear). By far the most common pANCA target is myeloperoxidase (MPO), a neutrophil granule protein whose primary role in normal metabolic processes is the generation of oxygen radicals. This type of ANCA can be found in patients with microscopic polyangiitis and Churg-Strauss syndrome. With the cANCA pattern, binding of ANCA to antigen targets throughout the neutrophil cytoplasm takes place. The most common protein target in patients with a cANCA pattern is proteinase 3 (PR3). PR3 is the most common antigen target of ANCA in patients with granulomatosis with polyangiitis.

Anti-Inflammatory and Immunomodulatory Therapy

Introduction

The isolation of cortisone (compound E) in 1935 by Edward Kendall, and the subsequent clinical demonstration of the dramatic beneficial effects of this drug in acute rheumatoid arthritis, was one of the major advances in the care of patients with ocular inflammatory diseases. Subsequently, Gordon extended the use of corticosteroids into ophthalmology in 1950. Roda-Perez reported the first case of uveitis treated with cyclophosphamide in 1951, and Wong and Hersh cited for the first time the use of methotrexate in the treatment of ocular inflammatory diseases in 1965.

In recent years, biologically engineered substances, such as monoclonal antibodies and aptamers, have been added to the treatment options in selected cases of stubborn ocular inflammatory disease when conventional immunomodulatory therapy is unsuccessful. However, despite the advances published in the past 55 years with the introduction of these non-steroidal drugs for the care of patients with ocular inflammatory disease, a considerable number of patients are not offered such therapy due to a slow evolution of ocular immunologist training in the use of immunomodulatory therapy and the lack of such specialists in most departments of ophthalmology resulting in each graduating class of residents having learned to treat uveitis only with corticosteroids. Regrettably, 10% of all blindness occurring in the United States alone results from suboptimal treatment of uveitis.

We reviewed the literature from the past 5 years regarding the most current immunomodulatory therapy and we include also in this review the new group of drugs known as biologic response modifiers. We will address our main indications for using each drug along with possible side effects. None of the medications described are FDA-approved for therapy of uveitis and as such medications are always used "off label."

Non-steroidal anti-inflammatory Drug

Systemic non-steroidal anti-inflammatory agents (NSAID) have long been used and proven effective for ocular inflammatory conditions, such as episcleritis and scleritis. Although, their use for treating non-infectious uveitic syndromes has been less documented, it is important to be aware of their usefulness in the treatment in this group of patients. The most important potential side effects of NSAIDs include gastrointestinal tract ulcerations, which are more likely to occur with the nonselective NSAIDs than with cyclooxygenase-2 (COX-2) selective inhibitors. Other potential side effects are: easy bruising, hypertension, headache, drowsiness, confusion, fluid retention, and allergic reaction. Case reports have demonstrated the efficacy of oral NSAIDs in intraocular inflammation in conditions, such as juvenile idiopathic arthritis (JIA) associated iridocyclitis, idiopathic uveitis, and surgery-associated cystoid macular edema (CME). Our experience with NSAIDs was in patients with recurrent, HLA-B27-associated uveitis, who were randomly placed on systemic NSAIDs while being tapered off corticosteroid eye drops, from 1986 to 2004.

We generally use the NSAID diflunisal (Dolobid®, Merck) 500 mg twice a day or the COX-2 selective NSAID celecoxib (Celebrex®, Pfizer U.S. Pharmaceutical) 100-200 mg twice a day. If uveitis relapses occur or the patient develops side effects, then we change the NSAID. This is continued for 6-12 months or a trial of three different oral NSAIDs before considering NSAID therapy a failure and moving on to immunomodulatory therapy.

Corticosteroids

At present, corticosteroids remain the mainstay of management of ocular inflammatory and immune-mediated disease. Corticosteroids act by controlling the rate of protein synthesis. Anti-inflammatory effects of corticosteroids include: induction of lymphocytopenia, neutrophilic leukocytosis, reduction of circulating eosinophils and monocytes, inhibition of macrophage recruitment, migration and bactericidal activity with consequent alterations in cell-mediated immune responses, stabilization of mast cell, basophilic and lysozomal membranes, inhibition of prostaglandin synthesis, reduction of capillary permeability, and suppression of fibroplasia. The primary effects appear to be mediated by suppression of proinflammatory transcription factors, most notably NF-KB, and by inhibition of phospholipase A2 production.

Topical corticosteroids (e.g. prednisolone acetate) are mainly used in non- infectious anterior uveitis. Topical application can be as frequent as needed (e.g. every 15 minutes while awake in an acute attack of anterior uveitis), but they are associated, if used for a long time, with well known side effects such as cataracts and secondary glaucoma. Patients with posterior uveitis will not respond to topical corticosteroids and oral, periocular, intraocular or intravenous administration is more suitable for patients with posterior uveitis.

Prednisone is the preferred oral corticosteroid, and is typically prescribed at 1-2 mg/kg/day and tapered off by a decrease of io mg every week. At 20 mg daily, further decrease is by 5 mg every week.

Methylprednisolone is a very effective intravenous corticosteroid and is used in patients with severe, vision or life-threatening ocular inflammation (e.g. severe acute anterior uveitis or Adamantiades-Behget's Disease (ABD)). It is delivered in intravenous pulses of 250-1000 mg. Methylprednisolone rapidly controls inflammation, but is associated with more acute side effects, such as severe hyperglycemia.

Systemic corticosteroids are associated with numerous potential side effects, some of which are guaranteed if used chronically (Table 1). The chronic use of systemic corticosteroids should be avoided in the case of patients with ocular inflammatory disease, unless doses of prednisone 5 mg or less a day can be employed. Such a dose is not associated with serious side effects in chronic use. If the patient requires more than 5 mg of prednisone, bone preservation strategies are advisable such as the use of calcium, vitamin D, and bisphosphonate or in the case of bisphosphonate contraindication, salmon calcitonin. Changes in lifestyle are also advised (e.g. increasing physical activities, diet, smoking cessation). Moreover, childbearing females should avoid pregnancy.

Table 1. NONOCULAR COMPLICATIONS OF CORTICOSTEROIDS THERAPY

Cardiovascular	Immunologic
Hypertension	Delayed tissue healing
Sodium and fluid retention	Impaired inflammatory response
Dermatologic	Metabolic
Acne	Hyperlipidemia
Hirsutism	Hyperosmotic, Hyperglycemic, or nonketonic coma
Striae	Secondary diabetes mellitus
Subcutaneous tissue atrophy	
Endocrine	Musculoskeleta
Adrenal insufficiency	Aseptic hip necrosis
Cushing's syndrome	Osteoporosis
Menstrual disorders	Vertebral compression fractures
Gastrointestinal	Neuropsychiatric
Gastric hemorrhage	Depression
Intestinal perforation	Insomnia
Pancreatitis	Mood swings
Peptic ulcer	Pseudotumor cerebri
	Psychosis

Immunomodulatory Therapy

In the past decade, there has been an important development of several modalities and effective treatment strategies for the management of ocular inflammatory disease. The goal of this therapy is to modulate the immune inflammatory response, whether it is due to trauma, surgery, infection, or response to foreign or self antigens, in an attempt to avoid ocular damage.

Immunomodulatory agents suppress at least one type of immune reaction. A common feature of this group of drugs is their ability to interfere with the synthesis of nucleic acids or proteins or both. The immunomodulatory drugs are used for the control of several ocular conditions that are shown by class in Table 2. Because of concerns regarding their low therapeutic index, immunomodulatory agents were reserved just for sight-threatening, steroid-resistant ocular inflammatory diseases. Currently these drugs are not only used as steroid-sparing agents, but they are often used as first-line therapy in life/sight threatening disease such as granulomatosis with polyangiitis, Adamantiades-Behget's disease, sympathetic ophthalmia, and Vogt-

Table 2. Immunomodulatory Therapy Drug by Class

Adjuvant	**Biologic**
Bromocriptin	Adalimumab
Colchicin	Alemtuzumab
Ketoconazole	Daclizumab
	Infliximab
Alkylating Agent	Interferon
Chlorambucil	Intravenous immunoglobulin
Cyclophosphamide	Rituximab
Antimetabolite	**Signal Transduction Inhibitors**
Azathioprine	Cyclosporine
Methotrexate	Sirolimus
Mycophenolate Mofetil	Tacrolimus

Koyanagi- Harad disease. Lists of specific immunomodulators used are summarized in Table 3. The safe use of these drugs begins with exclusion of infectious, mechanical, or other treatable causes of ocular inflammation. Informed consent must be obtained and documented, once the treating physician explained thoroughly all the potential risk and benefits of the immunomodulatory therapy. The potential side effects of immunomodulatory therapy are summarized in Table 4.

The choice of the immunomodulatory agent must be individualized for each patient and depends on a variety of factors, such as underlying disease, patient's age, sex, and general health status. The clinician who is going to be involved in the management of immunomodulatory therapy has to be familiarized and to be an expert in the use of these agents and in the recognition and treatment of potential serious adverse effects. If the ophthalmologist in charge does not have the experience in the management of these agents, collaboration with a chemotherapist is advised. Patients have to be followed each 6 weeks with total blood count and liver function testing in addition to other specific tests, if required, during immunomodulatory therapy.

The goal of immunomodulatory therapy is to achieve drug-free durable remission. In our experience we keep treating our patient free of inflammation and consider tapering the drug(s) in most patients after 2-year relapse-free period. In conclusion, immunomodulatory therapy is useful for the treatment of chronic, recalcitrant, and steroid-resistant inflammatory disease with acceptable side effects that can be minimized by careful monitoring and awareness.

Table 3. Main indications for specific immunosuppressive drugs

Drug	Indication
Adalimumab	Adamantiades-Behget's disease, Juvenile idiopathic arthritis-associated uveitis
Alemtuzumab	Adamantiades-Behget's disease
Azathioprine	Adamantiades-Behget's disease, juvenile idiopathic arthritis-associated uveitis, granulomatosis with polyangiitis, systemic lupus erythematosus, scleritis, ocular cicatricial pemphigoid
Chlorambucil	Adamantiades-Behcet's disease, sympathetic ophthalmia, juvenile idiopathic arthritis-associated-uveitis
Cyclophosphamide	Granulomatosis with polyangiitis, polyarteritis nodosa, rheumatoid arthritis-associated necrotizing scleritis, relapsing polychondritis-associated sclertis, sympathet ic ophthalmia, Adamantiades-Behcet's disease, ocular cicatricial pemphigoid
Cyclosporine	Birdshot choroidoretinopathy, Adamantiades-Behcet's disease, sarcoidosis-associated uveitis, Vogt-Koyanagi-Harada syndrome, sympathetic ophthalmia
Daclizumab	Idiopathic posterior uveitis, scleritis
Infliximab	Adamantiades-Behget's disease, Juvenile idiopathic arthritis-associated uveitis, posterior idiopathic uveitis
Interferons	Adamantiades-Behget's disease, serpiginous choroiditis
Intravenous immunoglobulin	Ocular cicatricial pemphigoid, posterior idiopathic uveitis, idiopathic panuveitis
Methotrexate	Sympathetic ophthalmia, scleritis, juvenile idiopathic arthritis-associated uveitis, sarcoidosis-associated uveitis, Vogt-Koyanagi Harada
Mycophenolate mofetil	Juvenile idiopathic arthritis-associated uveitis, systemic lupus erythematosus, birdshot choroidoretinopathy, orbital pseudotumor
Sirolimus	Adjunct to cyclosporine
Tacrolimus	Adamantiades-Behcet's disease, idiopathic posterior uveitis

Table 4. Potential side effects of immunomodulatory therapy

Drug	Side effect
Adalimumab	Injection site discomfort, opportunistic infections
Alemtuzumab	Anaphylaxis, leukopenia, pneumonitis, liver toxicity, pancreatitis
Azathioprine	Bone marrow suppression, nausea, secondary infections
Bromocriptine	Postural hypotension, methemoglobinemia, nausea, mononucleosis-like syndrome, blurred vision
Chlorambucil	Bone marrow suppression, gonadal dysfunction, secondary malignancies
Colchicine	Nausea, vomiting, diarrhea, bone marrow suppression
Cyclophosphamide	Sterile hemorrhagic cystitis, bone marrow suppression, alopecia (reversible), secondary malignancies, transient blurry vision
Cyclosporine	High blood pressure, osteoporosis, gingival hyperplasia, nephrotoxicity, hyperglycemia, liver toxicity, nausea vomiting
Daclizumab	Gastrointestinal upset, liver toxicity, fatigue, skin rash, leukopenia
Infliximab	Lupus induced syndrome, tuberculosis infection reactivation, opportunistic infections, anaphylaxis, sepsis
Interferon	Fever, arthralgias, antinuclear antibodies, depression, leukopenia
Intravenous immunoglobulin	Headaches, high blood pressure (transient), nausea, vomiting, tachycardia
Ketoconazole	Liver toxicity, endocrine abnormalities, gastrointestinal upset
Methotrexate	Liver toxicity, ulcerative stomatitis, bone marrow suppression, diarrhea, sun light sensitivity, pneumonitis
Mycophenolate mofetil	Diarrhea, vomiting, gastrointestinal upset, leukopenia, hair loss, secondary infection
Sirolimus	Skin rash, hypercholesterolemia, gastrointestinal upset
Tacrolimus	High blood pressures (less likely than cyclosporine), headache, electrolytes disturbances

References:

1) Roda-Perez E: Sobre un case se uveitis de etiologia ignota tratando con mostaza introgenada. *Rev Clin Esp* 1951;40:265-267
2) Wong VG, Hersh EM: Methotrexate in the therapy of cyclitis. *Trans Am Acad Opthalmol Otolaryngol* 1965;69:279-293
3) Teasley L, Christen W, Foster CS. Oral non-steroidal agents in the treatment of chronic or recurrent non infectious uveitis. *Contemporary Ophthalmology* (in press).
4) Cunningham ETJ: Diagnosis and management of acute anterior uveitis. *In Focal Points.* Edited by Ophthalmology AAO; published by The American Academy of Ophthalmology, San Francisco, CA, 2002.
5) Rothova A: Corticosteroids in uveitis. *Ophthalmol Clin North Am* 2002, 15:389-394.
6) Carnahan MC, Goldstein DA: Ocular complications of topical, periocular, and systemic corticosteroids. *Curr Opin Ophthalmol* 2000, 11:478-483.
7) Monnet D, Moachon L, Dougados M, Brezin AP. Severe uveitis in an HLA-B27-positive patient with ankylosing spondylitis.*Nat Clin Pract Rheumatol.* 2006 Jul;2(7):393-7.
8) Wakefield D. Methylprednisolone pulse therapy in severe anterior uveitis. *Aust N Z J Ophthalmol.* 1985 Nov;13(4):411-5.
9) Reed JB, Morse LS, Schwab IR. High-dose intravenous pulse methylprednisolone hemisuccinate in acute Behcet retinitis. *Am J Ophthalmol.* 1998 Mar;125(3):409-11.
10) Wakefield D, McCluskey P, Penny R. Intravenous pulse methylprednisolone therapy in severe inflammatory eye disease. *Arch Ophthalmol.* 1986 Jun;104 (6): 847-51.
11) Jabs DA, Rosenbaum JT, Foster CS, et al.: Guidelines for the use of immunosuppressive drugs in patients with ocular inflammatory disorders: recommendations of an expert panel. *Am J Ophthalmol* 2000, 130:492-513.
12) Picado C, Luengo M. Corticosteroid-induced bone loss. Prevention and management. *Drug Saf* 1996;15:347-59.
13) Jabs DA, Rosenbaum JT, Foster CS, Holland GN, Jaffe GJ, Louie JS, Nussenblatt RB, Stiehm ER, Tessler H, Van Gelder RN, Whitcup SM, Yocum D. Guidelines for the use of immunosuppressive drugs in patients with ocular inflammatory disorders: recommendations of an expert panel. *Am J Ophthalmol.* 2000 OCT; 130(4) 492-513 .

Adamantiades-Behcet's Disease

Definition: Adamantiades-Behget's disease (ABD) is a recurrent systemic inflammatory disorder of unknown etiology characterized by oral and genital ulcerations, skin lesions, and recurrent uveitis. The vascular system, central nervous system (CNS), gastrointestinal tract, kidneys, lungs and joints may also be affected.

History: This condition has been recognized since ancient times. Hippocrates first and some other authors later described some of the symptoms of the disease. However, it was in the twentieth century when two independent doctors, one from Greece in 1931 (Benedictos Adamantiades) and another from Turkey in 1937 (Hulusi Behget), gave an accurate description of ABD, and were the first to consider it as an individual entity among the inflammatory disorders.

Epidemiology: ABD has a worldwide distribution, but it is most prevalent in the Middle and Far East, along the latitudes 30 to 45 degrees north in Asia and the Mediterranean Basin, which corresponds to the old Silk Route used by traders from the Far East to Europe. In Turkey, .008% to .003% of the population is affected, where it has the highest prevalence. Elsewhere, the prevalence of ABD among patients with uveitis ranges from 0.2 to 0.4% in United States to more than 20% in Japan.

Clinical Features:

Systemic manifestations: Recurrent oral aphthae is the most frequent finding in ABD, producing a significant discomfort. Cutaneous involvement is also frequent in ABD with a wide spectrum of manifestations including erythema nodosum, superficial thrombophlebitis, skin eruptions or pathergy (development of sterile pustules at sites of spontaneous or induced trauma). Although vasculitis as the presenting symptom is rare, vessels of any size may be affected. Four types of vascular lesions are recognized: arterial occlusion, aneurysms, venous occlusion, and varices. Nervous system involvement, either caused by primary neural parenchymal lesions (neuro-ABD) or by major vascular involvement (vasculo-ABD), is one of the most serious features of ABD. There may be genitourinary, gastrointestinal, pulmonary and joint problems that may arise due to the systemic nature of this disease.

Ocular manifestations: Ocular involvement occurs in 43% to 72% and loss of sight occurs in 25% of ABD patients. Nongranulomatous inflammation with necrotizing obliterative vasculitis may be found either in the anterior or the posterior segment, or, more commonly, in both.

Anterior segment: Anterior non-granulomatous uveitis may be the only ocular manifestation of ABD. The classic iridocyclitis with hypopyon is present in only 19% to 31% of cases. Other less common anterior segment findings are episcleritis, keratitis, conjunctival ulcers and subconjunctival hemorrhages.

Posterior Segment: Vitritis is always present during the acute phase of ABD. The essential retinal finding is severe obliterative vasculitis (affecting both the arteries and veins) with marked infiltration of leukocytes in and around blood vessels and into retinal tissues. Retinal vasculitis can affect macular and/or peripheral blood vessels and may lead to ischemic retinal changes because of vascular occlusion. Bleeding into the vitreous cavity can lead to organization with membrane formation. Atrophy of the retinal pigment epithelium can be observed as well. Other findings are retinal edema (especially in the macula), sheathing of the veins (which often precedes sheathing of the arterioles) and choroidal vascular involvement. The optic nerve is affected in at least one-fourth of ABD patients, and papillitis is observed quite frequently. Recurrent episodes of inflammation may lead to progressive optic atrophy.

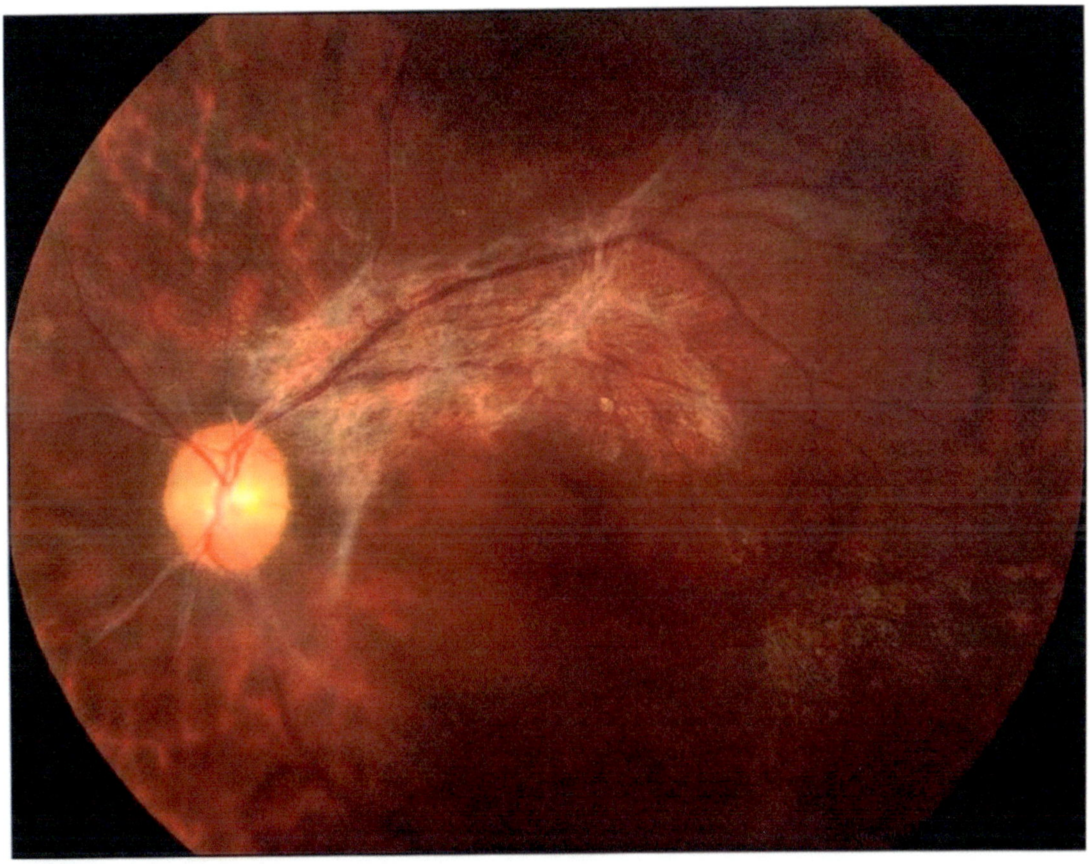

Figure 7: Perivascular fibrosis along the superior arcade as a result of previous inflammation caused by ABD. The visual acuity was 20/60.

Pathology/Pathogenesis: ABD is primarily an inflammatory disorder involving small blood vessels, particularly venules. The cause of ABD remains unknown. Environmental factors, infectious agents (as herpes simplex virus type 1) and genetic factors (HLA B51 is the major disease susceptibility gene for ABD). Although there are disagreements as to whether ABD should be considered an autoimmune disease, autoimmune mechanisms are truly implicated in the pathogenesis of ABD. The early lesions resemble a delayed-type hypersensitivity reaction, whereas the late lesions resemble an immune complex-type reaction.

Diagnosis: Diagnosis of ABD is based on clinical observation. Therefore, the criteria defined either by the International Study Group of Behget's disease or the Japanese Research Committee of Behget's disease should be applied. There are no specific tests for ABD, but some are helpful for evaluation.

Fluorescein Angiography(FA) and Indocyanine Green Angiography(ICG): FA is mandatory in the study and longitudinal care of patients with ocular ABD. FA shows marked dilatation and occlusion of the retinal capillaries in patients with ABD. During acute inflammation, there is diffuse fluorescein leakage from the retinal capillaries, the larger engorged vessels, and the optic disc. Persistent diffuse dye leakage is seen even with resolution of inflammatory episodes. Macular alterations such as edema or gliosis may also be observed. Some abnormalities of the choroidal vasculature are revealed only with ICG.

Electrophysiology: Flash electroretinography (ERG) plus pattern visually evoked potentials may be helpful not only in monitoring, but also in predicting visual prognosis.

- Serologic studies: Elevation of some acute-phase reactants, such as erythrocyte sedimentation rate or C-reactive protein during the acute phase of ABD may be helpful for diagnosis and monitoring.

- Posterior segment changes may resemble those seen in sarcoidosis, viral retinitis, polyarteritis nodosa, systemic lupus erythematosus, Whipple's disease, Crohn's disease, and relapsing polychondritis.

Treatment: ABD is categorically a blinding disease. The goal of therapy should be not only to suppress inflammation, but also to reduce the frequency and severity of recurrences, trying to minimize the potentially devastating visual consequences. Immunosuppressive therapy (IMT) is required for the effective treatment of patients with ocular ABD and it is of utmost importance to initiate this treatment without delay. Prompt treatment is the key to preservation of vision. Systemic corticosteroids have a rapid and definite antiinflammatory effect in all phases of ocular ABD (especially the acute).

Unfortunately, these drugs fail to prevent long term visual deterioration. Oral or intravenous administration probably is the most appropriate route, although topical and regional could also be used as adjuvants of the systemic treatment. It is important to stress that these patients must be put on high-dose systemic corticosteroids and IMT immediately. Chlorambucil, cyclophosphamide and azathioprine are currently used in the treatment of ocular ABD. Other immunosupressive agents that have been successfully used are cyclosporine, tacrolimus and tumor necrosis factor alpha (TNF-á) inhibitors, such as infliximab. Interferon-á has also been used effectively. Other drugs, such as colchicine or thalidomide are used in the treatment of mucocutaneous disease, but have no effect on ocular manifestations of ABD. In summary, the best therapeutic results are obtained with a combination of drugs. Treatment requires long-term care and must be closely monitored. Eye surgery is sometimes necessary. However, this is only indicated whenever visual improvement can be expected and the eye has been free of inflammation for a minimum of 3 months.

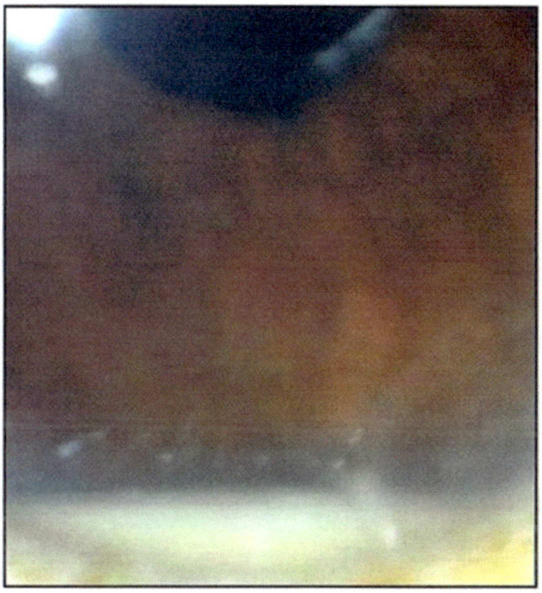

Figure 8: Hypopyon in a patient with ABD.

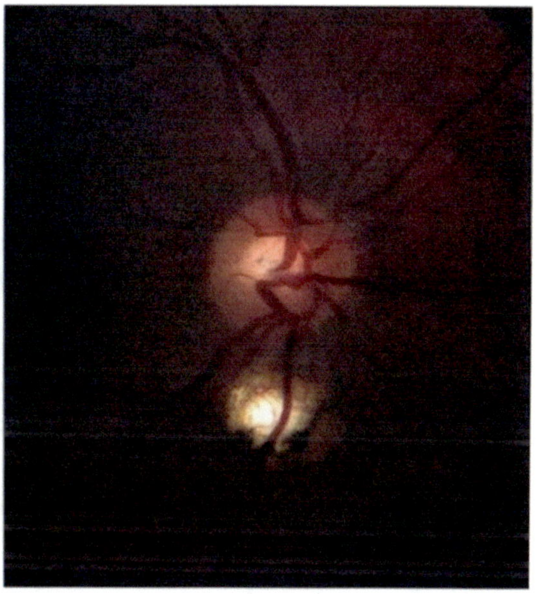

Figure 9: Chorioretinal scar in ABD that could easily be mistaken for an inactive toxoplasmosis scar.

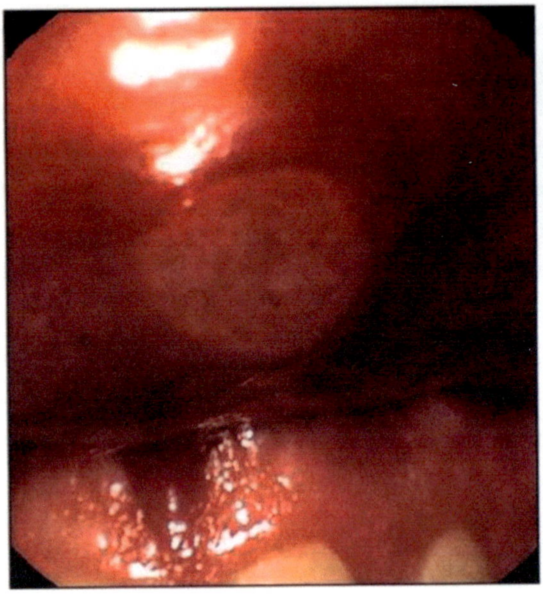

Figure 10: Mouth sore as seen in a patient with ABD.

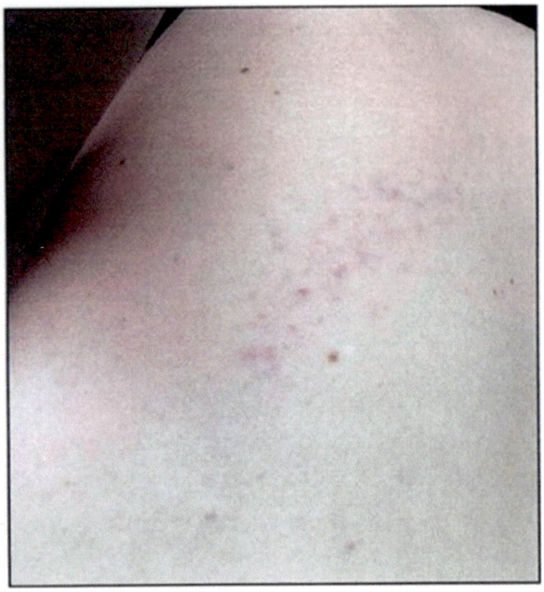

Figure 11: Characteristic reddish-purple nodules of erythema nodosum as seen in a patient with ABD.

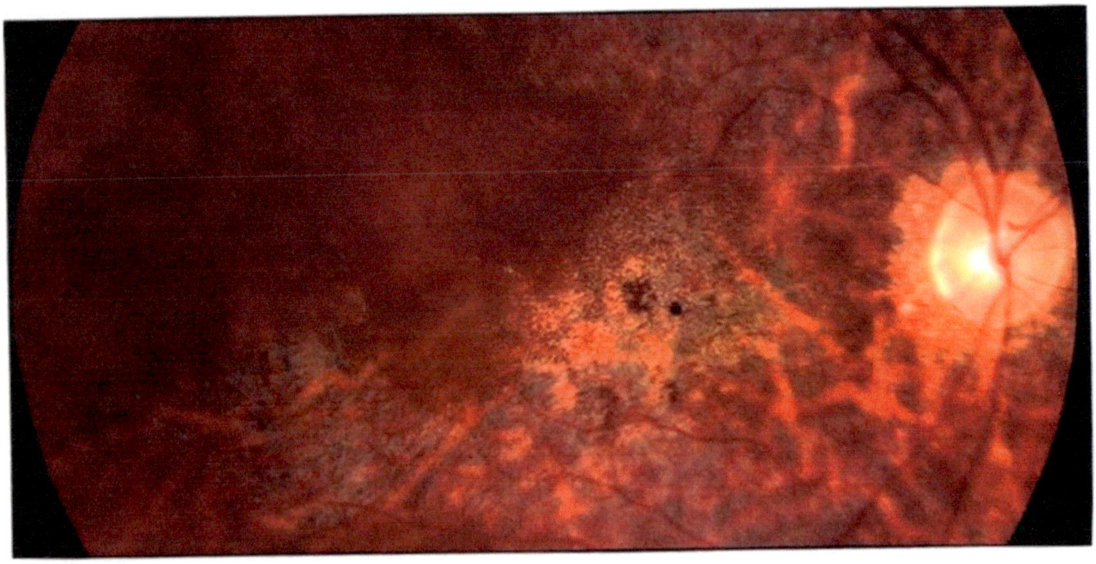

Figure 12: RPE atrophy in a 42 year-old female with ABD. Note the area of atrophy spreading from the optic nerve and along the arcades with RPE clumping. The visual acuity was 20/400.

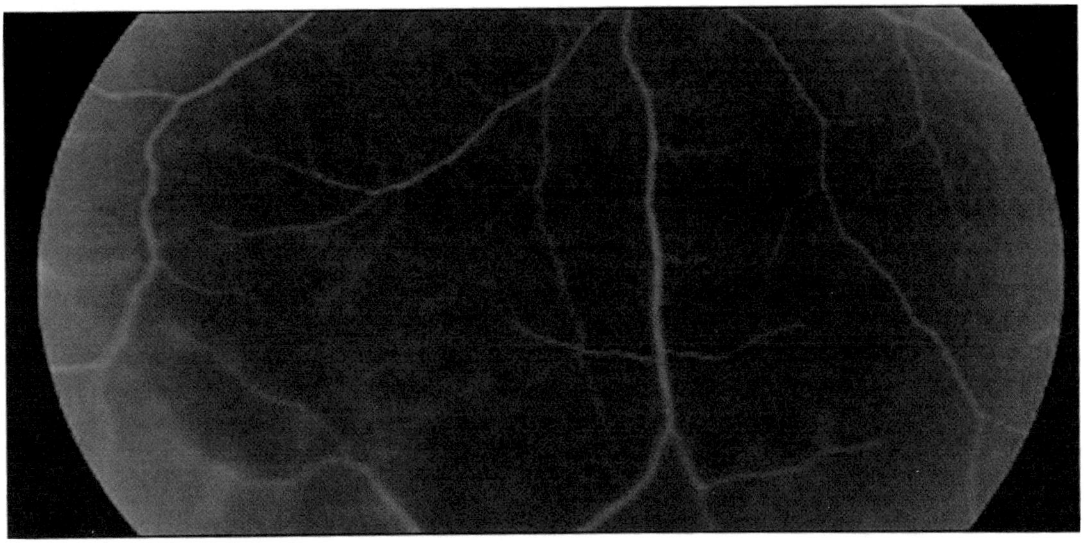

Figure 13: Fluorescein angiogram (FA) in a 25 year-old affected by ABD. Active retinal vasculitis in the inferior periphery represented by diffuse dye leakage from the retinal capillaries. The image also shows marked dilation with partial obstructions of the retinal veins.

References:

1) Zafirakis P, Foster CS. Adamantiades-Behcet disease; in: Foster CS, Vitale AT. *Diagnosis and Treatment of Uveitis*. Saunders. Philadelphia 2002. 632-52
2) Klisovic DD, Foster CS. Adamantiades-Behget disease. *Contemp Ophthalmol.* 2006; 5(10):1-8.
3) Zierhut M, Mizuki N, Ohno S, et al. Human genome and diseases: Review. Immunology and functional genomics of Behget's disease. *Cell Mol Life Sci.* 2003; 60:1903.
4) International Study Group for Belicet's Disease. Criteria for diagnosis of Behget's disease. *Lancet.* 1990; 335: 1078.

ANCA associated Pauci-immune Retinal Vasculopathies

Introduction

Churg-Strauss syndrome, microscopic polyangiitis, and granulomatosis with poly-angiitis collectively form part of the small-vessel pauci-immune vasculopathies. Anti-nuclear cytoplasmic antibodies (ANCA) are useful diagnostic serological markers, but its specificity does not allow one to distinguish diverse forms of necrotizing vasculitis. The incidence of the pauci-immune vasculopathies may be underestimated due to the under-recognition of systemic involvement in patients with retinal vasculitis. The recognition of these associated systemic clinical features cannot be over emphasized so that significant morbidity if not mortality can be prevented.

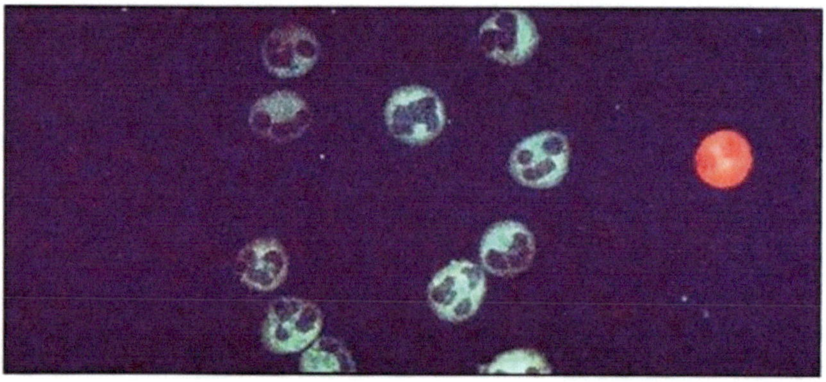

Figure 14: Indirect immunofluorescence demonstrating a negative ANCA of staining.

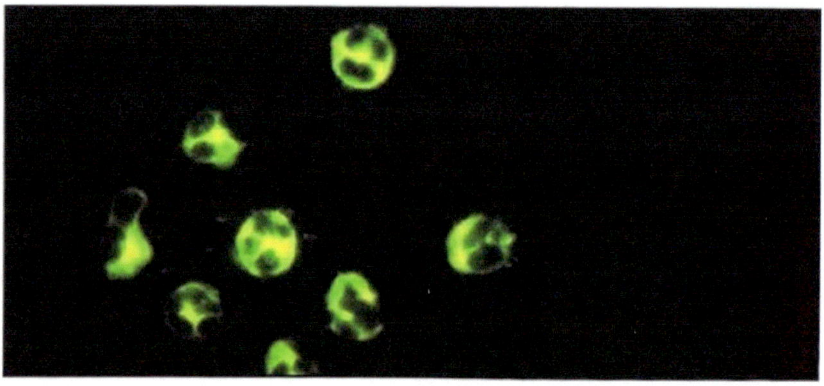

Figure 15: Positive c-ANCA (cytoplasmic) pattern of staining on ethanol fixed neutrophils by indirect immunofluorescence as seen in this photomicrograph.

Microscopic Polyangiitis

Introduction: Microscopic polyangiitis (MPA) is a now recognized pauci-immune systemic vasculitis with small vessel involvement as the definitive diagnostic criterion for diagnosis.

Epidemiology: MPA has an incidence of approximately 1:100,000 with a slight female predominance. The mean age of patients affected is 50 years, although any age group may be affected. The disease is commoner than polyarteritis nodosa but less common than granulomatosis with polyangiitis.

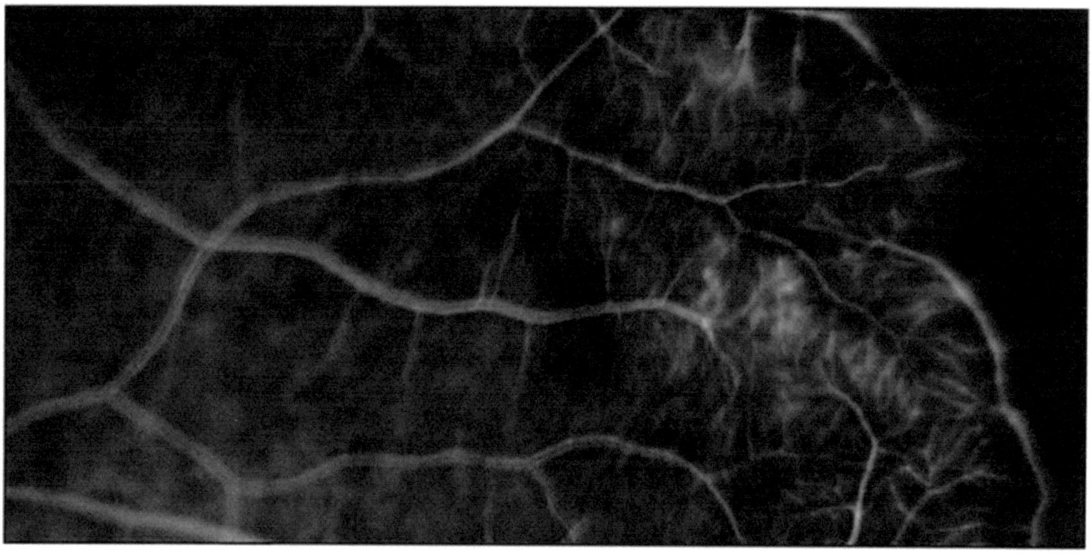

Figure 16: Peripheral vasculitis with ischemia secondary to MPA.

Clinical Features: MPA most commonly affects the kidneys and the skin with lesser involvement of the gastrointestinal, pulmonary, and central nervous system. The clinical course is usually indolent with heterogeneity of clinical signs which may cause delay in diagnosis and treatment. The eye when involved manifests as a retinal vasculitis with secondary retinal ischemia and neovascularization.

Pathogenesis: The pathophysiological relevance of ANCA has been studied extensively. It has been demonstrated that IgG fractions from ANCA positive sera, are capable of inducing tumor necrosis factor primed neutrophils to release lysosomal enzymes and produce reactive oxygen species inducing vascular injury.

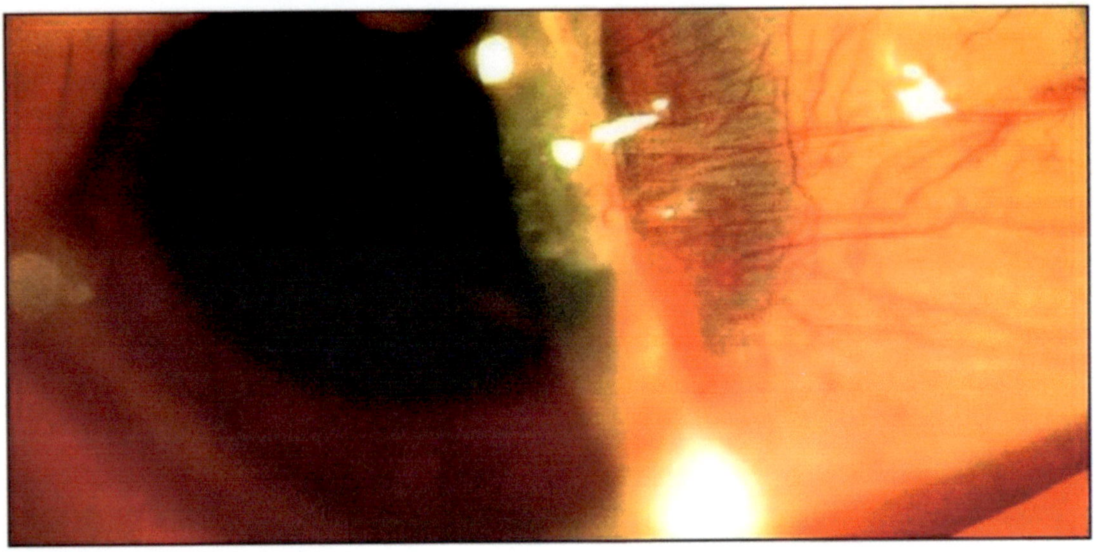

Figure 17: MPA-associated PUK with secondary pseudopterygium.

Diagnosis: We recommend adherence to the International Consensus Statement on testing and reporting of ANCA in conjunction with the presenting clinical features. Serum ANCA specificity is 40% for PR3-ANCA (c-ANCA), and 50% for MPO-ANCA (p-ANCA) in untreated disease

Treatment: The recommended treatment for MPA is initial high-dose corticosteroids in conjunction with immunomodulation with cyclophosphamide. Serum ANCA titers are useful in monitoring disease response to treatment.

Granulomatosis with Polyangiitis

Definition/History: Granulomatosis with polyangiitis is a systemic disease of unknown etiology characterized by granulomatous inflammation of the upper and lower respiratory tract, necrotizing vasculitis, and nephritis. It is a systemic vasculitis of the medium and small arteries, venules, arterioles, and, occasionally, large arteries. The classic criteria for the diagnosis of granulomatosis with polyangiitis are based on the pathologic findings of Godman and Churg in their paper of 1954[1].

Epidemiology: Granulomatosis with polyangiitis is a rare disease. Estimates of granulomatosis with polyangiitis frequency vary from about 0.8 to 15 per 1,000,000 yet these figures are likely underestimated because of incorrect diagnosis. The disease typically manifests in the fourth and fifth decades, although its occurrence at ages ranging from 7 to 75 has been reported.[2,3] The disease can affect either sex, with some of the larger series revealing a preponderance of males in a ratio as high as 1.5:1.[4] Granulomatosis with polyangiitisoccurs most commonly in white patients but has been reported in blacks and Hispanics. A higher frequency of HLA-DR1, DR13 and DR6 in patients with granulomatosis with polyangiitis has been reported.[5,6] A retrospective study by Booth et al from 2003 demonstrated a cumulative 5-year survival rate of 76% and a 1-year mortality rate of 18%.[7]

Pathology/Pathogenesis: The earliest lesion of this disorder is injury and necrosis of the vessels that evolves into a necrotizing and palisading granuloma without inflammation. Tissue injury in granulomatosis with polyangiitis is a result of interaction between the inflammatory cascade and the pathogenic immune response to the neutrophil granule proteins. Antibodies to cytoplasmic antigens within neutrophils (antineutrophilic cytoplasmic antibody [ANCA], designated C-ANCA for diffuse cytoplasmic staining and P-ANCA for perinuclear staining by immunofluorescence) suggest an important humoral component of the disease. The expression of proteinase-3 (PR3) on endothelial cell membranes provides a possible role of ANCA-endothelial interactions in the pathogenesis of ANCA-associated vasculitis.

Clinical Features:

Systemic Manifestations: Patients may present with a wide range of clinical manifestations, defined chiefly by the primary anatomic site of involvement. The first symptoms of granulomatosis with polyangiitis are often vague, but most often involve the upper respiratory tract. Fatigue, weight loss, fevers, shortness of breath, bloody sputum, joint pains, and sinusitis are common complaints. Nasal ulcerations and even blood nasal discharge can occur. Other areas of the body that can also become inflamed in patients with granulomatosis with polyangiitis include the eyes, the nerves (neuropathy), the middle ear (otitis media) and the skin resulting in skin nodules or ulcers. Arthralgias and nondeforming arthritis are common in granulomatosis with polyangiitis. Skin involvement occurs in 45 percent of patients and can take the form of papules, vesicles, palpable purpura, ulcers, or subcutanous nodules.

Ocular Manifestations: The ocular manifestations of granulomatosis with polyangiitis can be divided into two categories: contiguous and focal. Contiguous disease arises from contiguous granulomatous sinusitis of long duration and results in severe orbital pseudotumor, orbital abscess or cellulitis, or nasolacrimal duct obstruction. Focal disease in granulomatosis with polyangiitisis defined as focal vasculitis, involving the anterior, posterior, or both segments of the eye and possibly the orbit, unrelated to any upper airway disease.[8] In all of these series, the most common ophthalmic manifestation of granulomatosis with polyangiitis was orbital inflammation with proptosis. Of the focal manifestations of granulomatosis with polyangiitis, conjunctivitis and episcleritis are most common.

Corneal or scleral involvement is not benign and takes the form of peripheral ulcerative keratitis or scleritis. The scleritis may be diffuse, nodular, or necrotizing. Peripheral ulcerative keratitis and necrotizing scleritis are the two most malignant ocular manifestations of granulomatosis with polyangiitis; each can result in ocular perforation, leading to blindness and possibly to loss of the eye. Localized conjunctivitis or episcleritis usually occurs before the onset of peripheral ulcerative keratitis or scleritis. Given that ocular signs and symptoms are often part of the presentation of granulomatosis with polyangiitis, the patient may first seek medical attention from an ophthalmologist. It is notable that it is not unusual for the active, generalized phase of granulomatosis with polyangiitis to be heralded by an episode of "red eyes."

Diagnosis:

Clinicopathologic Criteria

Classic Diagnostic Triad For Granulomatosis With Polyangiitis[9]

1.Necrotizing granuloma of the upper or lower respiratory tract Typically, mucosal inflammation and ulceration in the respiratory tract; mucosal inflammation characterized by foci of epithelioid cells, multinucleated giant cells, and fibrillar organization with secondary necrosis of fibrillar tissue; tissue eosinophilia common

2. Vasculitis involves both arteries and veins and is of a focal, necrotizing variety; is granulomatous in nature, featuring multinucleated giant cells; typically seen in lung tissue and variably present elsewhere

3. Nephritis: focal, necrotizing glomerulitis with fibrinoid necrosis and thrombosis of capillary loops, sometimes extending beyond Bowman's capsule; neutrophils usually present; granulomatous inflammation with giant cells only occasionally seen

Treatment: The treatment protocol may be summarized as follows: oral cyclophosphamide for a maximum of 1 year and oral prednisone. Plasmapheresis is not considered a standard therapy in classic granulomatosis with polyangiitis. High-dose intravenous immune globulin therapy has been used in systemic vasculitides such as Kawasaki's disease and rheumatoid vasculitis, but any benefit in granulomatosis with polyangiitis has been transient.[10]

References:

1) Godman GC, Churg J: Wegener's granulomatosis. Pathology and review of the literature. *Arch Pathol* 58:533, 1954-
2) McDonald TJ, DeRemee RA: Wegener's granulomatosis. *Laryngoscope.* 93:220, 1983.
3) DeRemee RA, McDonald TJ, Harrison EG et al: Wegener's granulolmatosis. Anatomic correlates, a proposed classification. *Mayo Clin Proc* 51:777, 1976.
4) Niffennegger JH, Jakobiec FA, Raizman MB, et al: Pathological diagnosis of very limited (ocular or orbital) Wegener's granulomatosis.
5) Carruthers DM, Watts RA, Symmons DP, et al: Wegener's Granulomatosis-increased incidence or increased recognition? *Br J Rheumatol* 35:142, 1996.
6) Fauci AS, Haynes BF, Katz P, Wolff SM: Wegener's granulomatosis: prospective clinical and therapeutic experience with 85 patients for 21 years. *Ann Intern Med* 98:76, 1983.
7) Booth AD, Almond MK, Burns A: Outcome of ANCA-associated renal vasculitis: a 5-year retrospective study. *Am J Kidney Dis* 2003; 41 (4): 776-84.
8) Straatsma BR: Ocular manifestations of Wegener's granulomatosis. *Am J Ophthalmol* 44:789, 1957.
9) Raynauld JP, Bloch DA, Fries JF: Seasonal variation in the onset of Wegener's granulomatosis, polyarteritis nodosa and giant cell arteritis. *J Rheum* 20:1524, 1993-
10) RA. Empiricism and Wegener's granulomatosis [editorial]. *N Engl J Med* 1996; 335:54-55.

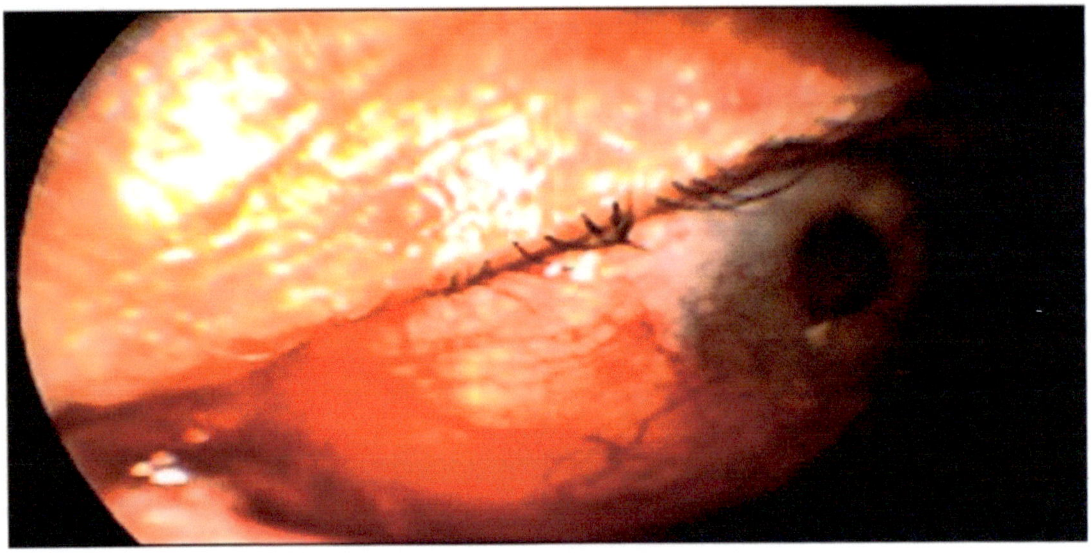

Figure 18: Proptosis secondary to granulomatosis with polyangiitis.

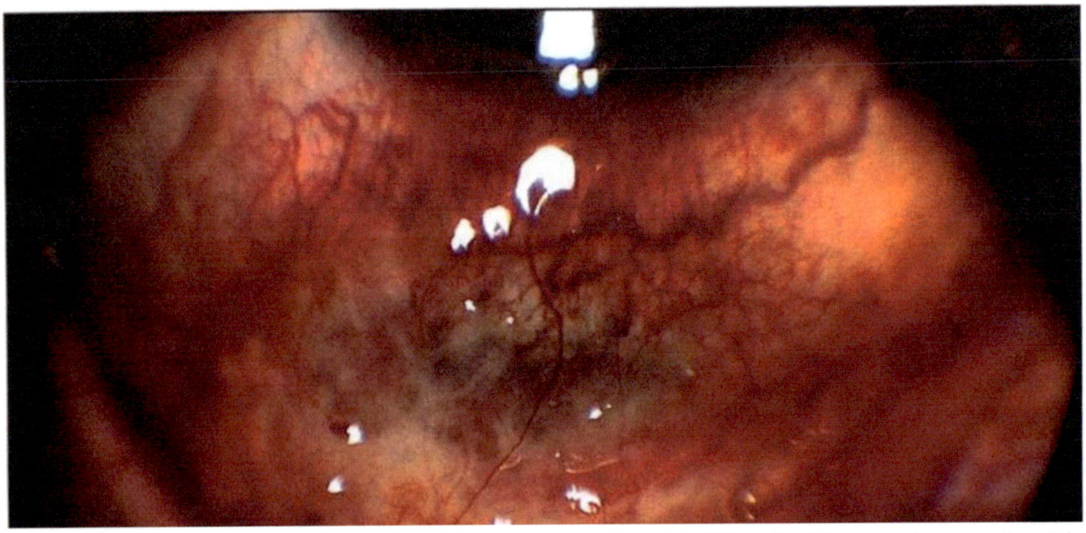

Figure 19: Ischemic scleritis in an African-American female afflicted with granulomatosis with polyangiitis.

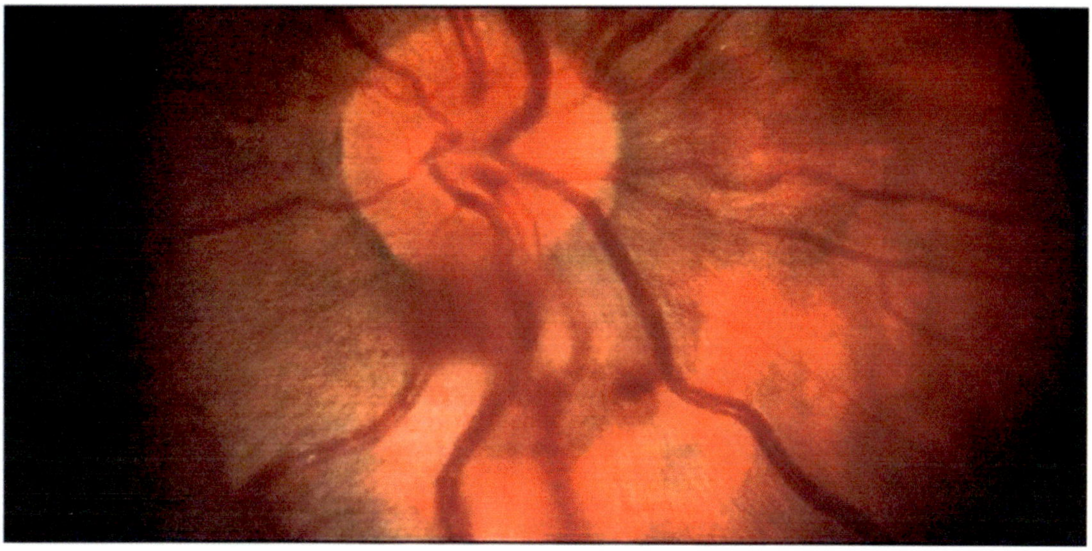

Figure 20: Peripapillary hemorrhage in the context of granulomatosis with polyangiitis.

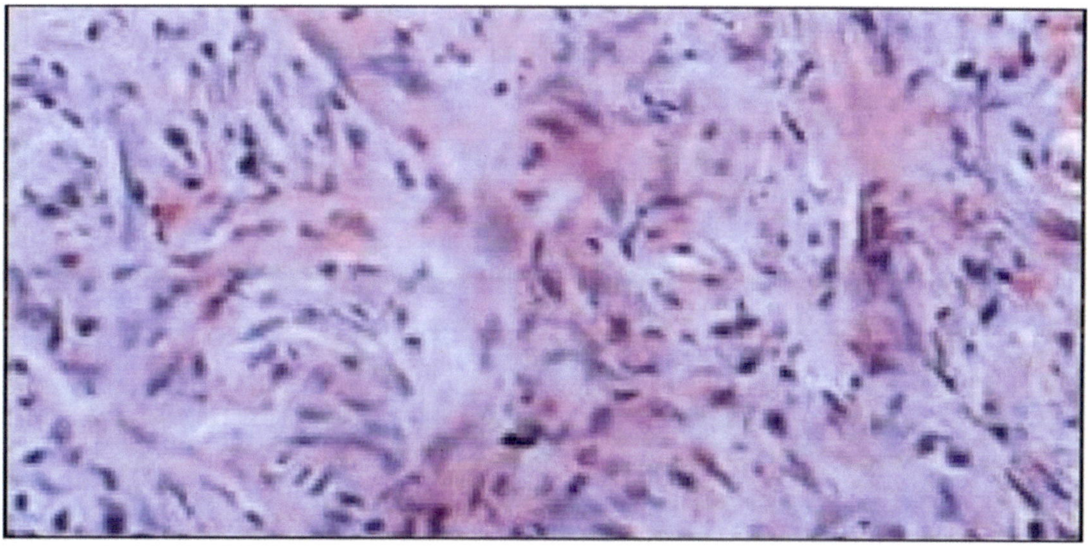

Figure 21: Epithelioid cells and eosinophils in the histopathologic specimen from a patient with granulomatosis with polyangiitis.

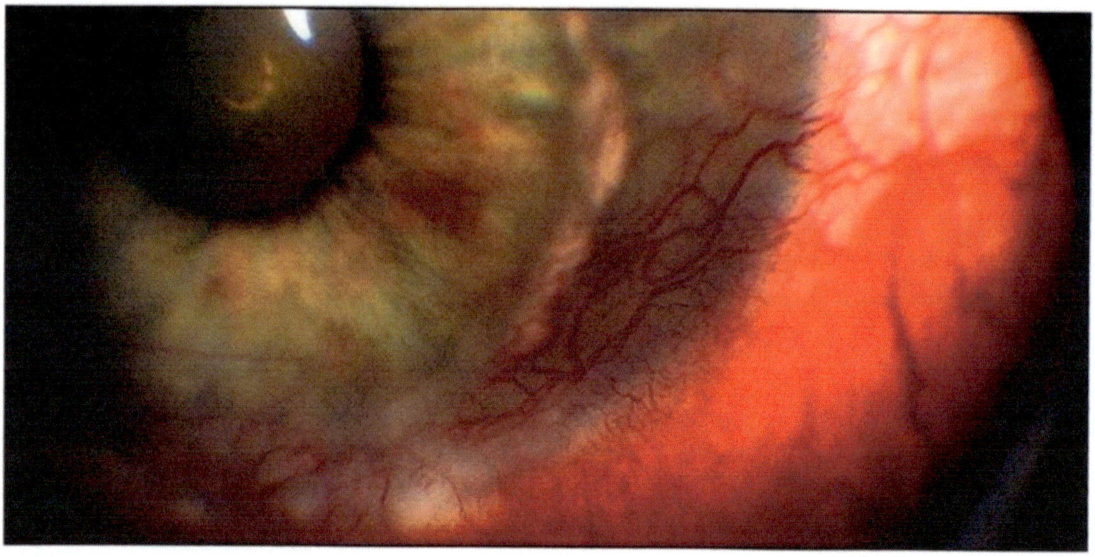

Figure 22: Corneal neovascularization spreading to an area of old peripheral ulcerative keratitis in a seventy-two year old patient with granulomatosis with polyangiitis.

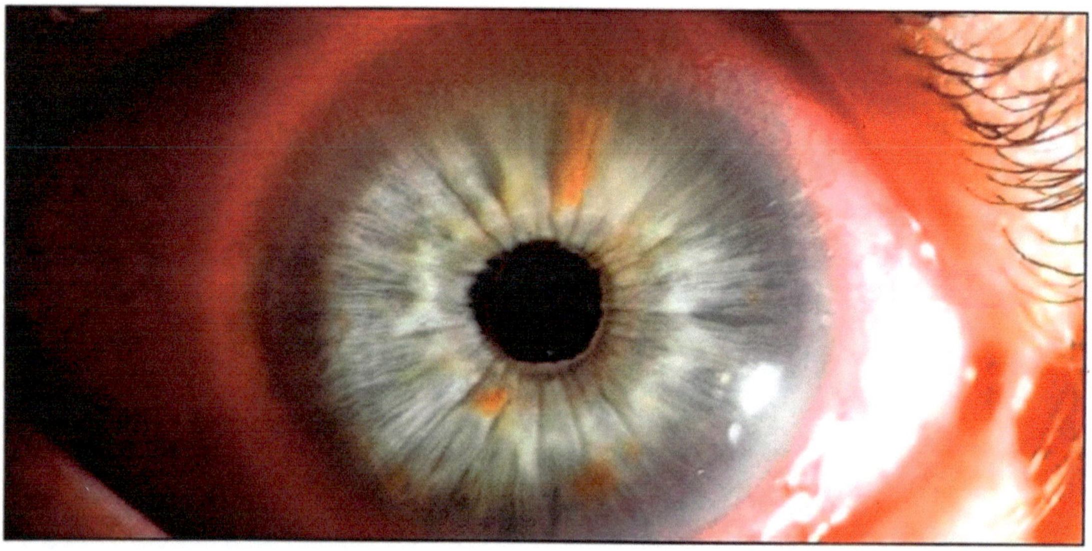

Figure 23: Scleritis in a patient with a granulomatosis with polyangiitis and relapsing polychondritis overlap syndrome.

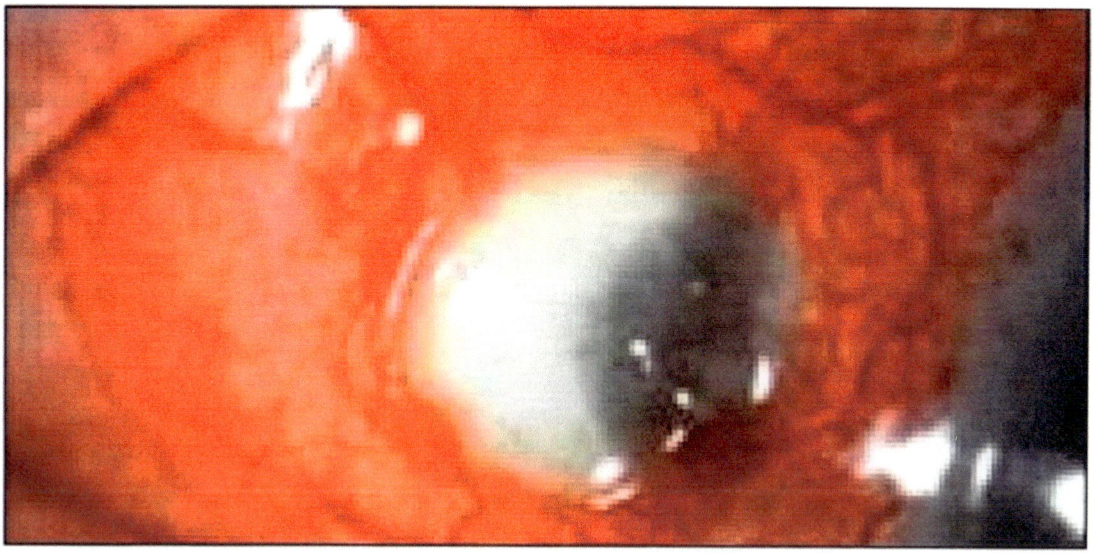

Figure 24: Scleral performation and choroidal show secondary to granulomatosis with polyangiitis.

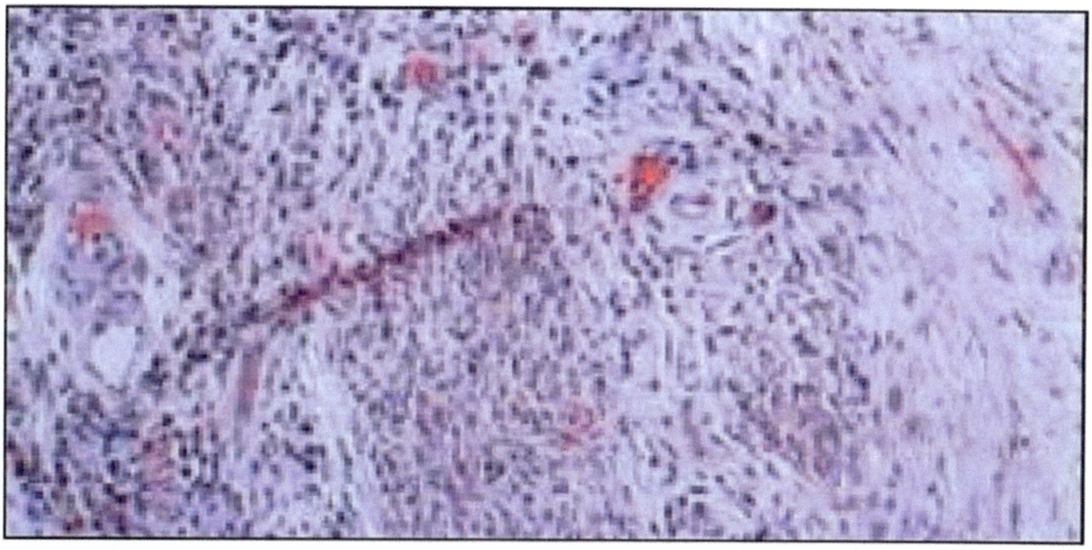

Figure 25: Histopathology of a large conjunctival mass revealed vasculitis with micro-abscesses in a patient who was subsequently diagnosed with granulomatosis with polyangiitis.

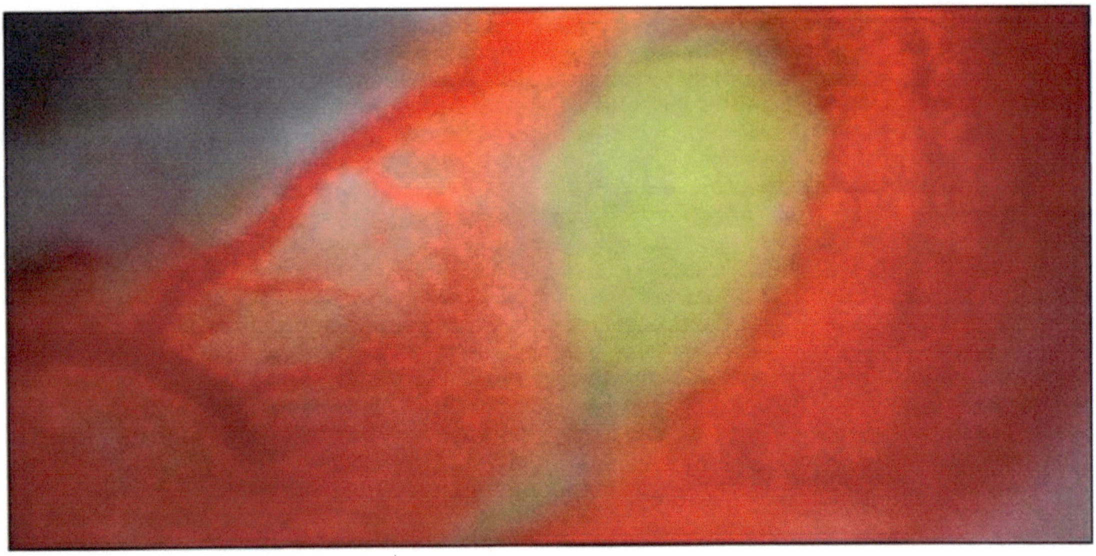

Figure 26: Inferotemporal corneal neovascularization with an area of active necrotizing scleritis in the left eye of a patient with granulomatosis with polyangiitis that necessitated a scleral patch graft.

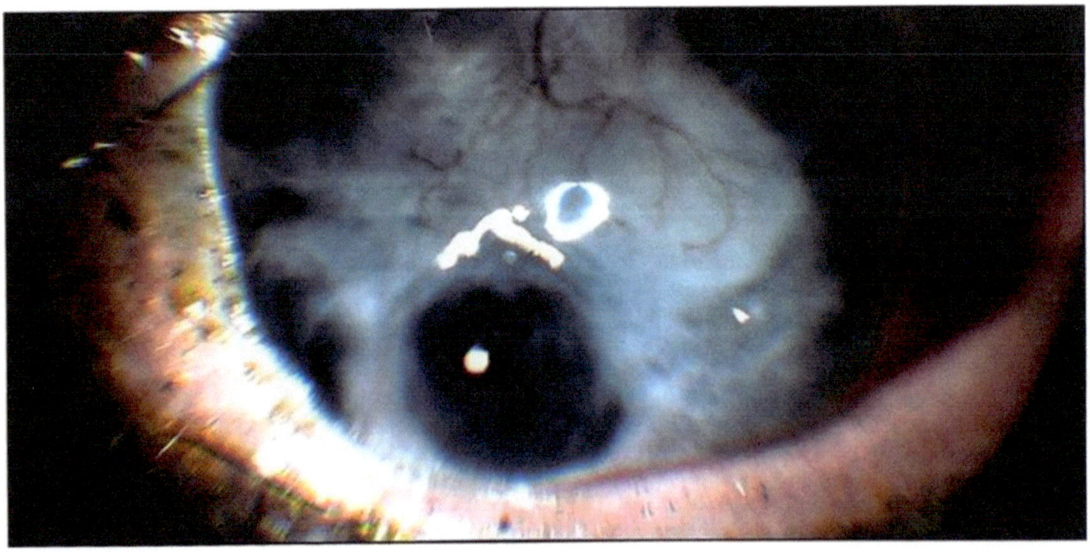

Figure 27: Bulging of the uvea from prolonged inflammation. Note the scleral thinning of this 30 year old Hispanic female.

Antiphospholipid syndrome

Definition: Antiphospholipid syndrome (APS) is a hypercoagulable disorder with extremely variable symptoms including ocular manifestations and characterized by the triad of arterial or venous thrombosis, recurrent abortions caused by placental vascular insufficiency, and thrombocytopenia associated with elevated levels of antiphospholipid antibodies (aPL) which are the serological markers of this clinical entity. Clinically, the most important aPL are anticardiolipin antibodies (aCL) and Lupus anticoagulant (LAC). Antiphospholipid syndrome may be associated with an underlying systemic autoimmune disorders, particularly systemic lupus erythematosus (SLE) and "lupus-like" syndromes or may appear isolated without manifestations of systemic disease (primary antiphospholipid syndrome).

History: Despite several attempts to characterize this condition during the 20th century, in 1993, G.R. Hughes gave an accurate description of this syndrome, thus being the first to consider it as an individual entity.

Epidemiology: The low incidence of this condition and the poor standardization of diagnostic tests make it very difficult to have clear data about its epidemiology. Moreover, the aPL are not specific for AP. The prevalence of aCL in the general population is less than 5%. The frequency of LAC and aCL in SLE is considerably higher.

Clinical Features: This disease is a multisystemic disorder involving almost any organ system.

Systemic manifestations: The presentation varies from the subacute form (migraine, visual disturbance, occasional dysarthria, and possible deep thrombosis or recurrent early miscarriages) to the acute (accelerated cardiac valve failure, thrombocytopenia, cerebrovascular accident, and widespread thrombosis).

Ocular manifestations: Ophthalmologic manifestations described in association with the existence of aPL include episodes of amaurosis fugax, transient diplopia and visual field loss, ischemic optic neuropathy, retinal and choroidal vascular occlusions, and peripheral proliferative retinopathy. In addition, retinal abnormalities have been found in 88% of patients with primary APS. Anterior segment involvement is usually mild and relatively uncommon.

Pathology/Pathogenesis: The aPL antibodies are a group of immunoglobulins (IgG, IgM, IgA, or a mixture of these three) with varying affinities for phospholipid-protein complexes. Included in this family are aCL, LAC, and antibodies, which cause a false-positive serologic test for syphilis. There is no clear explanation for the immune response which leads to the development of aPL. T-lymphocytes are known to play an important role in autoantibody production and disease pathogenesis. Complexes formed by aPL and antigens involved in the maintenance of normal hemostasis can also be in-vivo immunogens and lead to the autoimmune response.

Diagnosis: This is based on both clinical and laboratory criteria. Definite APS is considered if at least one of the clinical, and one of the laboratory criteria are present.

Clinical criteria:

1) Vascular thrombosis (confirmed by imaging, Doppler studies, or histopathology, with the exception of superficial venous thrombosis).
2) Pregnancy morbidity:
   a. One unexplained death of a morphologically normal fetus
   b. One premature birth (because severe preeclampsia or eclampsia, or severe placental insufficiency)
   c. Three or more unexplained consecutive abortions

Laboratory criteria:

3) CL antibody (IgG or IgM) in blood, detected on two occasions, at least 6 weeks apart using standardized ELISA.
4) LAC present in plasma on two or more occasions, at least 6 weeks apart, detected according to the guidelines of the International Society on Thrombosis and Hemostasis.

Treatment: Current management varies considerably and is based on disease manifestations. In patients who are positive for aPL without any clinical history of APS it is important to emphasize the need to reduce other risk factors for thrombosis, such as obesity and smoking among others. Hydroxychloroquine and/or aspirin (or other antiplatelet agents) have also been used to prevent thrombotic events in these patients.

In APS, patients who have had thrombotic events require anticoagulants (like warfarin) immediately. Thrombocytopenia has to be carefully managed in these patients and treated only in severe cases with corticosteroids and/or intravenous immunoglobulins. In pregnancy, warfarin is contraindicated and should be substituted by a combination of subcutaneous heparin and aspirin.

In patients with ocular complications (especially vaso-occlusive pathology), anticoagulant therapy should be initiated. The duration of this therapy remains controversial, but it is probably prudent to continue it for many years after the occurrence of the vasculopathy. Corticosteroids and/or other immunomodulatory agents should be given only if the thrombopathy persists despite adequate anticoagulation and antiplatelet therapy. Laser photocoagulation may be indicated in eyes with profuse peripheral retinal neovascularization and vitreous hemorrhages.

References

1) Miserocchi E, Foster CS. Antiphospholipid syndrome; in: Foster CS, Vitale AT. *Diagnosis and treatment of uveitis*. Saunders. Philadelphia 2002:683-92.
2) Lima Cabrita FV, Foster CS. Anticardiolipin antibodies and ocular disease. *Ocul Immunol Inflamm.* 2005 Jul-Aug;13(4):265-70.
3) Behbehani R, Sergott RC, Savino PJ. The antiphospholipid antibody syndrome: diagnostic aspects. *Curr Opin Ophthalmol.* 2004 Dec;15(6): 483-5.

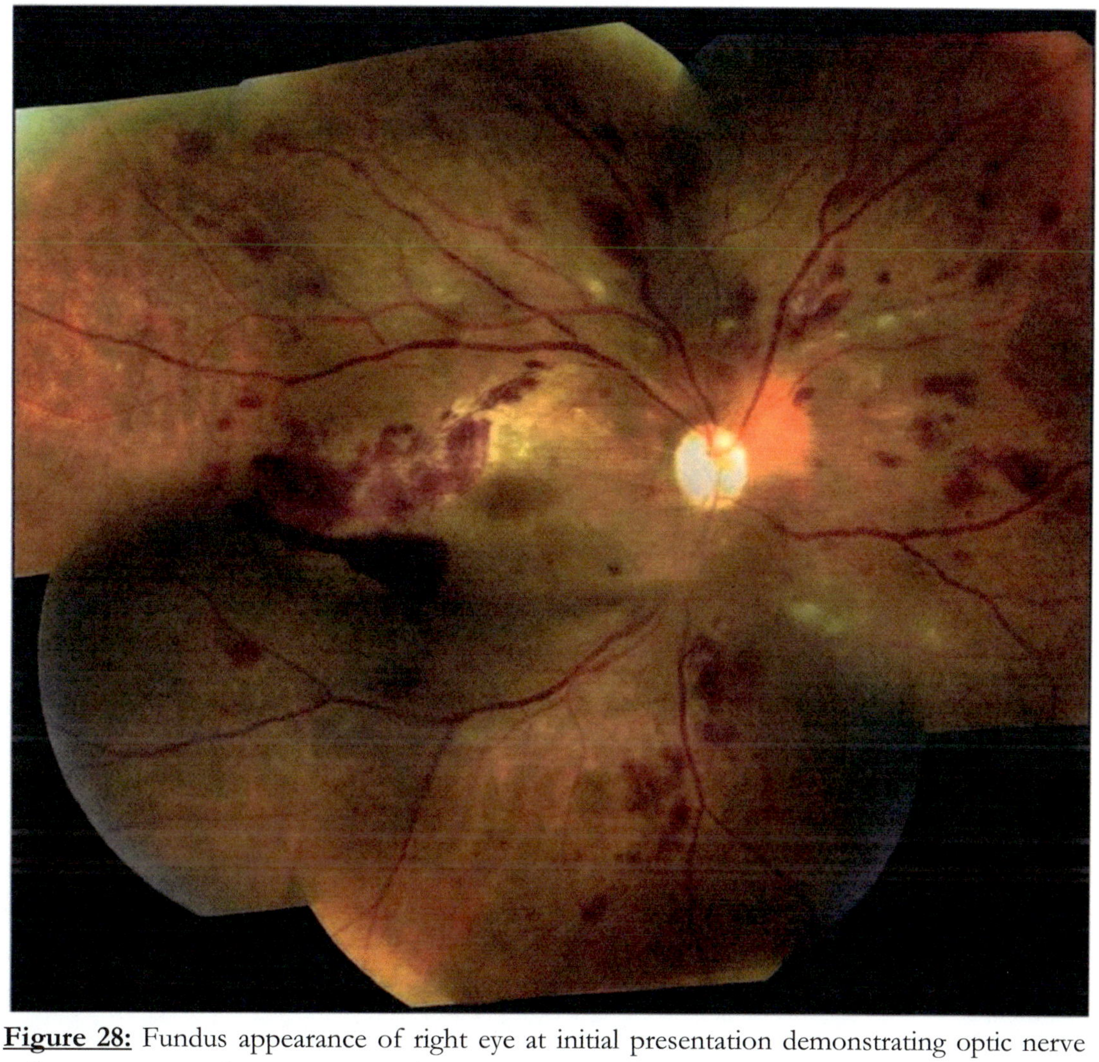

Figure 28: Fundus appearance of right eye at initial presentation demonstrating optic nerve pallor, cotton wool spots, scattered intraretinal hemorrhages, vessel segmentation, and preretinal hemorrhages in antiphospholipid syndrome.

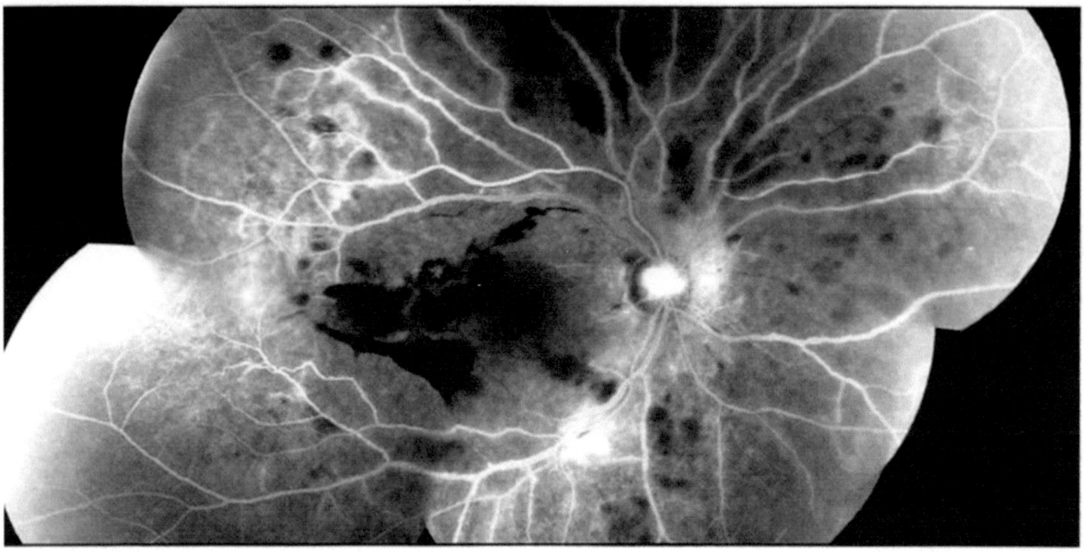

Figure 29: Same patient as in Figure 28. On fluorescein angiography there is severe and diffuse retinal vasculitis with small vessel occlusion, neovascularization of the disc, capillary nonperfusion and prominent venous segmentation.

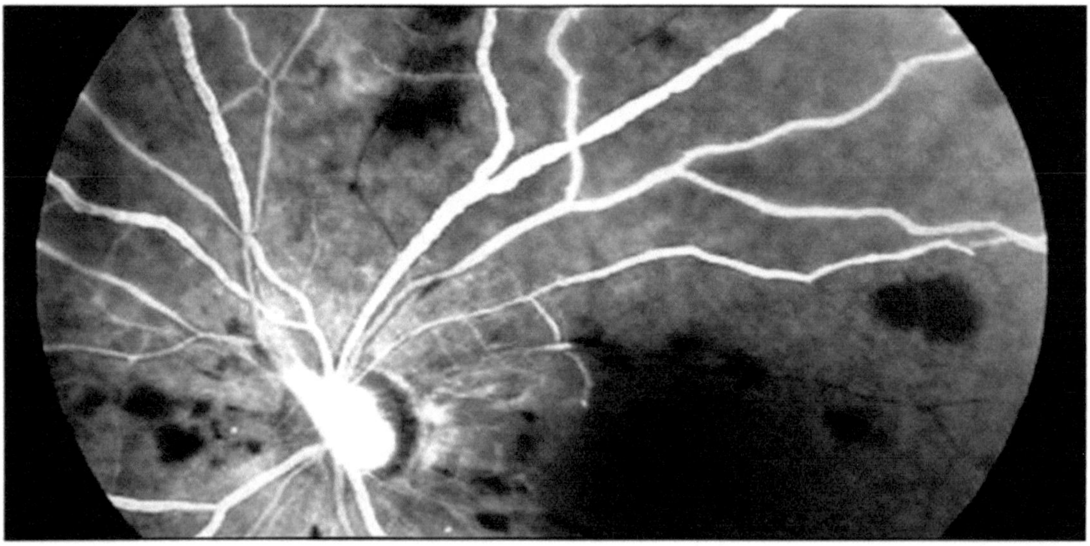

Figure 30: Same patient as in Figure 28. Angiographic view of a vaso-occlusive retinopathy in an eye affected by antiphospholipid syndrome. Note the macular ischemia and profuse retinal hemorrhages.

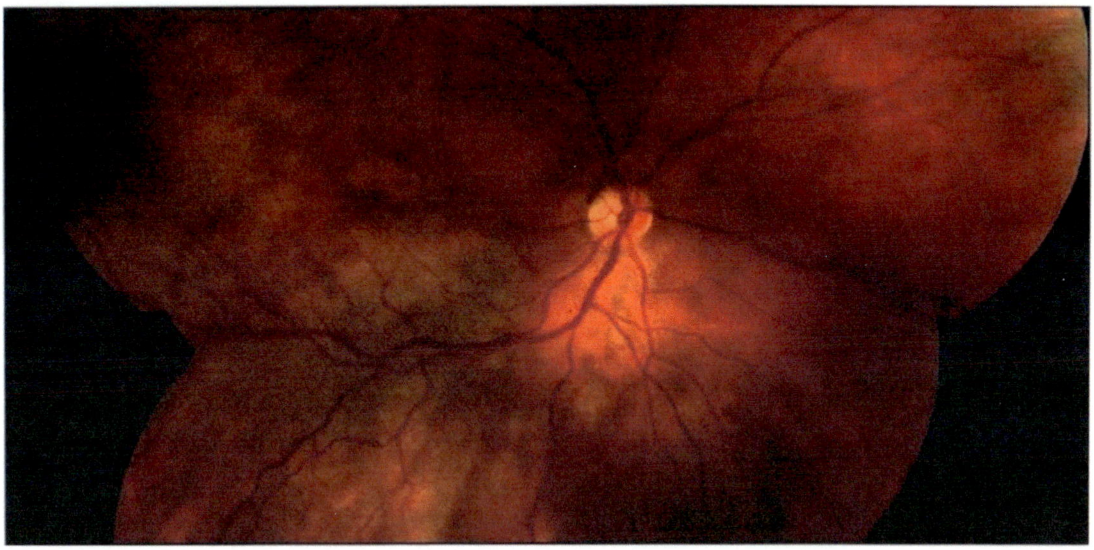

<u>Figure 31.</u>: Fundus photo montages of massive choroidal infarcts and hypopigmentation in a 39 year-old female with a flare-up post-pregnancy.

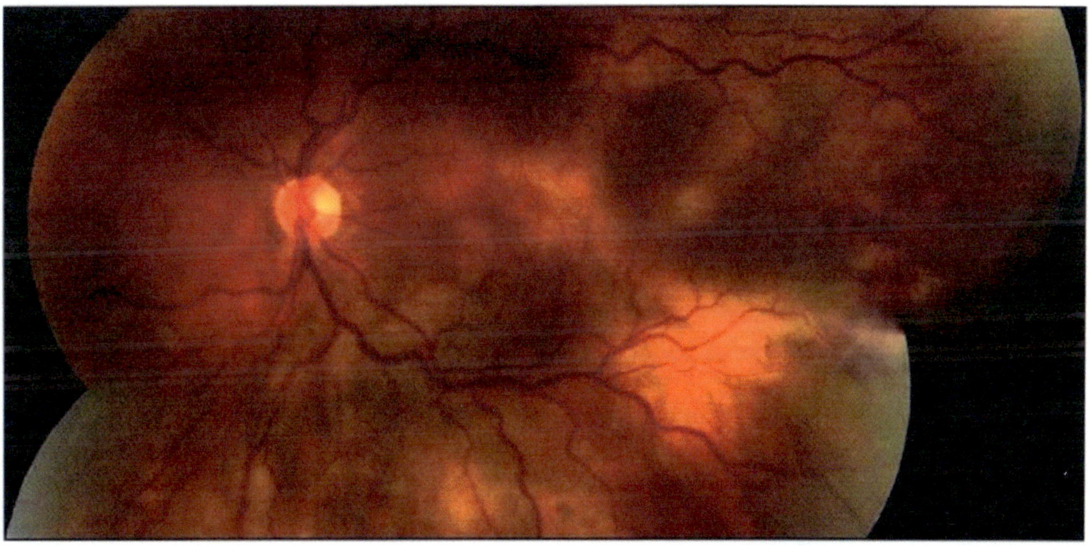

<u>Figure 32:</u> Same patient as in Figure 31. Note the scattered hemorrhages located temporally and inferiorly in the left eye.

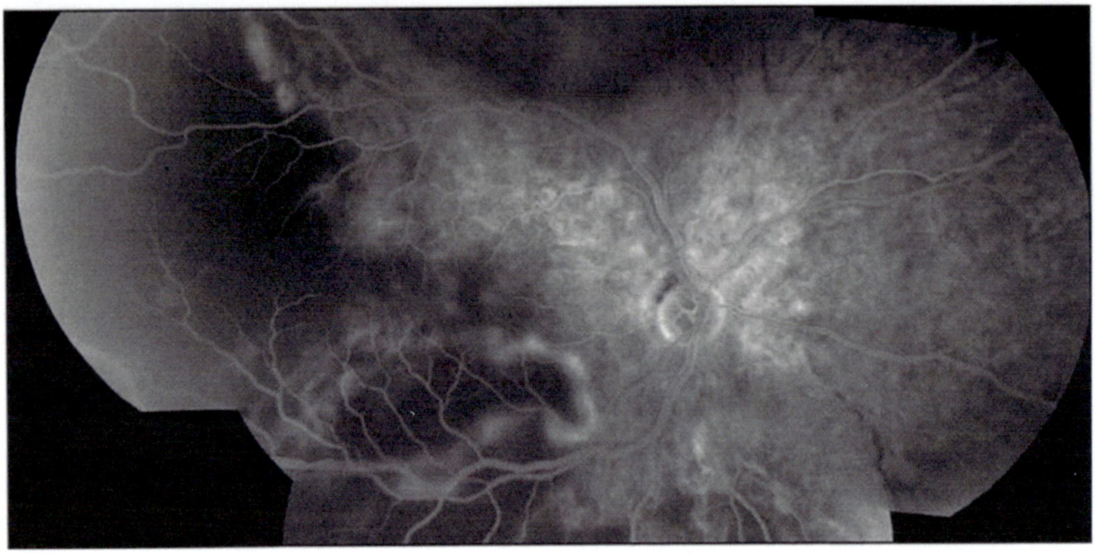

Figure 33: Same patient as in Figure 31. There is choroidal ischemia inferiorly, temporally, and superiorly, which is well-delineated on FA. Nasally, the choroidal vessels are perfused normally.

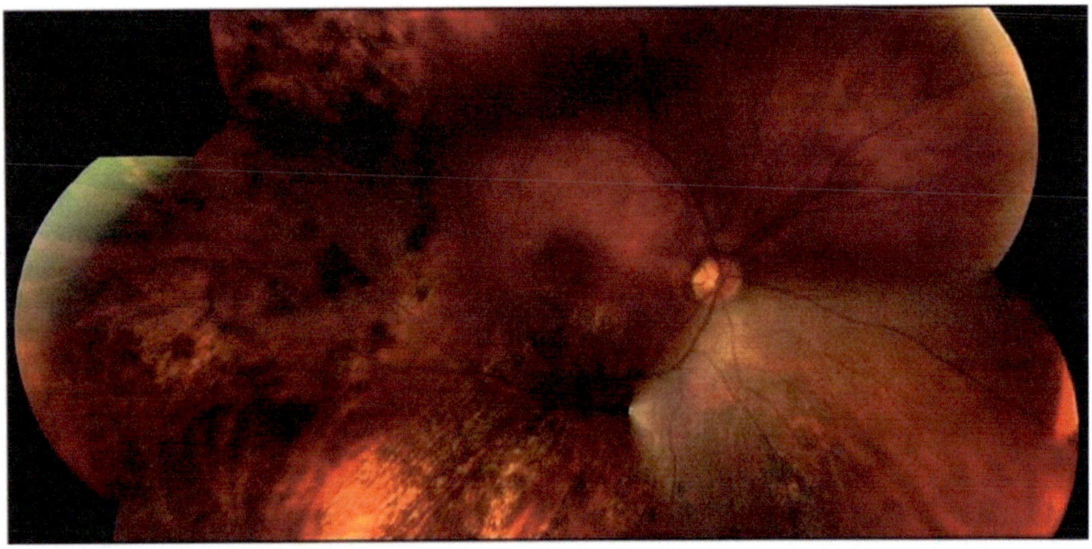

Figure 34: Same patient as in Figure 31. Inactive anti-phospholipid syndrome with peripheral scarring status-post intravenous rituximab treatment as seen in the right eye.

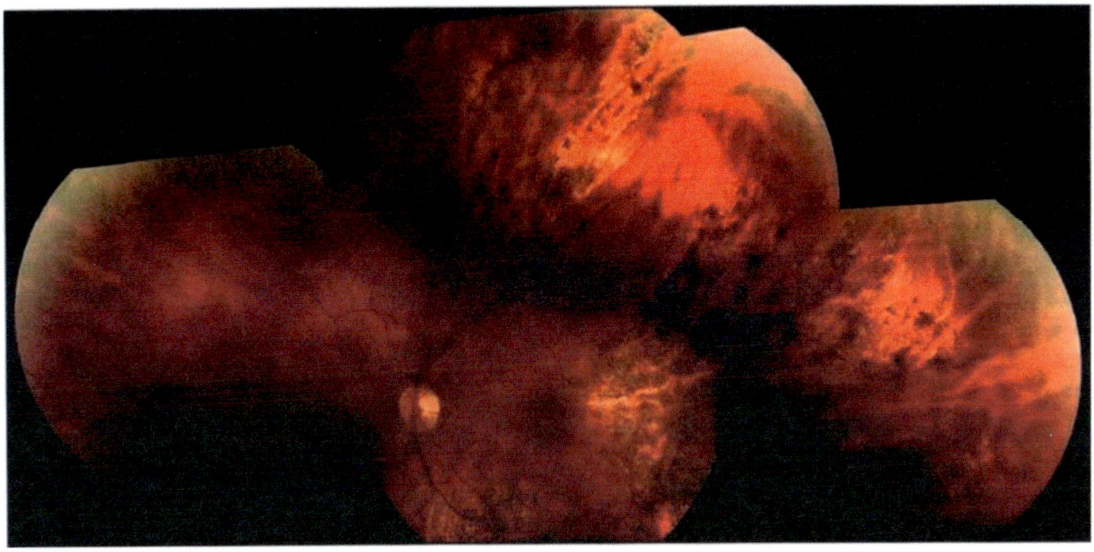

Figure 35: Same patient as in Figure 31. Left eye with similar appearance.

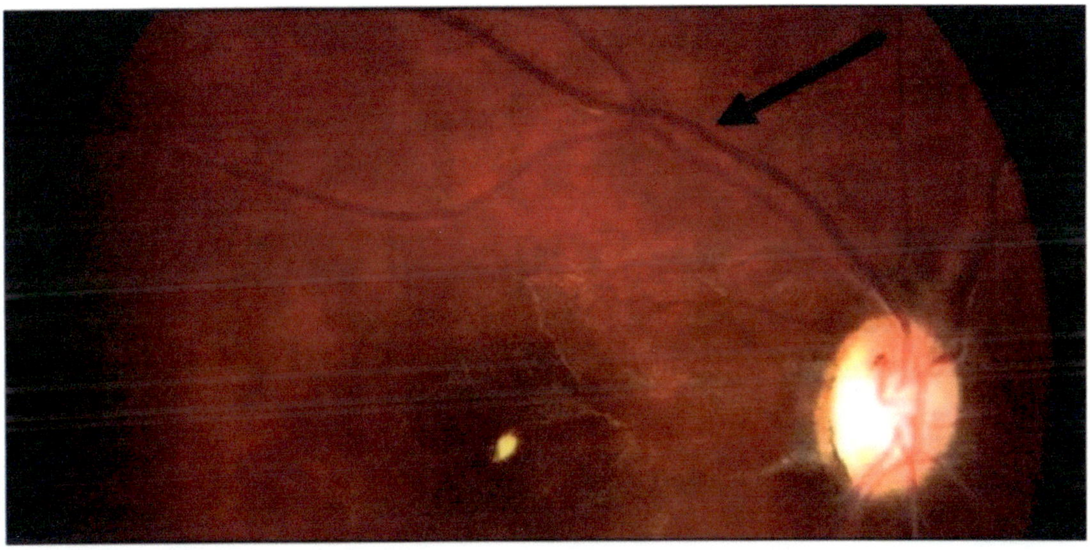

Figure 36: Cilioretinal artery plaque and optic nerve pallor as a result of recalcitrant inflammation in anti-phospholipid syndrome. Note the vascular sheathing along the superior arcade.

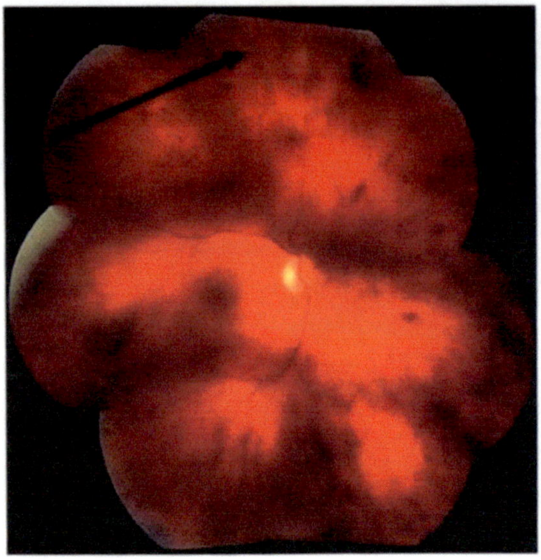

Figure 37: Superior area of vascular sheathing secondary to anti-phospholipid syndrome in the right eye

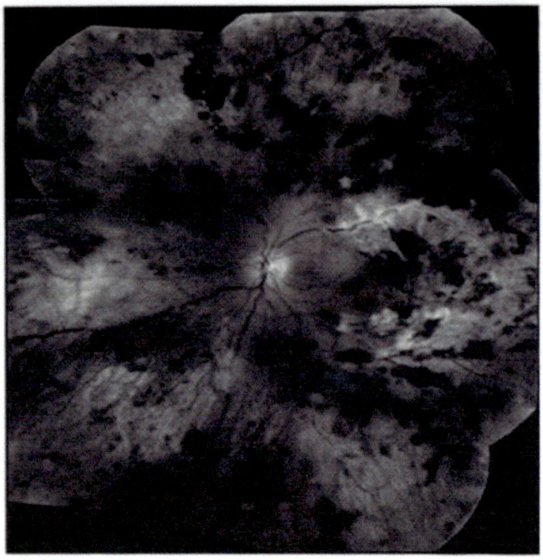

Figure 38: Diffuse retinal hemorrhages in the periphery of the left eye in patient afflicted by anti-phospholipid syndrome.

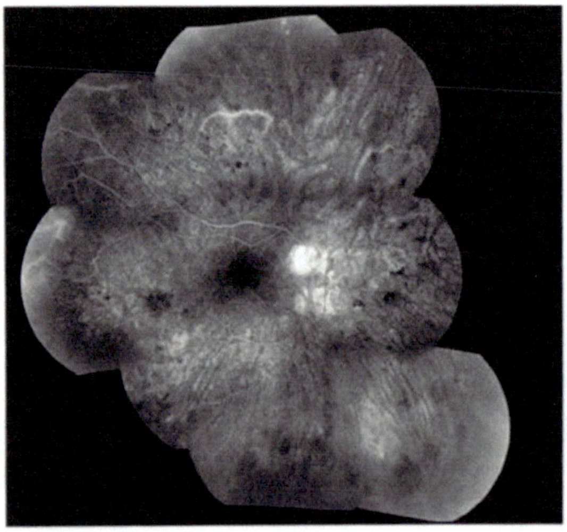

Figure 39: Extensive peripheral neovascularization and vasculitis in this patient with anti-phospholipid syndrome.

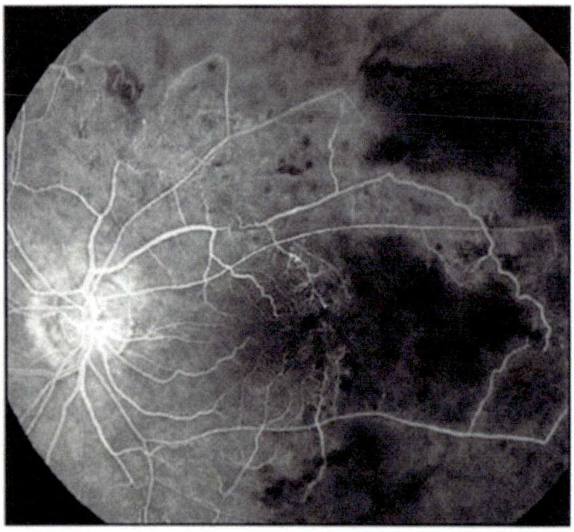

Figure 40: Diffuse macular hemorrhages with widespread capillary dropout.

Part Two:

External Diseases

Episcleritis

Definition: Episcleritis is an acute, benign, self-limiting condition of the episclera that is rarely associated with systemic disease. It can be further subdivided into diffuse and nodular forms.

Epidemiology: Episcleritis is more prevalent in females, and occurs most frequently in young and middle-aged adults, but affects all age groups. It is usually idiopathic, but may be associated with a number of systemic diseases:

- Diffuse episcleritis may occur in association with seronegative arthropathies (such as Reiter's syndrome and enteropathic arthritis) and any of the vasculitides.

- Nodular episcleritis is most frequently idiopathic, but may be associated with any of the rheumatic conditions, particularly rheumatoid arthritis; such patients account for approximately 6 percent of all cases of episcleritis.

Clinical Features: Episcleritis is abrupt in onset, with the eye becoming red within an hour of the start of the attack. The main symptom is mild discomfort or irritation. It is always localized to the eye and does not radiate. Unlike scleritis, there is no tenderness to palpation of the globe, and frank pain is uncommon. The main sign is redness, which may range from a mild pinkish hue to fiery red, with injection and dilation of the superficial episcleral blood vessels. Episcleritis is bilateral in approximately one-third of cases, although both eyes are not usually affected simultaneously. Recurrences are common over a period of years, decreasing in frequency after the first 3 to 4 years. Vision is usually not affected, but mild tearing and mild to moderate photophobia may be present.

Diagnosis: The ocular examination in sclera diseases must include an episcleral and scleral examination in addition to a general ophthalmologic examination. The episcleral examination should be performed under conditions of daylight and with the slit-lamp, employing diffuse, white light, the narrow slit beam, and red-free illumination. Slit-lamp examination under conditions of diffuse illumination helps to detect congested vessels, nodules, or avascular areas with sequestra or uveal show. It also helps to differentiate the configuration of vessels; in episcleritis, congested vessels follow the usual radial pattern, whereas in scleritis, the pattern is altered, and new abnormal vessels are formed. Slit-lamp examination with the narrow slit beam helps to detect the depth of inflammation, indicating which network of vessels is predominantly affected. In episcleritis, maximum congestion is in the superficial episcleral network, with no changes in the deep episcleral network. The edema is localized to the episcleral tissue. Topical application of 10% phenylephrine renders the eye white, as its vasoconstrictor effect is greater on the superficial episcleral plexus with no significant effect on the deep episcleral vessels.

Anterior segment fluorescein angiogram demonstrates that the speed of circulation is very rapid in the affected area, with the whole transit of dye being completed within three seconds as opposed to the normal 11 to 15 seconds. There is also extensive leakage, mainly into the episcleral nodule in nodular episcleritis, with no changes in the normal vascular pattern. ICG angiography also demonstrates extremely rapid filling and short transit time, although there is no leakage.

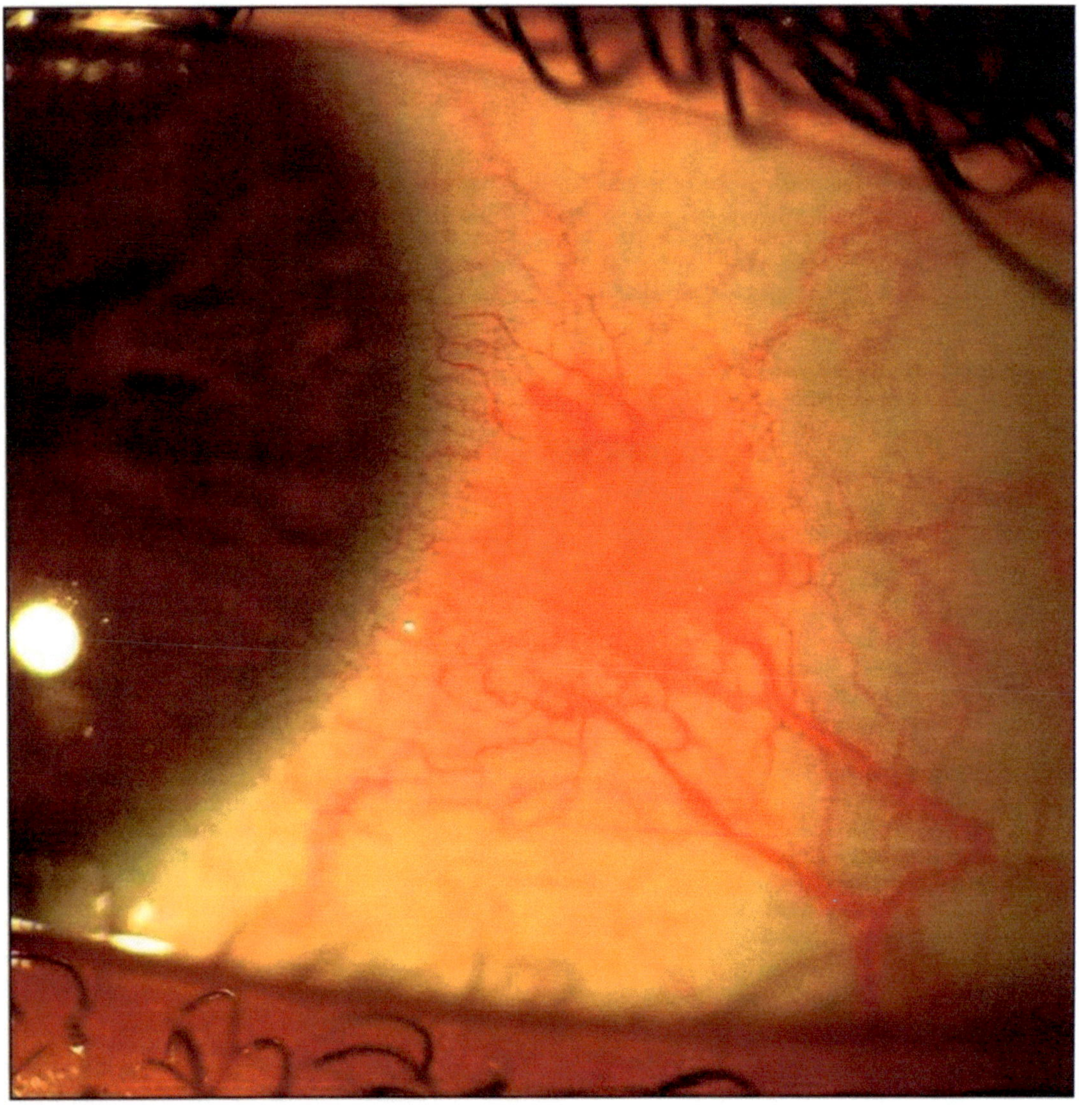

Figure 41: Nodular episcleritis in a 10 year-old male.

Treatment: Episcleritis is a benign self-limiting process and apart from palliative therapy with cool compresses and iced lubrication, may be left untreated. Topical NSAIDs appear to be ineffective. Topical corticosteroids speed up the resolution process, but significant side effects such as elevated intraocular pressure and cataract formation may occur. Recurrences of the episcleritis are common on cessation of the corticosteroids. Patients with nodular episcleritis with persistent episodes or frequent recurrences require oral NSAIDs, Episcleritis associated with rosacea, atopy, gout, or herpetic disease should be treated with specific therapy for each disease.

References:

1) C. Stephen Foster and Maite Sainz de la Maza. *The Sclera.* New York: Springer -Verlag, 1994:95 -137
2) Episcleritis and Scleritis. De la Maza. *Contemporary Ophthalmology.* Vol 5#9 2006:1-2

Acute Allergic Conjunctivitis

Immune-Mediated Conjunctivitis: The eye is a very intricate organ which may be affected by any immunologic process. Understanding the mechanism of a particular patient's inflammatory problem is importance if one is to develop a rational treatment regimen. Allergic conjunctivitis encompasses a variety of disorders characterized by immunologic hypersensitivity reactions directed against allergens. Atopic (out of place, inappropriate) phenomena are responsible for the ocular allergies. These are usually categorized into acute or chronic disease, the former including seasonal (SAC) and perennial allergic conjunctivitis (PAC). Chronic ocular surface allergic phenomena include giant papillary conjunctivitis (GPC), vernal keratoconjunctivitis (VKC), and atopic keratoconjunctivitis (AKC).

Definition/History: Allergic conjunctivitis is characterized by swelling and redness of the mucous membrane that lines the inner surface of the eyelids (palpebral conjunctiva) and the front part of the sclera (bulbar conjunctiva). The term "allergy" was coined by the Austrian pediatrician Clemens Pirquet who defined it as a harmful hypersensitivity. The word allergy is derived from the Greek words "allos," meaning different or changed and "ergos," meaning work or action. It was first used in 1905 to describe the adverse reactions that occurred in children that had been vaccinated with horse serum.

Epidemiology: Seasonal (SAC) and perennial allergic conjunctivitis (PAC) are the most commonly reported types of ocular allergy. SAC may affect up to 33% of individuals in a given population. A positive history of atopy with an obvious seasonal influence is a hallmark of this entity. PAC presents similarly, but with year-round symptoms. Common allergens including pollen, grass, and weeds in both conditions. Household dust, mites, and animal dander, year-long offenders are distinctive provocateurs in PAC.

Pathology/Pathogenesis: Acute allergic conjunctivitis is by the most part a type I (immediate) hypersensitivity reaction in which IgE antibodies are produced when a previously sensitized individual comes in contact with an allergen. Mast cells are central to this process, being upregulated after exposure to the offending antigen. Cross-linked IgE antibodies then interact with mast cells and basophils, causing the release of numerous pre-formed inflammatory mediators, such as histamine, prostaglandins and leukotrienes, into the conjunctival epithelium. Chemotactic and adhesion molecules provide continuous stimuli by recruiting eosinophils and neutrophils to the area, perpetuating this inflammatory cascade through the production of additional inflammatory molecules. These molecular changes translate into increased vascular permeability and characteristic conjunctival findings.

Clinical Features: Itching and tearing are classic symptoms in both SAC and PAC, and are usually bilateral. Vision is typically unaffected, an important feature which distinguishes acute from chronic allergic conjunctivitis. Allergic rhinitis and a positive history of atopy will be found in most patients. Physical examination reveals a hyperemic, edematous bulbar and/or tarsal conjunctiva without corneal findings. Erythematous, swollen eyelids may be observed. Purulent secretions should alert the physician of an underlying infectious rather than allergic etiology.

Diagnosis: Diagnosis is usually straight forward, based on the patient's history and physical examination. Conjunctival biopsy is not routinely performed, but when done, will reveal mast cells and eosinophils in the conjunctival epithelium. Increased levels of IgE and histamine in the patient's tears are to be expected.

Treatment:

Nonpharmacologic agents: The first step in treating allergic disorders is through allergen avoidance. To achieve this, the allergen(s) must be identified, usually through the patient's history, but many times with the help of an allergist. The expert allergist will become an invaluable resource, providing guidance in environmental control procedures and offering skin testing and/or allergen immunotherapy when deemed necessary. Physical measures, such as cool compresses and artificial tears, may suffice in controlling patients with mild disease.

Pharmacologic agents: These agents target various points in the allergic, inflammatory cascade. Treatment should be tailored in accordance to the patient's symptoms and findings. Vasoconstrictors (naphazoline, phenylephrine) will decrease ocular redness, but often cause a rebound injection once they are discontinued. Mast cell stabilizers (cromolyn sodium, lodoxamide, nedocromil sodium, and pemirolast potassium) prevent the release of allergic mediators, but only when used on a regular basis. They do not provide relief in acute episodes in which mast cell contents have already been released. Antihistamines (emedastine, levocabastine) reduce conjunctival injection and alleviate itching. Since they block histamine receptors in a reversible manner, their action is short-lived, limiting their use to controlling acute symptoms. Combined antihistamine/ mast cell stabilizers (olopatadine, epinastine, ketotifen) provide relief from both acute and chronic symptoms of the allergic reaction by decreasing the effects of both preformed and newly synthesized inflammatory molecules. This is the main reason why they are currently considered to be the mainstay of therapy. Nonsteroidal anti-inflammatory drugs (NSAIDs, ketorolac, bromfenac) may be used adjunctively and are useful in treating findings associated with vasodilatation. Corticosteroids are very effective, but long-term use of nonspecific anti-inflammatory drugs has been associated with varying degrees of ocular side effects, depending on their potency. Ophthalmologists should prescribe topical steroids in a regularly monitored setting.

Chronic Allergic Conjunctivitis

Definition/History: Chronic allergic conjunctivitis is perennial, occurring continuously or on and off year-round. *Vernal keratoconjunctivitis* (VKC) can affect the bulbar conjunctiva, the palpebral conjunctiva, or both. The limbal form of VKC was first described by Arlt in 1846, predating the description by von Graefe of the palpebral form by 25 years. *Atopic keratoconjunctivitis* (AKC) is associated with atopic dermatitis and was first described by Hogan in 1952. In 1974, Spring noticed that soft contact lens wearers developed an allergic reaction on the upper tarsal conjunctiva, presenting with complaints of contact lens intolerance and excessive mucus production. Three years later, Allensmith and coworkers provided a more detailed description of this disorder, calling it *giant papillary conjunctivitis* (GPC) because of the appearance of papillae in the upper tarsal conjunctiva.

Epidemiology: *Giant papillary conjunctivitis* is a well-known complication of chronic contact lens use. It is also seen in patients with ocular prosthesis, extruding scleral buckle retinal detachment surgery material, and corneal foreign bodies. In a retrospective study by Donshik and Porazinski, 21% of contact lens users who replaced their lenses at 4 weeks or longer developed GPC. They did not find a relationship between GPC and sex, age, contact lens material or fitting characteristics of the lens.

Vernal keratoconjunctivitis (VKC) is a disease that generally affects young men, with pronounced seasonal influence. Bonini reported that approximately 23% of patients have a perennial form of VKC and that 60% have additional recurrences during winter. It has a worldwide distribution, but is most common in the Mediterranean region and Central/South America. Past diagnosis of an atopic condition and a positive family history are present in the vast majority of affected individuals. One particularly well-known allergen in patients with VKC is the house dust mite and its feces. VKC may be further subdivided into palpebral and limbal forms, depending on the location of the papillae. The former exhibits the classic "cobble-stone papillae" in the tarsal conjunctiva. Limbal VKC is distinguished by the presence of large papillae at the corneoscleral limbus, with associated Horner-Trantas dots, collections of inflammatory cells at the papillaes' apices.

Atopic keratoconjunctivitis (AKC) presents most frequently in men, in their late teen years or early 20S, and may persist until the fourth or fifth decade of life. Between 25% and 40% of patients with atopic dermatitis have some type of ocular complication. Earlier disease onset is associated with greater ocular surface epithelial damage due to the effects of prolonged inflammation. Atopic keratoconjunctivitis is always bilateral and does not present with obvious seasonal variations.

Pathology/Pathogenesis: *Giant papillary conjunctivitis*- In addition to exhibiting the classic type I- hypersensitivity response of all allergic disorders, GPC appears to have mixed mechanisms. It seems to develop because of tarsal conjunctival sensitization to environmental allergenic material present on the surface of the contact lens, coupled with the trauma to the upper tarsal conjunctiva associated with the excursion of the eyelid over the lens. This irritation causes the release of neutrophil chemotactic factor and other inflammatory mediators.

Vernal keratoconjunctivitis-The histopathologic characterization of the tissues affected with VKC suggest that this entity results from a combination of both type I and type IV hypersensitivity reactions. The presence of the classic allergic mediators (mast cells and eosinophils) along with large collections of mononuclear cells, fibroblasts, and newly secreted collagen, explain the characteristic conjunctival findings. Leukotrienes may be largely responsible for chemosis, conjunctival injection, and increased mucus secretions. If unchecked, tarsal conjunctival remodeling and inflammation lead to corneal epithelial defects, and to the pathognomonic corneal "shield ulcer."

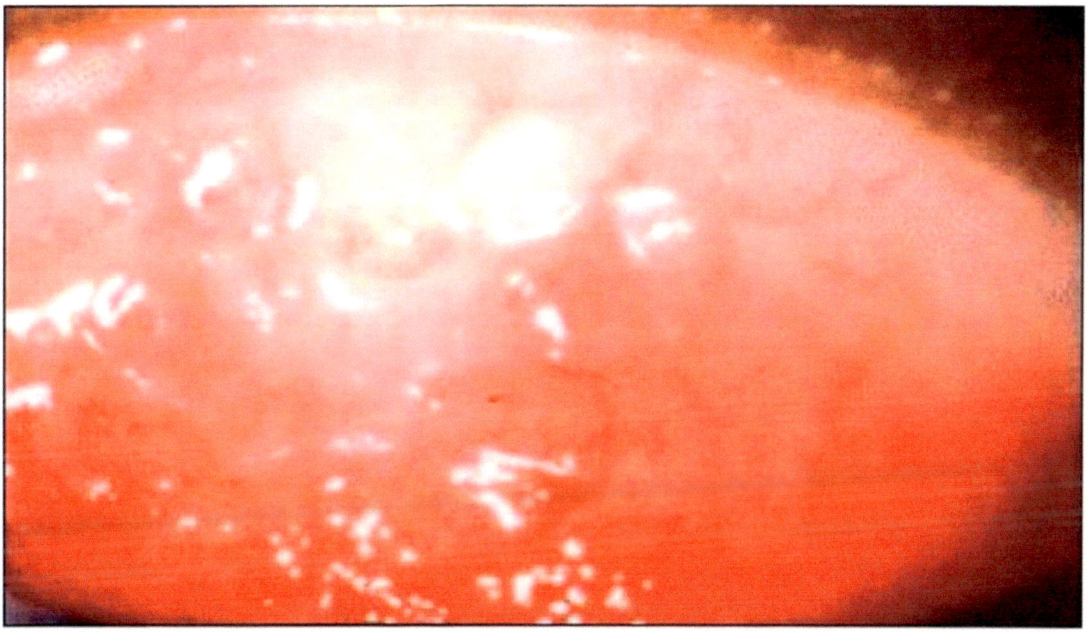

Figure 42: Mildy injected and edematous conjunctiva in a patient with allergic conjunctivitis.

Atopic keratoconjunctivitis-Type I hypersensitivity is only one of the mechanisms in the pathogenesis of AKC; in fact it is widely accepted that Th2 cells play an important role as well, a finding that is shared with VKC. Ocular surface disease in patients with atopic dermatitis is characterized by decreased goblet cells and conjunctival squamous metaplasia, which seem to worsen with increased number of flare-ups. Reduced goblet cells counts contribute to tear instability by limiting the secretion of mucin. Fibroblast activation, proliferation, and subsequent cicatrization result from chronic conjunctival inflammation in which T cells, macrophages, and mast cells collaborate. Giant papillary formation is essential in the pathogenesis of AKC.Conjunctival histopathologic examination of the excised papillae show elevated number of goblet cells, inflammatory leukocytes, and fibrotic tissue, along with evidence of angiogenesis. Upregulated interferon-gamma levels correlate with increased expression of ICAM-1 on conjunctival fibroblasts and the secretion of IL-6 and IL-8. When activated by IL-4 and TNF-alpha, corneal fibroblasts expressed ICAM-1 and VCAM-1 and increased eotaxin production, all leading to continued eosinophil adhesion to these molecules and persistent allergic keratopathy.

Clinical Features:

Giant papillary conjunctivitis- Patients will complain of progressive contact lens intolerance, foreign body sensation, and excessive mucus production. Visual symptoms may arise when there is a significant accumulation of mucus and/or protein underneath the lens or in advanced cases presenting with corneal pathology. Upon initial examination, mild bulbar conjunctival injection and deposition of mucus in tears and over the lens surface may be the only findings. Eversion of the upper eyelid discloses conjunctival hyperemia and tarsal papillae greater than 1 mm in diameter.

Vernal keratoconjunctivitis- The predominant symptom of VKC is itching. Excessive tearing, mucus production, photophobia, and foreign body sensation are common. The signs are mostly confined to the conjunctiva and cornea. The hallmark of VKC is the presence of giant papillae, usually in the upper tarsal conjunctiva, with an associated ropy mucus discharge found in the inferior fornix.Vision threatening complications of VKC occur in the cornea, usually in the form of mild epithelial keratitis, or in more severe cases, as "shield ulcers." Keratoconus may be seen in chronic cases, secondary to chronic eye rubbing.

Atopic keratoconjunctivitis- Patients with AKC often develop eyelid irritation, a finding mostly seen in AKC, not VKC. Ophthalmic symptoms include itching, photophobia, burning, foreign body sensation, excessive tearing, and an abundant mucoid discharge. Common signs in AKC are conjunctival injection, upper tarsal giant papillae, and blepharitis. Cicatrizing conjunctivitis, lid dermatitis, and chronic blepharitis with lid thickening and meibomian gland dysfunction are typical. In cases complicated by conjunctival scarring symblepharon, an aberrant adhesion between the bulbar and palpebral conjunctiva, may form. Superficial punctate keratitis may progress into persistent epithelial defects with associated herpes simplex or Staphylococcus aureus superinfections. Loss of vision occurs because of corneal scarring and neovascularization.

Diagnosis: Past medical and family history along with the patient's signs and symptoms should be enough to confirm the diagnosis. Further testing is warranted if the patient does not respond to standard therapy. IgE determination and skin testing are not considered useful because about half of the patients will have negative results. The histopathologic findings of the conjunctiva of patients with AKC are characterized by mast cell and eosinophil invasion of the epithelium, epithelial pseudotubule formation and increased goblet cells.

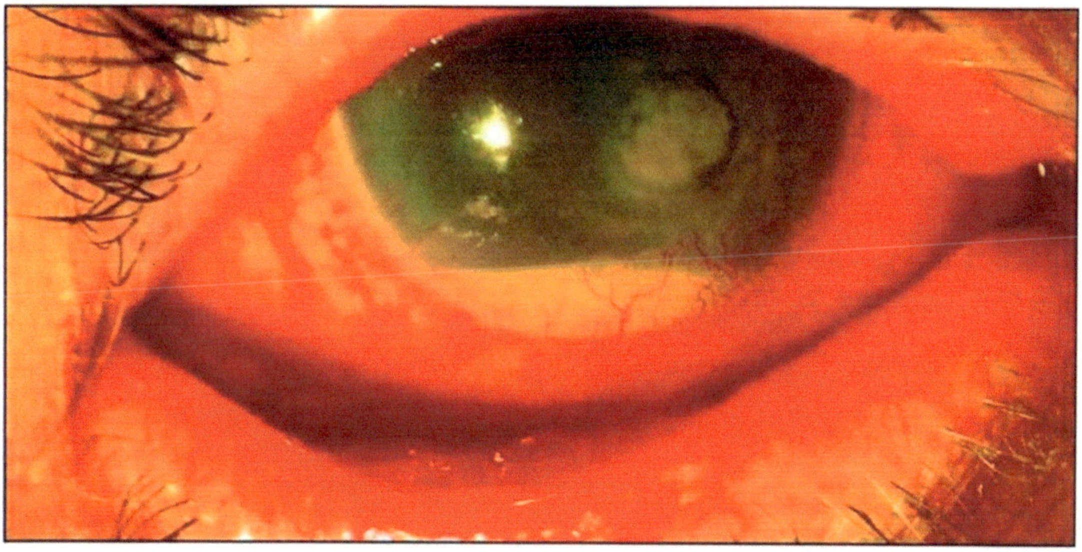

Figure 43: Severe conjunctival inflammation, corneal epithelial scar, and hypopyon in a patient with atopic keratoconjunctivis.

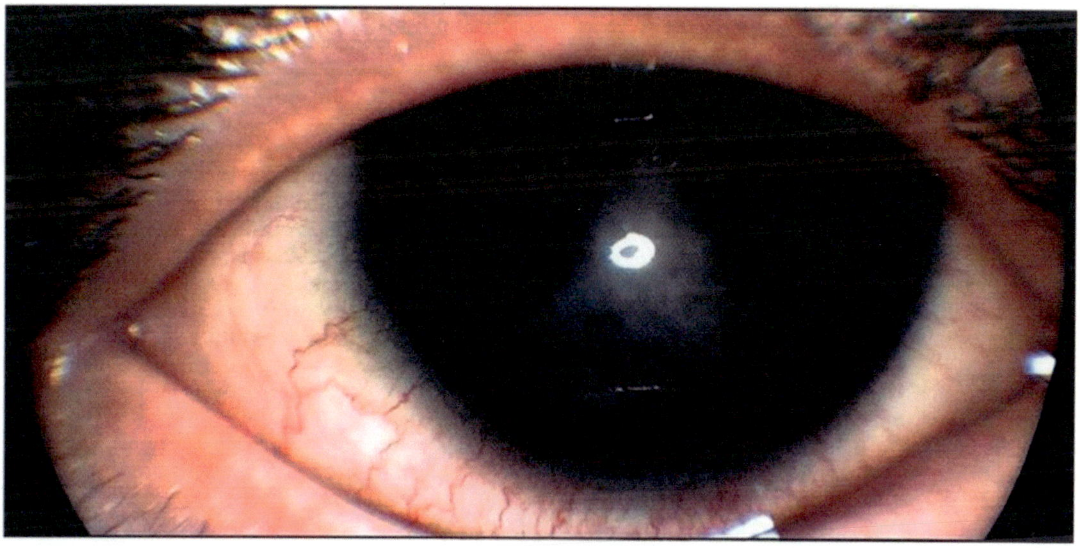

Figure 44: Central triangular corneal scar secondary to atopic keratoconjunctivitis.

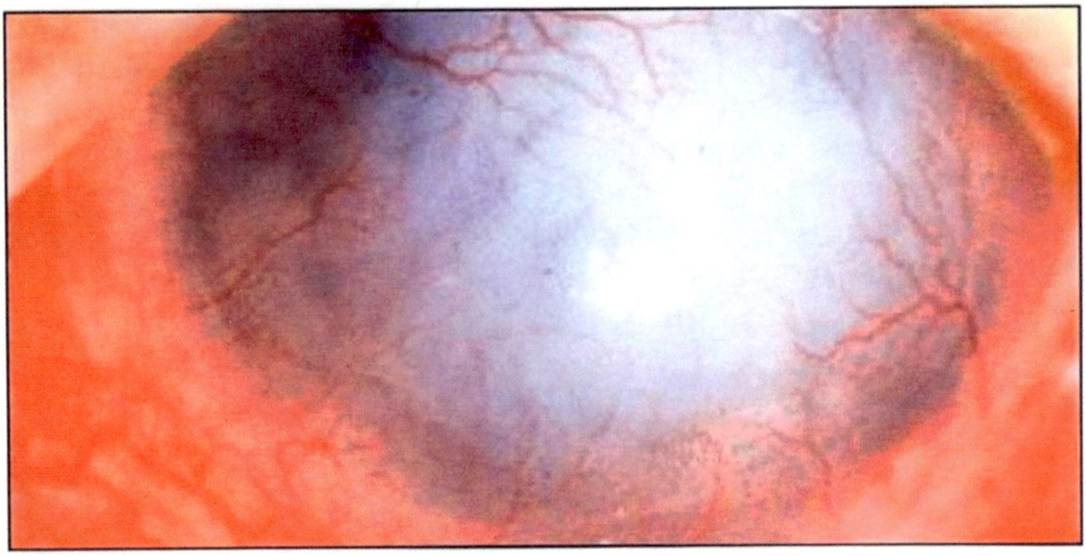

Figure 45: Corneal neovascularization in a severe case of atopic keratoconjunctivitis.

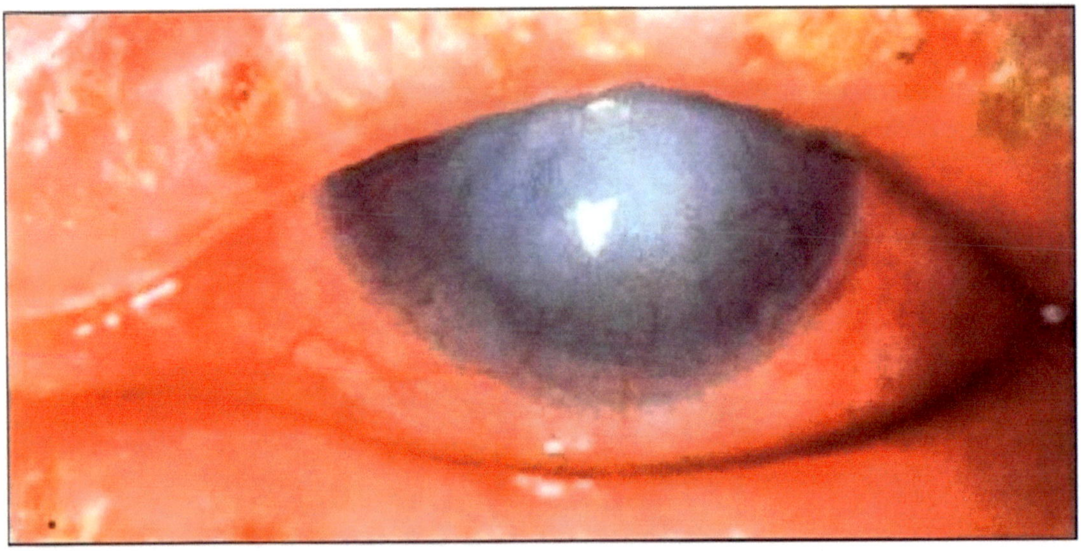

Figure 46: Erythematous lids, crusting, and scaling in atopic blepharoconjunctivitis.

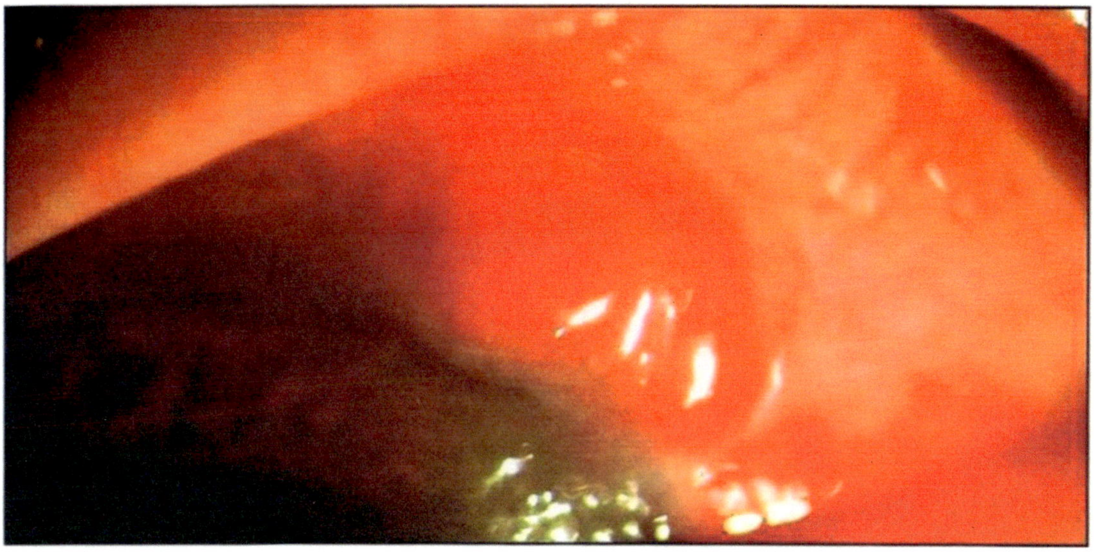

Figure 47: Conjunctival granuloma with vasculitic and atopic components in a patient with keratoconjunctivitis.

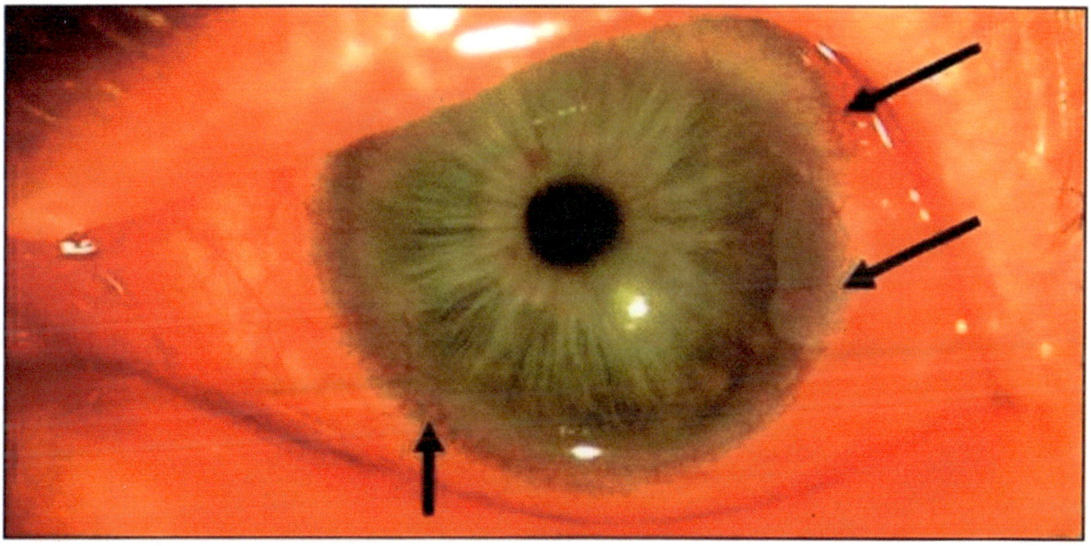

Figure 48: Pannus and limbal hypertrophy secondary to AKC.

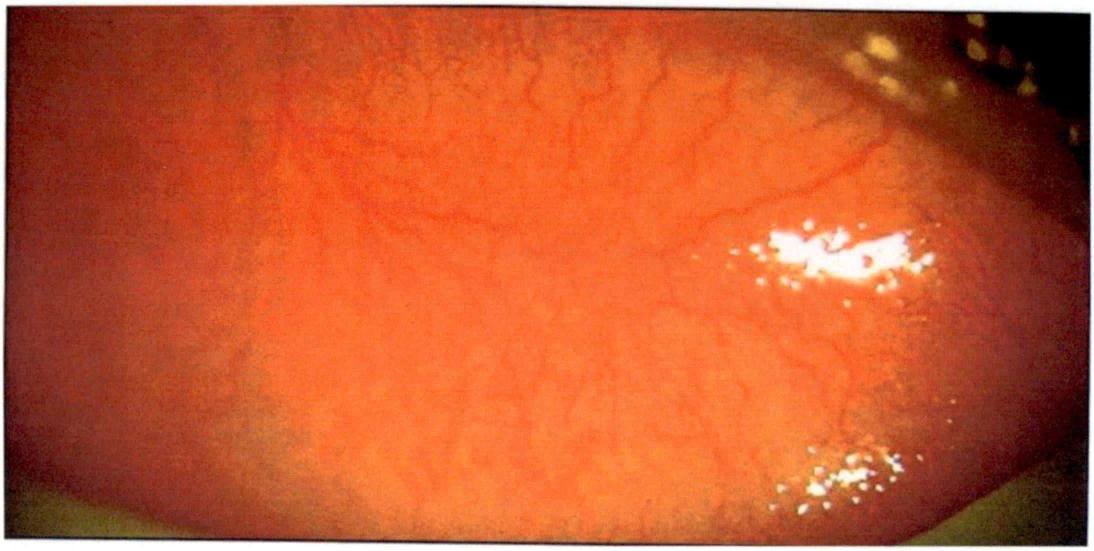

Figure 49: Conjunctival injection in a patient with fine papillae in giant papillary conjunctivitis.

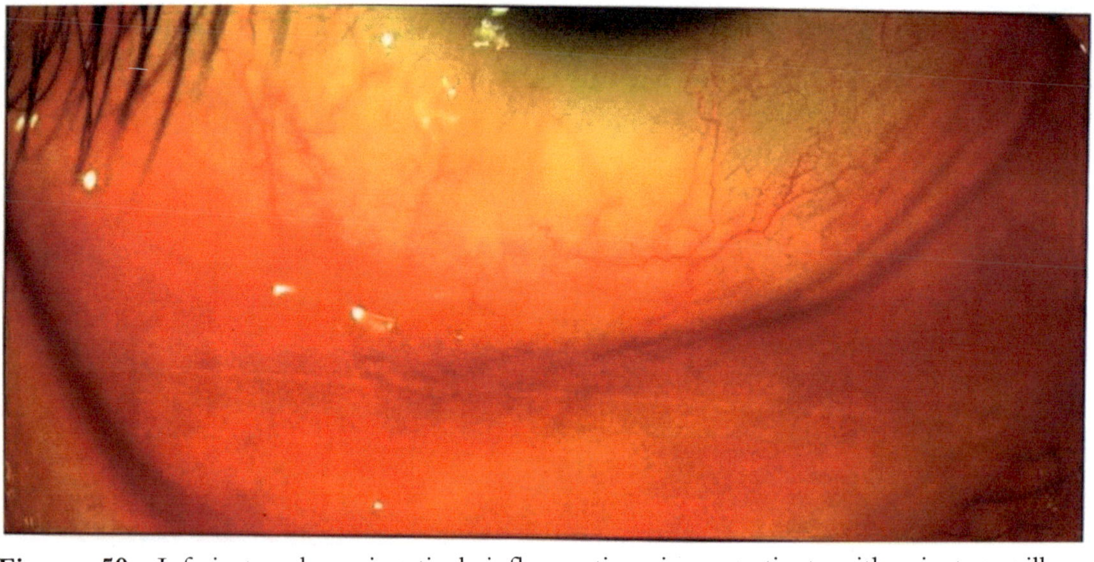

Figure 50: Inferiortorsal conjunctival inflammation in a patient with giant papillary conjunctivitis.

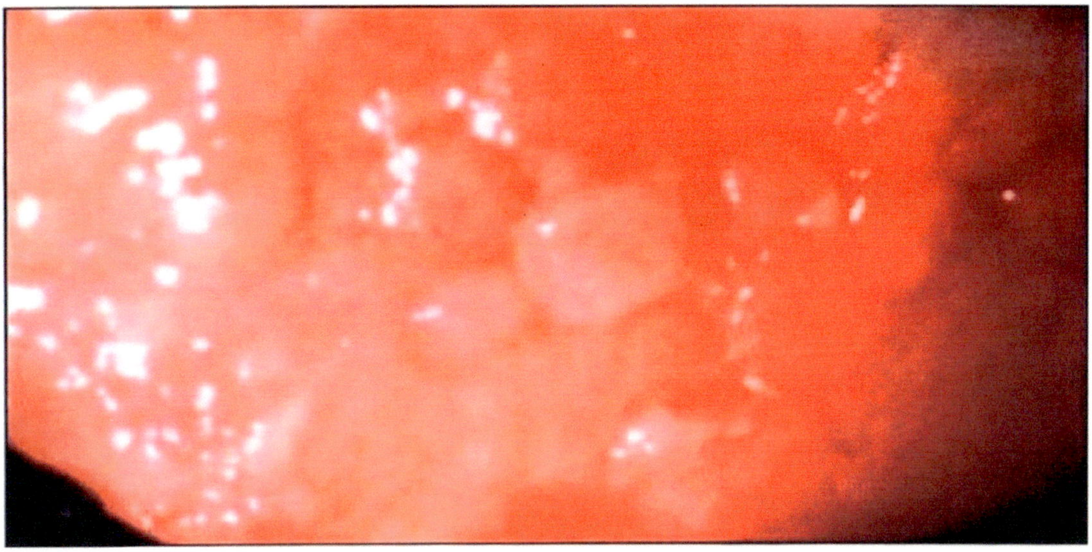

Figure 51: Characteristic finding of cobblestone-like giant papillae of the upper tarsal conjunctiva in VKC.

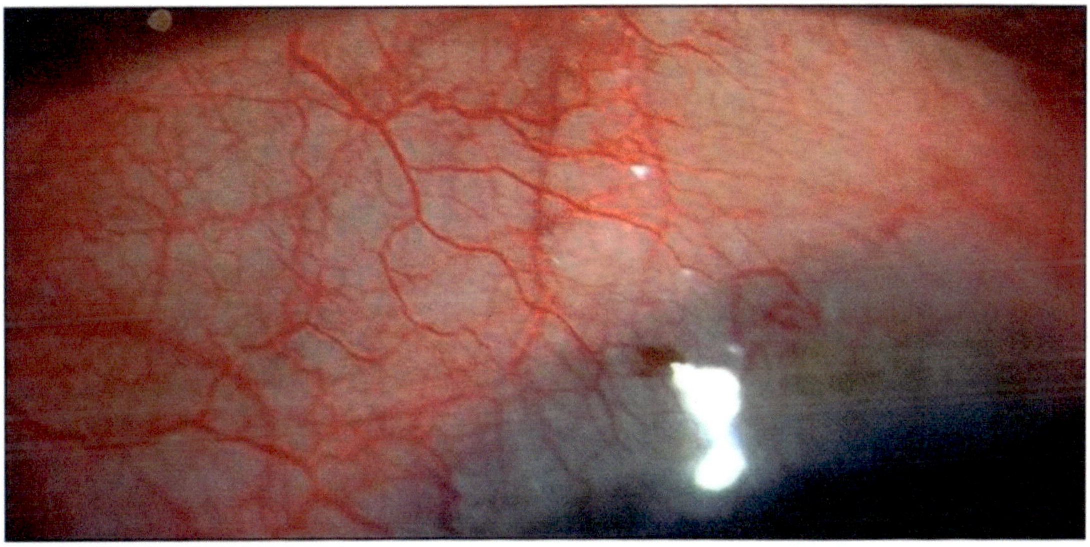

Figure 52: Conjunctival injection in a patient with vernal keratoconjunctivitis.

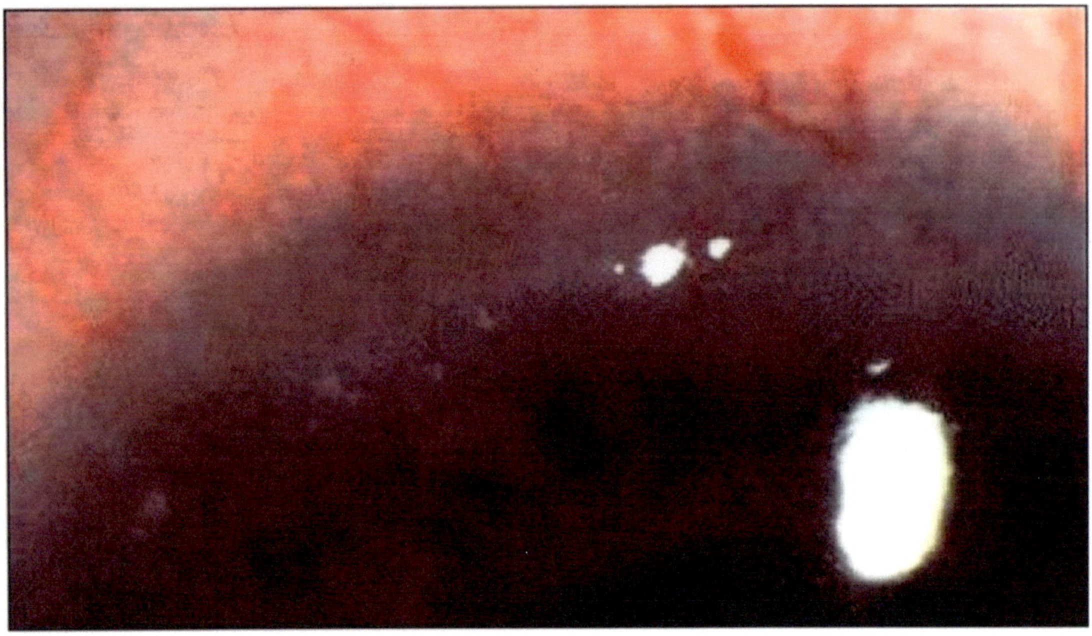

Figure 53: Limbal nodules and Trantas' dots as seen in VKC

Treatment:

Nonpharmacologic agents: As with acute conjunctivitis, identification and removal of the offending agent is crucial. Patients with GPC should limit the use of contact lenses, at times discontinuing their use altogether.

Pharmacologic agents: Topical combinations of mast cell stabilizers/antihistamines provide significant relief of symptoms and are currently the treatment of choice for chronic ocular allergy. Topical steroids may be used in acute episodes or to control breakthrough attacks after the patient has encountered a stimulating allergen. Adjunctive ocular therapy is required for secondary infection, for extreme mucus production and mucous plaque formation on "shield ulcers" and for persistent epithelial defects. Topical cyclosporine (Restasis) is well tolerated, and may be effective in reducing the signs and symptoms of VKC. N-acetylcysteine, a mucolytic agent used four times a day at 10-20% concentration, decreases mucus production, while bandage contact lenses aid heal epithelial defects. Systemic cyclosporine has been useful in controlling AKC through its inhibition of IL-2 and resultant reduction in T cell activation.

Surgical care: Surgical care is generally not employed except in advanced, refractory cases. Limbal cell transplants have been successful in patients in which previous amniotic membrane graft alone did not restore the ocular surface. Other surgical procedures such as cryoablation of giant papillae or surgical removal of papillae with mucosal grafting are generally not required, but may be helpful in extremely advanced cases.

References:

1) George du Toit. *Current Allergy & Clinical Immunology*, 2005 Vol 18, No.3.
2) Arlt F: Physiologisch and pathologisch anatomische Bemerkungen fiber die Bindehaut des Auges. *Prager Vierteljahrschrift* 1846; 4: 73.
3) von Graefe A: Klinische Vortrage fiber *Augenheilkunde*. Germany, Hirschberg, 1871, p 21.
4) Hogan, MJ. Atopic keratoconjunctivitis. *Trans Am Ophthalmol Soc* 1952; 50: 265- 81.
5) Spring TF: Reaction to hydrophilic lenses. *Med J Aust* 1974; 1:499.
6) Allansmith MR, Korb DR, Greiner JV, et al. Giant papillary conjunctivitis in contact lens wearers. *Am J Ophthalmol* 1977; 83: 697-708.
7) Friedlander MH. Conjunctivitis of allergic origin: Clinical presentation and differential diagnosis. *Surv Ophthalmol* 1993; 38 (suppl): 105-14.
8) Donshik PC and Porazinski AD. Giant papillary conjunctivitis in frequent-replacement contact lens wearers: a retrospective study. *Trans Am Ophthalmol Soc.* 1999; 97: 205-16; discussion 216-20.
9) Bonini S, Lambiase A, Marchi S, Pasqualetti P, Zuccaro 0, et al . Vernal keratoconjunctivitis revisited: a case series of 195 patients with long-term follow-up. *Ophthalmology*, 2000; 107: 1157-63.
10) Foster CS. Immunologic Disorders of the Conjunctiva, Cornea, and Sclera. *Principles and Practices of Ophthalmology:* Section VIII, Chapter 65, 2nd Edition. Philadelphia: WB Saunders Publishers, 1999; 803-828.
11) Garrity JA, Liesegang TJ. Ocular complications of atopic dermatitis. *Can J Ophthalmol* 1984; 19: 21-4.
12) Onguchi T, Dogru M, Okada N, Kato NA, Tanaka M, Takano Y, Fukagawa K et al. The impact of the onset time of atopic keratoconjunctivitis on the tear function and ocular surface findings. *Am J Ophthalmol* 2006; 141(3): 569-71.
13) Elgebaly SA, Donshik PC, Rahhal F, Williams W. Neutrophil chemotactic factor in the tears of giant papillary conjunctivitis patients. *Invest Ophthalmol Vis Sci* 1991; 32: 208-13.
14) Dogru M, Okada N, Asano-Kato N, Tanaka M, Igarashi A, Takano Y et al. Atopic ocular surface disease: implications on tear function and ocular surface mucins. *Cornea* 2005; 24(8 Supply: S18-S23.
15) Spencer, W.H., Zimmerman, L.E. Conjunctiva; Third Ed. *Ophthalmic Pathology: An Atlas and Textbook,* Vol 1. W.B. Saunders Company, Philadelphia, PA 1985. pp 109-228.
16) Volker, H.E., Naumann, G.O.H. Conjunctiva; *Pathology of the Eye,* First Ed. Springer-Verlag, Berlin 1985. pp 249-316.
17) Leonardi A, Fregona IA, Plebani M, Secchi AG, Calder VL. Thi- and The-type cytokines in chronic ocular allergy. Graefes *Arch Clin Exp Ophthalmol* 2006; [Epub ahead of print]
18) Okada N, Fukagawa K, Takano Y, Dogru M, Tsubota K, Fujishima H et al. The implications of the upregulation of ICAM-1/VCAM-1 expression of corneal fibroblasts on the pathogenesis of allergic keratopathy. *Invest Ophthalmol Vis Sci* 2005; 46(12): 4512-8.
19) Jay JL. Clinical features and diagnosis of adult atopic keratoconjunctivitis and the effect of treatment with sodium cromoglycate. *Br J Ophthalmol* 1981; 65: 335-4o.
20) Foster CS, Calonge M: Atopic keratoconjunctivitis. *Ophthalmology* 1990; 97: 992-1000.
21) Bonini S, Coassin M, Aronni S, Lambiase A. Vernal keratoconjunctivitis. *Eye* 2004; 18: 345-51.
22) Pucci N, Novembre E, Cianferoni A, Lombardi E, Bernardini R, Caputo R et al. Efficacy and safety of cyclosporine eyedrops in vernal keratoconjunctivitis. *Ann Allergy Asthma Immunol* 2002; 89(3): 298-303.
23) Sangwan VS, Murthy SI, Vemuganti GK, Bansal AK, Gangopadhyay N, Rao GN. Cultivated corneal epithelial transplantation for severe ocular surface disease in vernal keratoconjunctivitis. *Cornea* 2005; 24(4): 426-30.

Superior limbic keratoconjunctivitis

Definition/History: Superior limbic keratoconjunctivitis (SLK) is an inflammatory condition of the superior bulbar and tarsal conjunctiva and superior cornea. The condition was first described by Frederick H. Theodore in 1963.

Epidemiology: SLK is uncommon. It preferentially affects women ages 20-50, and 20-65 percent of patients with SLK have associated hyperthyroidism. Patients who have SLK and thyroid disease have a 90 percent probability of manifesting some kind of ophthalmopathy, about half being classified as severe.

Pathology/Pathogenesis: The cause of SLK is unknown. Most authors agree that the cause is likely mechanical. The superior bulbar conjunctiva in patients with SLK is abnormally mobile, becoming congested and edematous and bulky. The upper tarsal conjunctiva develops papillae, and together with the abnormal bulbar conjunctiva produce a vicious frictional cycle. The exposed abnormal surface epithelium stains with rose bengal and with lissamine green.

Clinical Features: Patients with SLK present with symptoms of foreign body and burning sensation, photophobia, and mucoid discharge. The degree of the patient's complaint may seem disproportionate to the objective findings. Subjective complaints of dry eye are common, and it is estimated that 25 percent of SLK patients do, in fact, have keratoconjunctivitis sicca. Slit lamp biomicroscopy reveals mild to moderate injection of conjunctival vasculature in a trapezoidal pattern in superior bulbar conjunctiva from limbus to varying extents posteriorly, from approximately 10 to 2 o'clock. This conjunctiva is thickened and is excessively mobile, as judged by watching its mobility as the examiner rubs the upper lid over the bulbar conjunctiva. The most diagnostic feature of the disease is found upon application of either rose Bengal or lissamine green dye, producing punctate staining of the superior bulbar conjunctiva. Papillae are also evident on the superior palpebral conjunctiva, giving it a velvety appearance, as this conjunctiva too is inflamed. The inferior palpebral conjunctiva is uninvolved. Corneal filaments occur in one-third of SLK patients (in those with more intense keratitis).

Diagnosis: SLK is typically bilateral but often asymmetric. The diagnosis of SLK is based solely upon the characteristic presentation. All patients presenting with SLK should undergo a systemic workup, including a serologic thyroid panel.

Treatment: SLK is chronic, recurrent and recalcitrant. And while it is not a threat to vision, it is commonly a significant source of aggravation and diminishes the patient's quality of life. While no treatment has yet been shown to be 100 percent effective, some modalities have been employed successfully. The most consistently effective therapies alter the relationship of the bulbar conjunctiva with the underlying sclera, such that the abnormal mobility of the conjunctiva is eliminated. Resection of the affected conjunctiva results in resurfacing of sclera with new conjunctiva which is tightly adherent. The same result can sometimes be achieved through the application of multiple points of cautery to the affected area. Continuous wear bandage soft contact lenses alleviate the mechanical irritation and the symptoms so long as the lenses are in place.

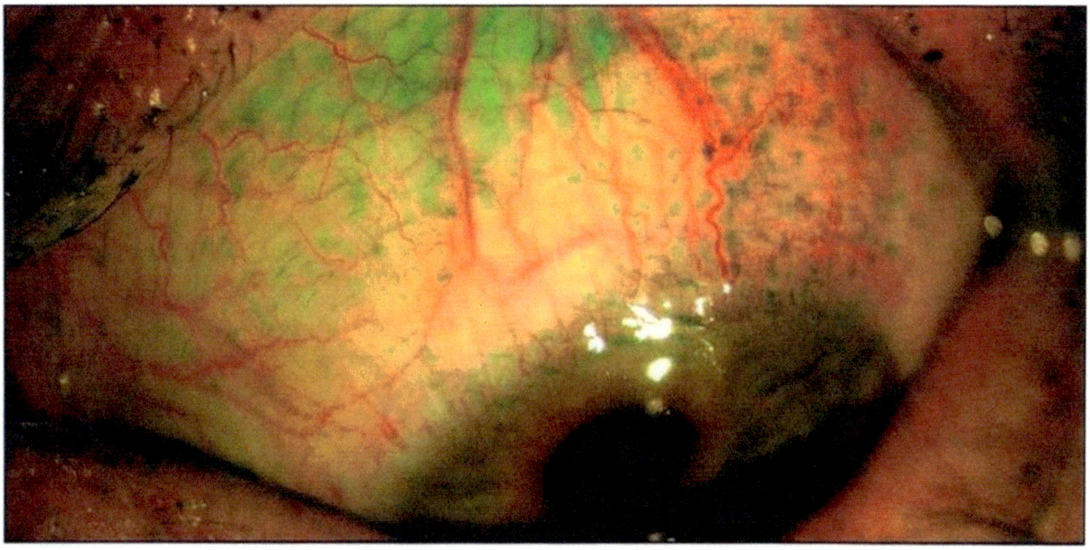

Figure 54: Superior limbic keratoconjunctivitis in patient with Sjogren's syndrome and lupus. Note the lissamine green-stained superior bulbar conjunctiva

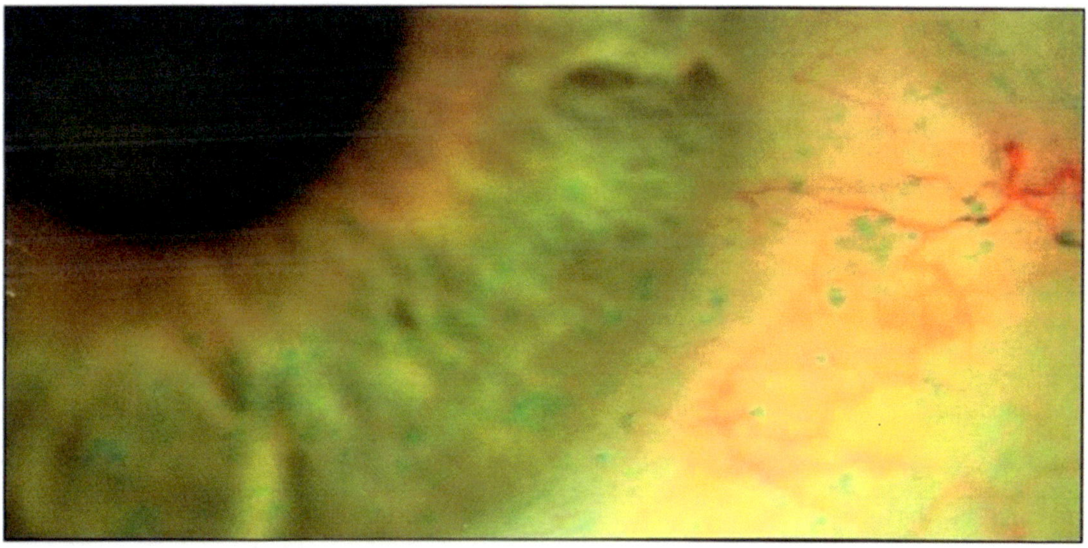

Figure 55: Inferior epithelial keratitis in the same patient with SLK.

Reference: Cher I. Blink-related microtrauma: when the ocular surface harms itself. *Clin Experiment Ophthalmol* 2003;3:183-90

Ocular cicatricial pemphigoid

Definition: Mucous membrane pemphigoid (MMP) is an immune-mediated disease characterized by autoantibodies to glycoproteins of the basement membrane zone of mucous membranes. The disease causes sub-epithelial scarring of these mucosae and hence its previous and still used name of cicatricial pemphigoid. Ocular cicatricial pemphigoid (OCP) is one subgroup of MMP. It is a chronic and progressive sight threatening condition. It may also be fatal as a consequence of serious complications such as tracheal and esophageal strictures. Systemic immunomodulatory therapy is essential in the care for patients with OCP; no topical therapy can ever put this systemic disease into remission. Early awareness and aggressive immunomodulatory therapy use is critical for the prevention of both ocular and systemic morbidity.

History: Lever was the first to make the clinical and histopathologic distinction between pemphigoid and pemphigus, but OCP has existed since ancient times. Lever and Talbott credit Hippocrates with the first use of the word pemphigoid. Hippocrates described different types of fevers including pemphigoid fever, *pemphigodes pyretoi*, which was probably a fever associated with blisters; the original connotation of the root word pemphix was air, puff, or perhaps swelling or blister.

Epidemiology: OCP is a relatively rare disease with an estimated incidence of 1 in 20,000 to 1 in 46,000 ophthalmic cases. Such processes typically last for several years and can ultimately lead to blindness. Approximately 80% of patients with mucous membrane pemphigoid or cicatricial pemphigoid have ocular involvement.

Pathogenesis: OCP is an autoimmune chronic cicatrizing conjunctivitis (CCC) associated with the linear deposition of immunoglobulin and complement on the conjunctival BMZ in vivo. Abnormal regulation of the immune system is a key feature of OCP. Patients with OCP have an increased expression of macrophage colony stimulating factor, heat shock protein 47 (HSP47), and transforming growth factor β1 (TGF-(β1)

Clinical Features: ***Systemic Manifestations:*** Cicatricial pemphigoid can affect the skin, scalp, oral mucosa, nasal mucosa, pharynx, larynx, esophagus, vagina, urethra and anus. Scarring of the vagina, urethral and anal mucosa can produce progressive stricture. Cicatricial pemphigoid can be fatal as a result of asphyxiation secondary to lodging of a food bolus in an esophageal stricture, and asphyxiation due to tracheal scarring and mucus accumulation. The skin lesions can present as recurrent vesiculobullous lesions similar to but smaller than those seen in bullous pemphigoid (which heal with no significant scarring) or erythematous plaques of the head and neck that evolve into pruritic blisters which rupture and leave atrophic scars (Brusting-Perry dermatitis).

Ocular Manifestations: A slow progression from chronic conjunctivitis to subepithelial fibrosis, fornix foreshortening, symblepharon, and ankyloblepharon formation with ocular surface keratinization are characteristic ocular manifestations. Dry eye syndrome due to loss of goblet cells and reduced tear production as a consequence of chronic inflammation is the rule during the pre-end-stage disease course. Another important complication of chronic OCP is trichiasis. Trichiasis was present in 86% of stage III eyes. Conjunctival keratinization is also a complication which can lead to chronic mechanical corneal surface damage.

Diagnosis: The diagnosis of OCP is based on clinical suspicion and immunohistopathology of conjunctival biopsy. Chronic conjunctivitis is the most common referral diagnosis in our experience. The subepithelial fibrosis that accompanies OCP leads to the ocular sequelae. The symblepharon appear as vertical folds between the bulbar and palpebral conjunctiva. During late stages of the disease, destruction of mucus-producing goblet cells in the conjunctiva decrease lacrimal tear quality. Severe cases can progress to corneal perforation.

Linear deposition of immunoreactants at the BMZ of inflamed conjunctiva is necessary for definitive diagnosis of OCP. If multiple mucous membranes are involved, the initial biopsy should be from one of the non-ocular mucous membranes. To date there is no sensitive and specific laboratory test to either establish the diagnosis or monitor the response to therapy.

Staging: We described our staging system in 1982. We defined 4 main stages that can describe the progressive destructive sequence of events during the natural course of the disease.

Stage .1: Conjunctival inflammation, mucous discharge, small patches of rose bengal-staining conjunctival epithelium, and conjunctival subepithelial fibrosis are the main initial features of the initial stages of the disease.

Stage 2: Include the presence of shortening of the conjunctival fornix. Within stage 2, the letters (a) through (d) describe the degree of fornix shortening: A. 0 to 25%, B. 25% to 50%,C. 50% to 75% and E. 75% to 100%.

Stage 3: At this stage the progressive subepithelial bands of connective tissue end up with symblepharon formation. As in stage 2, stage 3 is also subdivided (a) through (d) based on the percentage of horizontal involvement by symblepharon. Ocular pathology may be present as corneal vascularization, keratopathy, trichiasis, dystichiasis and severe dry eye.

Stage 4: Is the end stage of the disease which is characterized by ocular surface keratinization and ankyloblepharon.

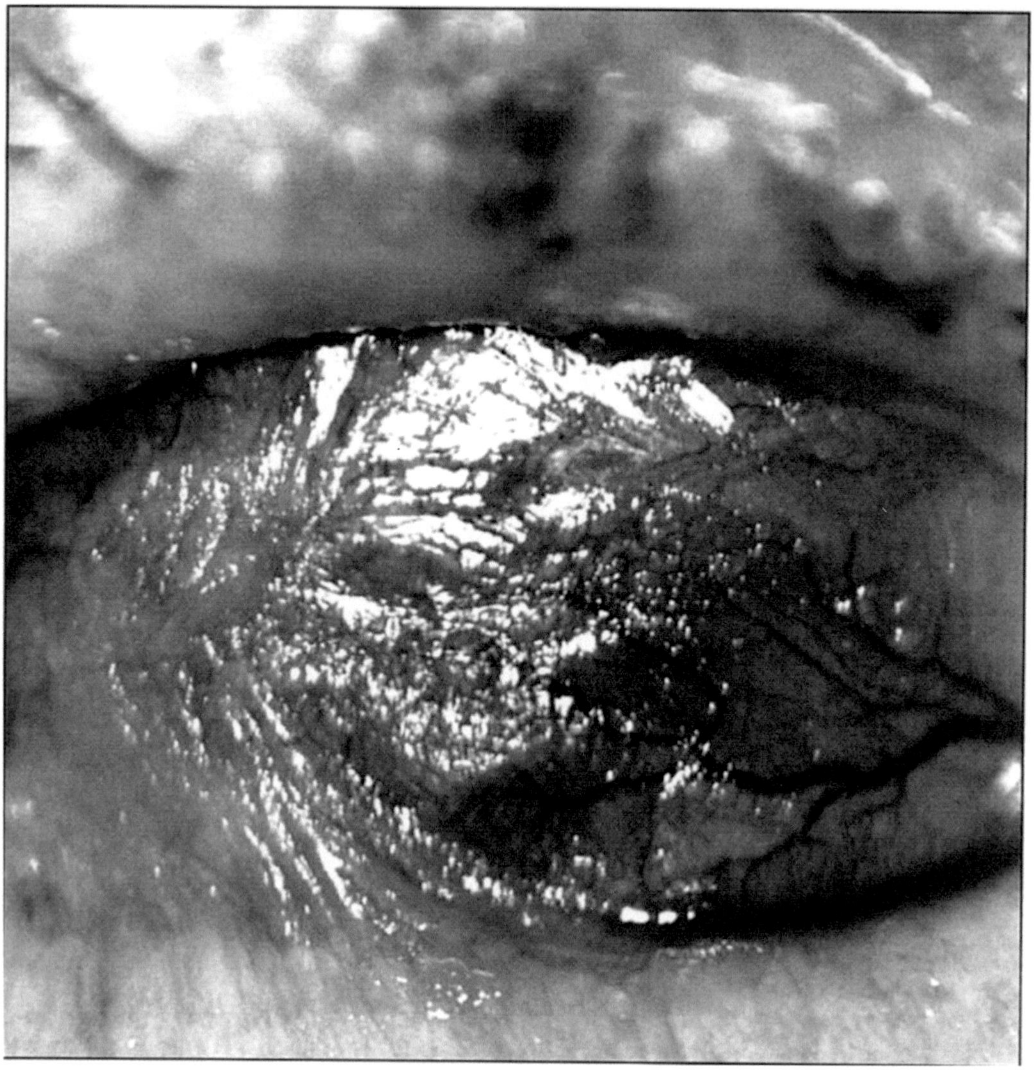

Figure 56: Conjunctivalization and keratinization of the entire surface of the cornea and ankyloblepharon in a patient with Stage IV OCP.

Treatment: High-dose oral prednisone can control scarring, but is ineffective for control induction and remission induction. Steroid-sparing agents are a preferable treatment strategy due to its low potential adverse effect that can be prevented with close monitoring of toxicity. We had previously demonstrated the effectiveness of immunomodulatory therapy decreasing the risk of progression of OCP in a prospective, nonrandomized, controlled study. Surgical approaches for patients with OCP include lid surgery to correct trichiasis and lid margin abnormalities, and symblepharon. Conjunctival restoration can be done by mucous membrane transplantation. Corneal surface can be treated with amniotic membrane transplantation, limbal stem cell transplantation, and lamellar keratoplasty/penetrating keratoplasty. And the last resource is implantation of a keratoprosthesis.

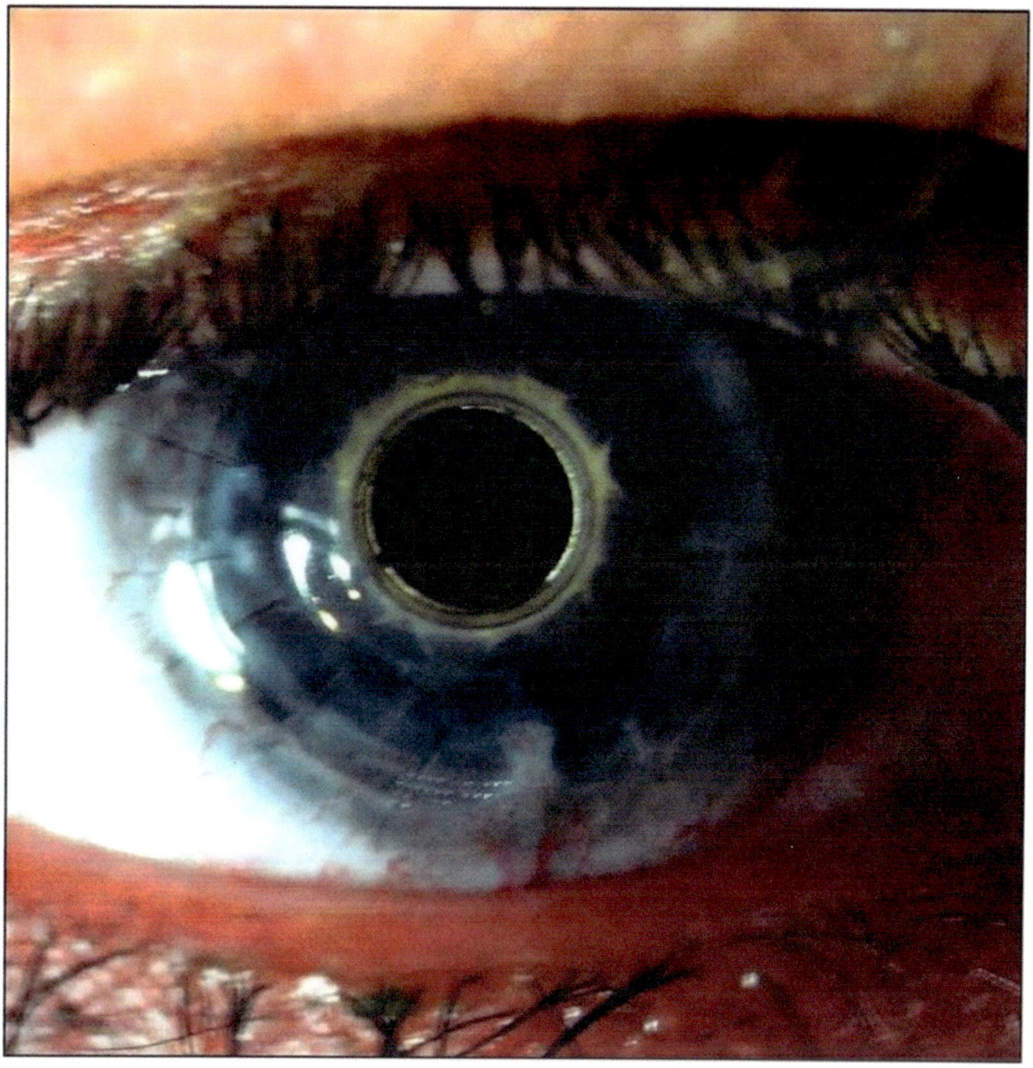

<u>Figure 57:</u> Type I Boston Keratoprothesis.

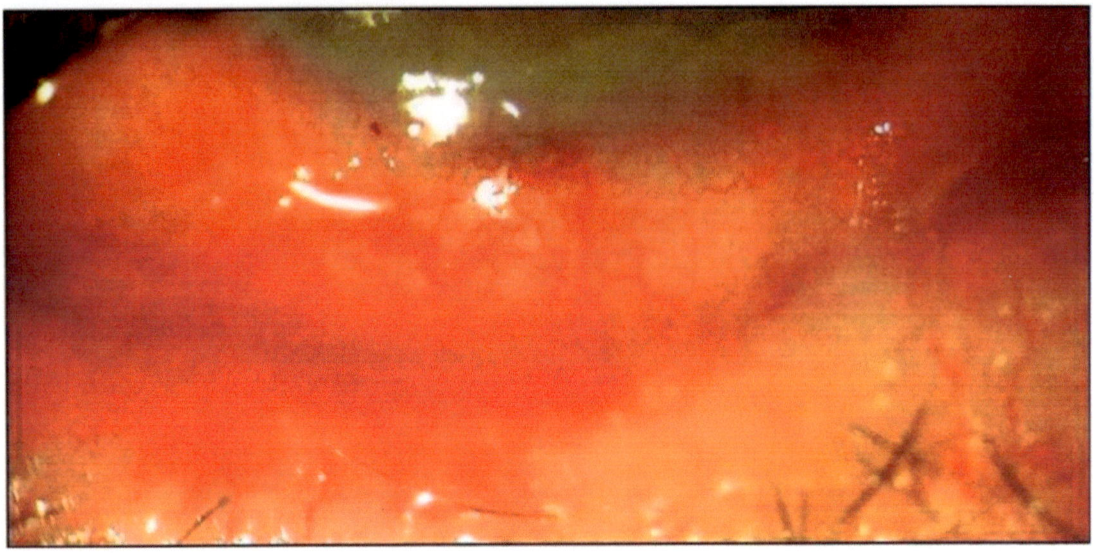

Figure 58: Ankyloblepharon, corneal scarring, and meibomian gland dysfunction in stage III OCP.

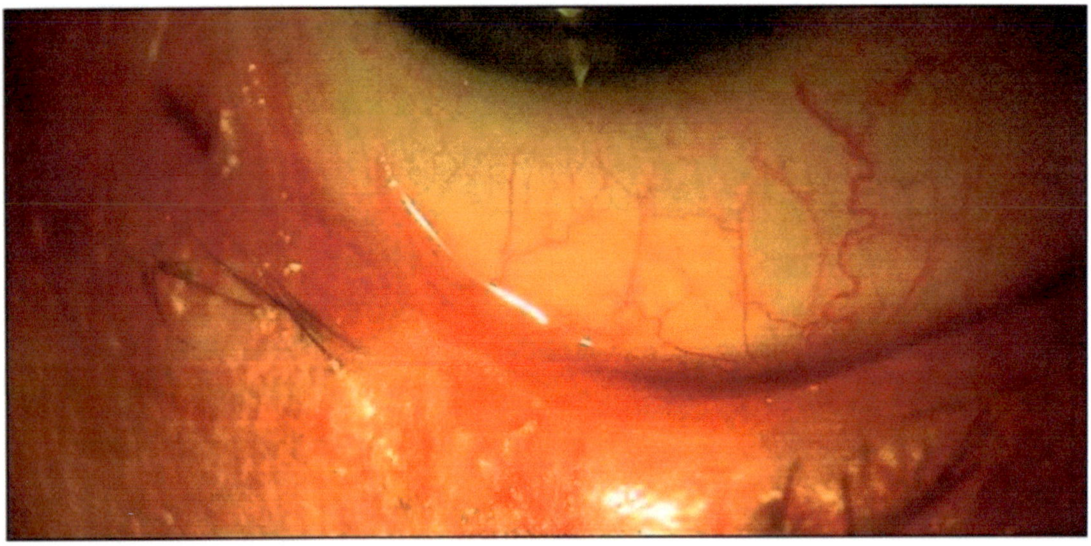

Figure 59: Stage II OCP, active, up-gaze showing temporal symblepharon.

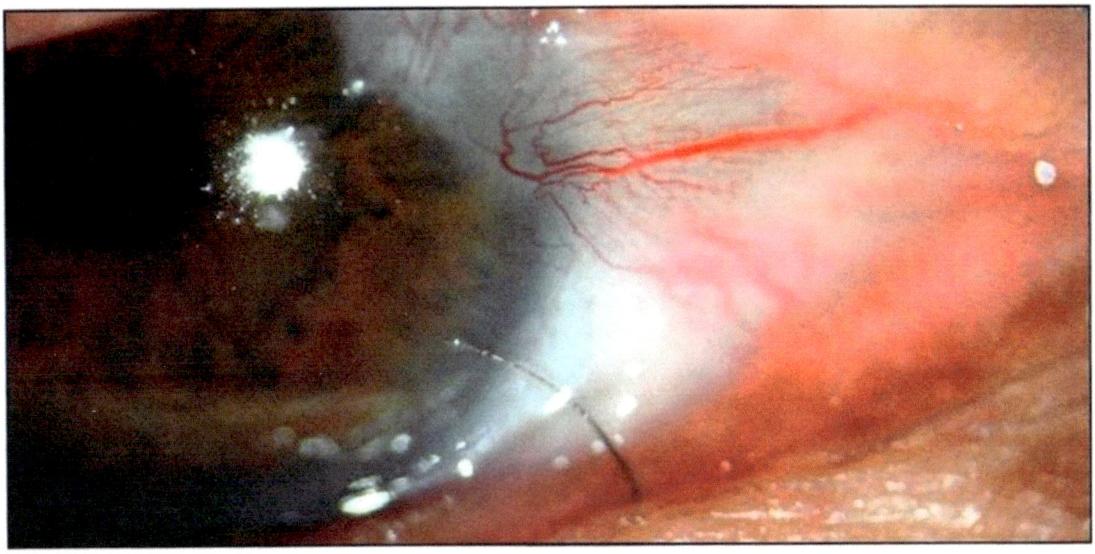

Figure 60: Pannus and trichitic lash on the inferior eyelid in a patient with quiet Stage III OCP.

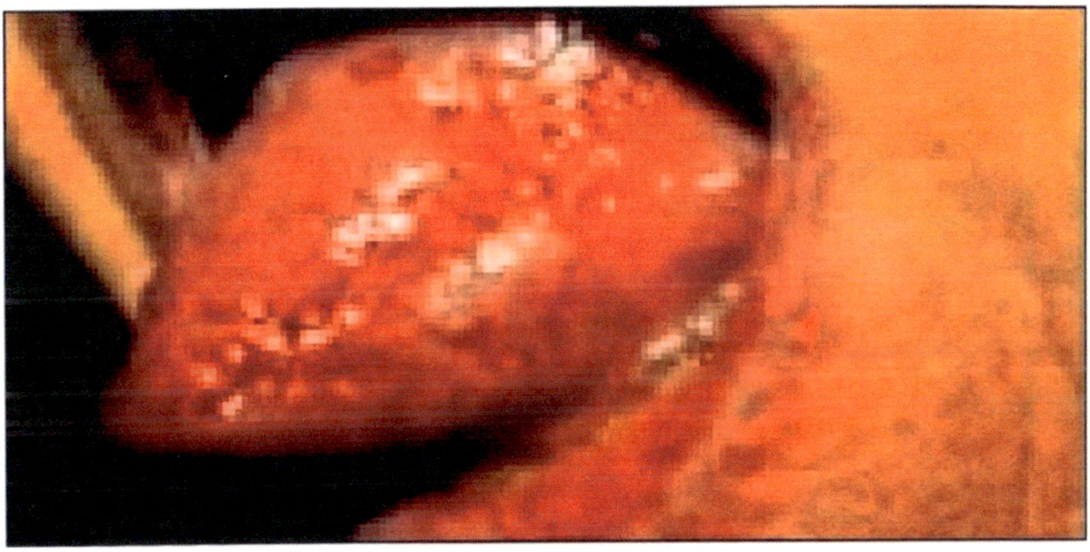

Figure 61: Tongue lesions in a patient with OCP.

Table 1. Differential diagnosis of chronic cicatricial pemphigoid

Atopic keratoconjunctivitis
Bullous pemphigus
Chemical burn
Cicatricial pemphigoid
Corynebacterium diphtheriae conjunctivitis
Epidermolysis bullosa acquisita
Irradiation damage
Linear IgA disease
Ocular rosacea
Pemphigus vulgaris
Pseudo-ocular cicatricial pemphigoid
Scleroderma
Squamous cell carcinoma
Sarcoidosis
Stevens-Johnson syndrome
Toxic epidermal necrolysis
Trauma

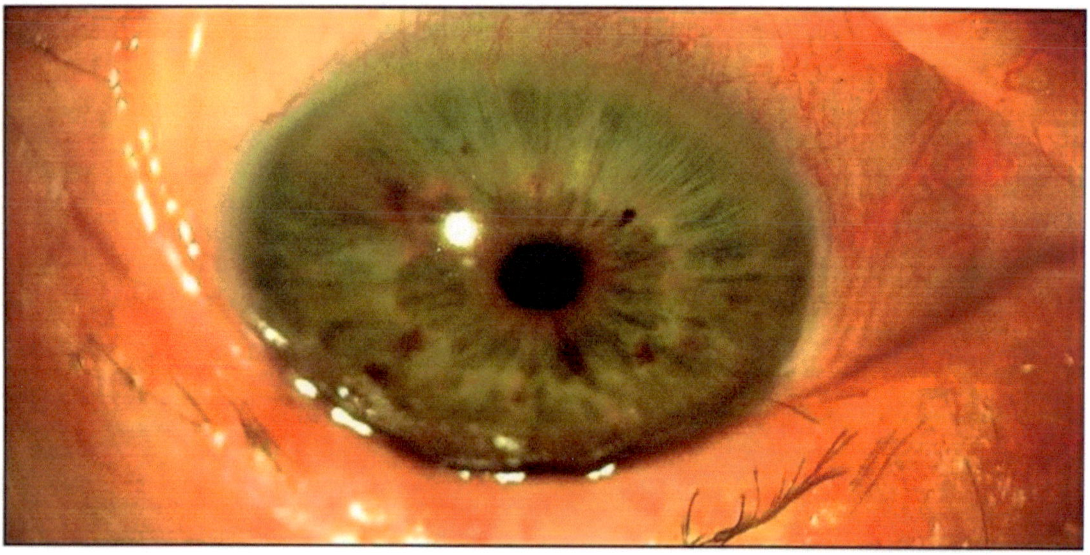

Figure 62: Down gaze image of patient with ocular cicatricial pemphigoid in whom the inferior bulbar and palpebral conjunctivae were white and quiet. However, note the continuing inflammation in the superior conjunctiva.

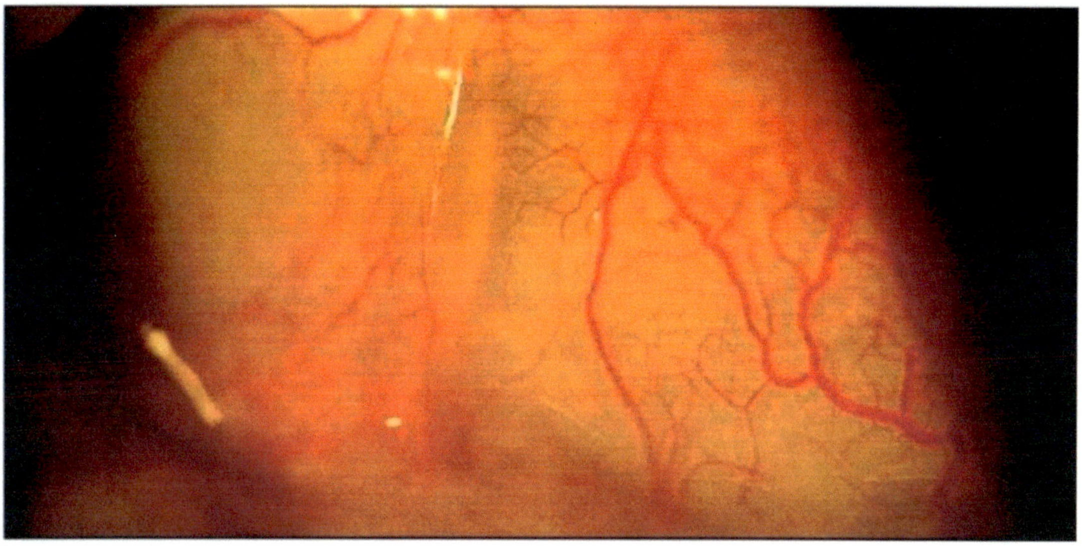

Figure 63: Fornix foreshortening seen in a patient with Stage II OCP.

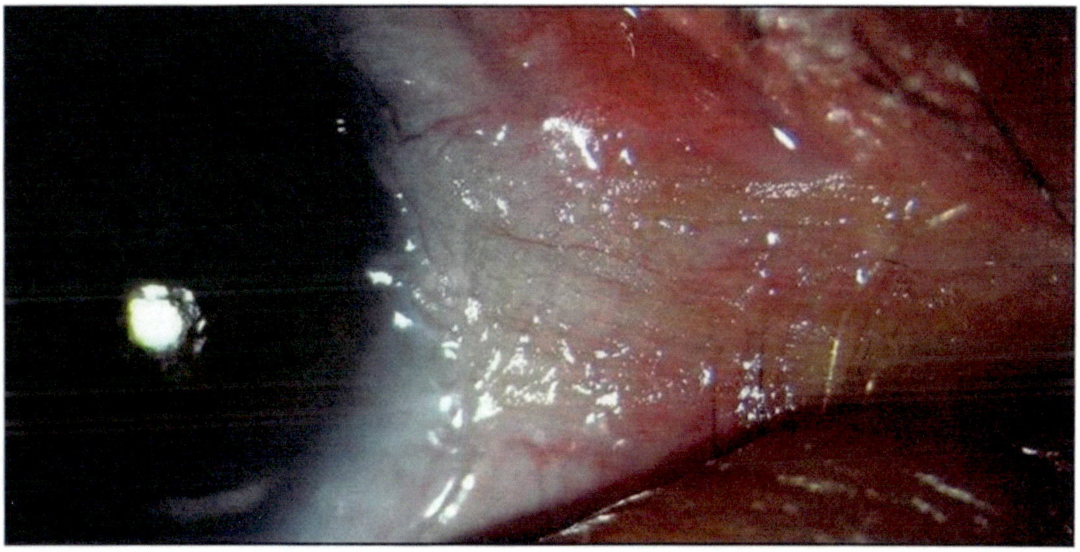

Figure 64: Stage III OCP with nasal ankyloblepharon and symblepharon

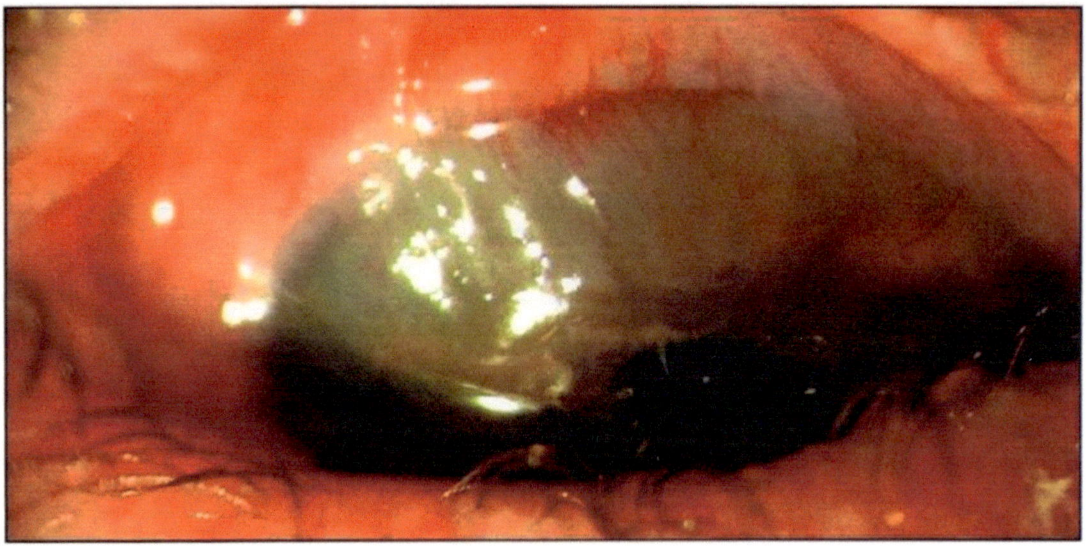

Figure 65: Peripheral corneal scarring and neovascularization in active Stage III OCP

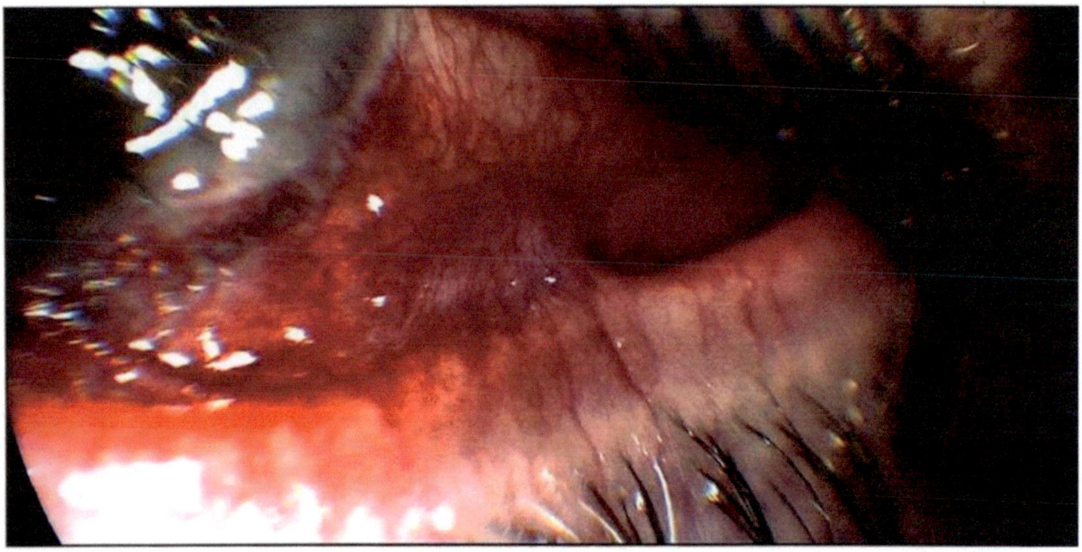

Figure 66: Ankyloblepharon in a patient with active Stage III OCP, which is rapidly progressing to Stage IV.

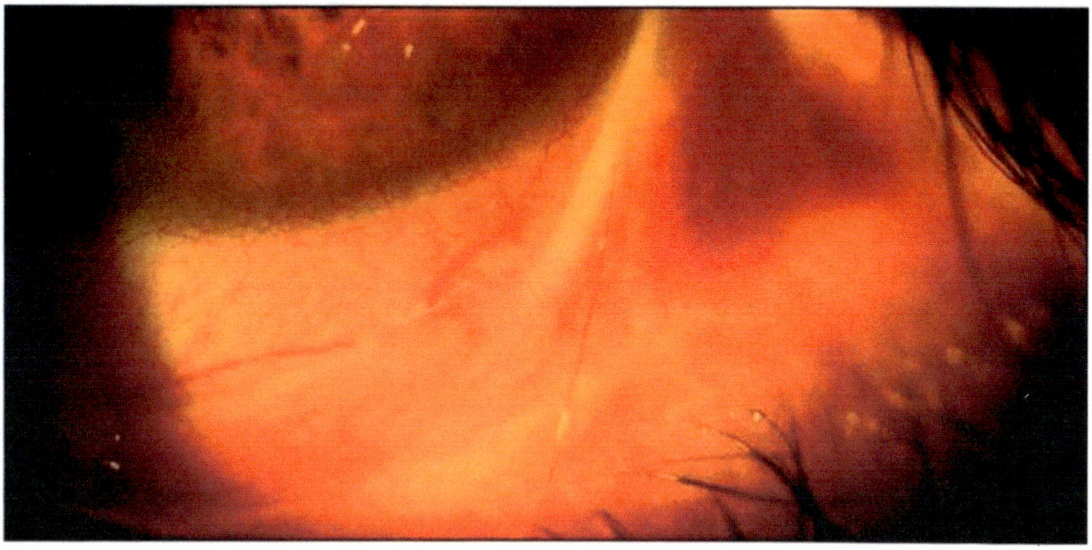

Figure 67: Trichitic lash with temporal symblepharon in quiet Stage III OCP.

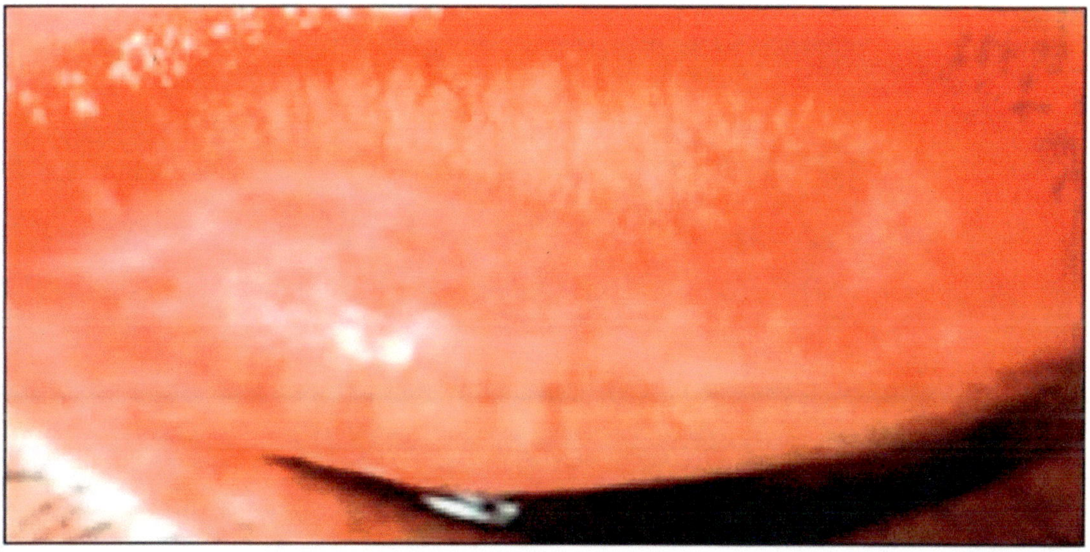

Figure 68: Subepithelial fibrosis with 2+ conjunctival injection as seen in Stage I OCP. This patient had normal fornices though as one can see examination of the tarsal conjunctiva is very important.

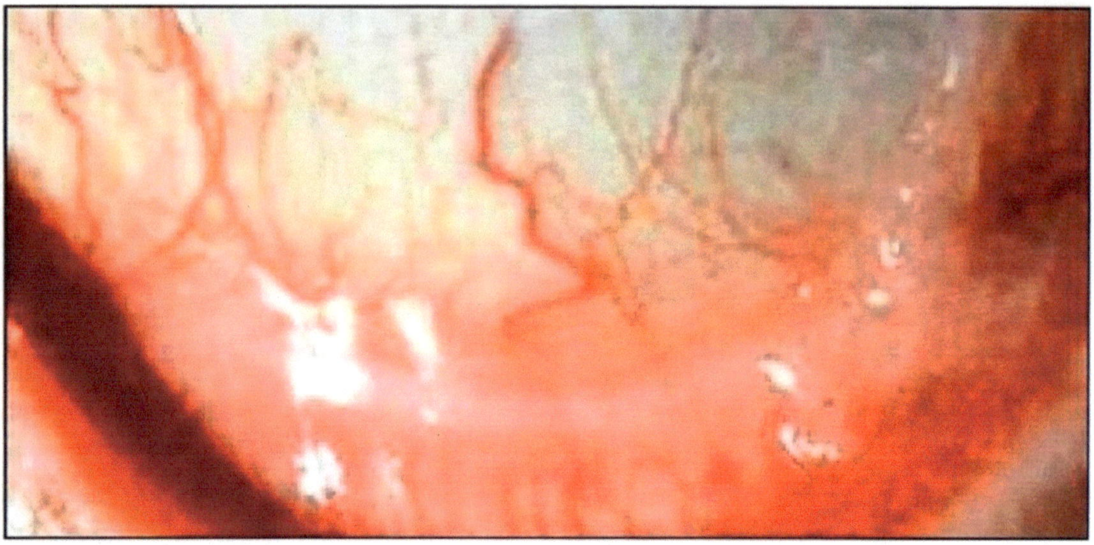

Figure 69: Fornix foreshortening seen in a patient with Stage II OCP

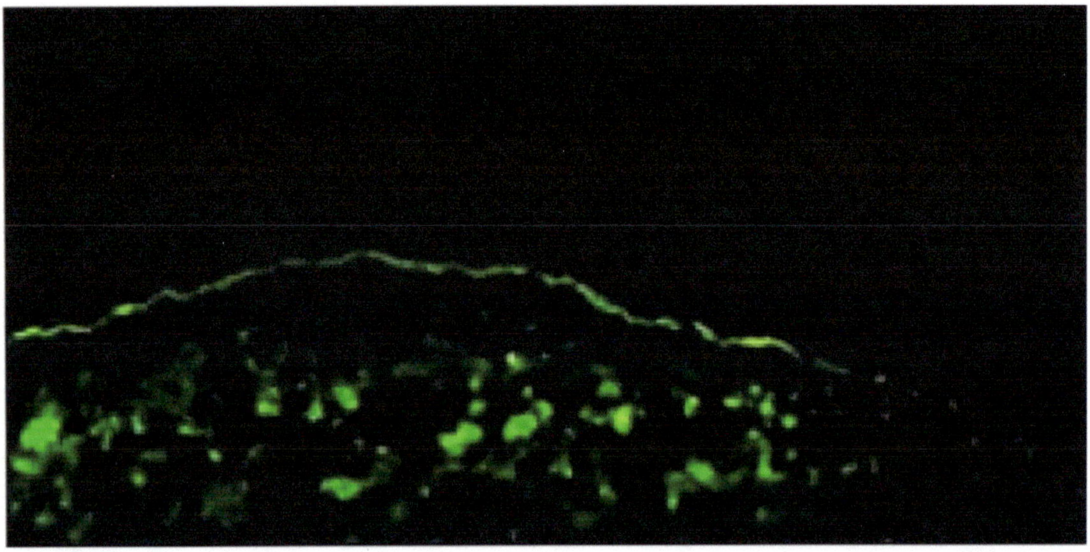

Figure 70: Immunohistochemistry in OCP. Linear IgA deposition at the BMZ correlates with primary subepidermal bullous disease in a high percentage of patients, but reflects a heterogenous group of blistering disorders (adult linear IgA bullous dermatosis, chronic bullous disease of childhood, CP, BP, EBA) with or without IgG deposition.

Figure 71: Positive immunofluorescence staining showing a linear deposition of Ig on the conjunctival BMZ, the sine qua non for definitive diagnosis of the disorder.

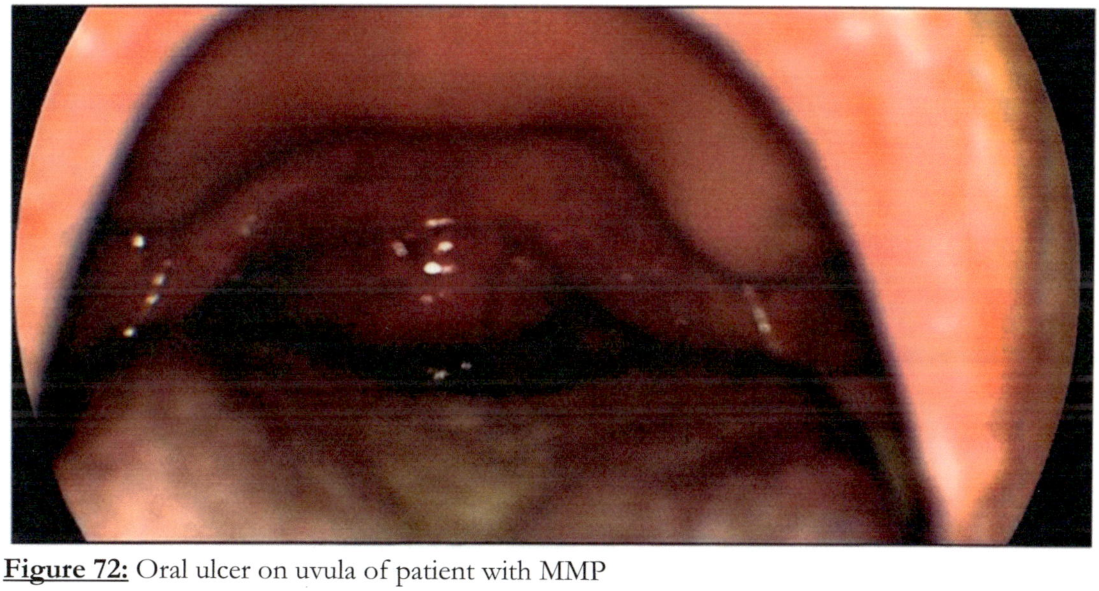

Figure 72: Oral ulcer on uvula of patient with MMP

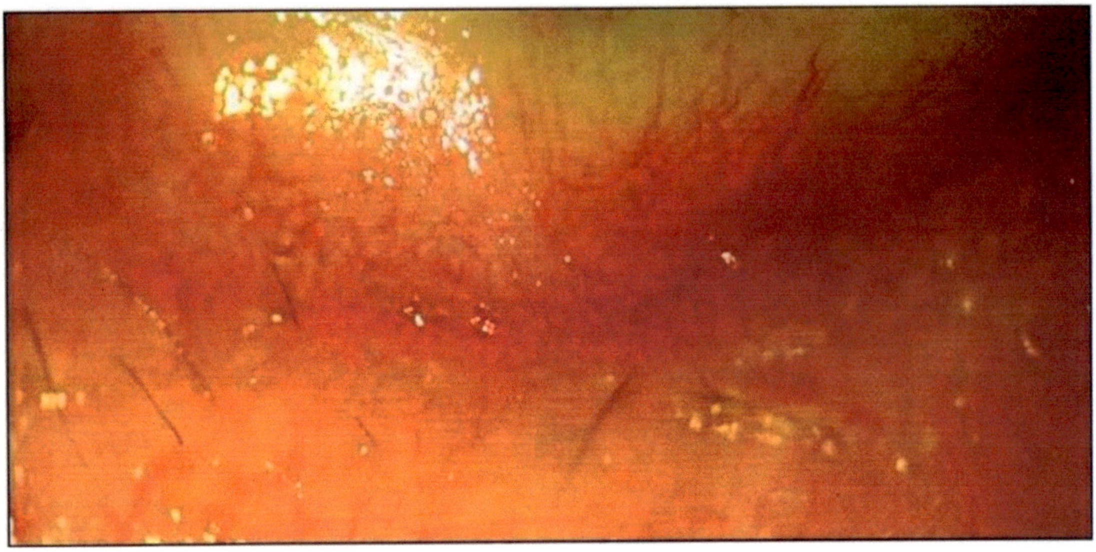

Figure 73: Stage III OCP: Complete fornix foreshortening with ankyloblepharon.

References:

1) Lever WF. Pemphigus. *Medicine* 1953: 32:1-23.
2) Lever WF, Talbott JH. Pemphigus: A historical study. *Arch Dermatol Syph* 942;00: 800-823.
3) Hippocrates. Hippocrates population liber sixtus, in JA van der Linden (ed): *Opera Omnia. Apud Gaasbeekius,* 1665, vol 1, p 798.
4) Duke-Elder S, (ed.), 1965. Diseases of the outer eye. Conjunctiva. *System of Ophthalmology.* Vol. 8. Part. I. St. Louis, CV Mosby, pp. 506.
5) Razzaque MS, Foster CS, Ahmed AR. Role of enhanced expression of m-CSF in conjunctiva affected by cicatricial pemphigoid. *Invest Ophthalmol Vis Sci* 2002; 43:2977-2983.
6) Mondino BJ, 1990. Cicatricial pemphigoid and erythema multiforme. *Ophthalmology* 97,939-952.
7) Foster CS, 1986. Cicatricial pemphigoid. *Trans. Am. Ophthalmol.* Soc. 84, 527-663.
8) Foster CS, Wilson LA, Ekins MB, et al. 1982. Immunosuppressive therapy for progressive ocular cicatricial pemphigoid. *Ophthalmology* 89,340-353

Orbital Myositis

Definition: Orbital myositis is defined as a non-specific inflammatory enlargement of the extraocular muscles involving the entire length of the muscle from the origin to insertion.

History: This entity was first described in 1905 by Birch-Hirschfield as part of the entities included in the idiopathic inflammatory pseudotumors.

Epidemiology: Orbital myositis is a disease of both pediatric and adult populations. It is more common in females than males (2:1). The average age of onset is 30-40 years old (range 3-84). Muscles commonly involved are the medial rectus (43%), Superior rectus (19%), Lateral rectus (17%), and Obliques/Inferior rectus (5% to 10%).

Clinical Features: In the acute phase, the main finding is paresis of one or more of the extraocular muscles with or without pain. Chronic disease may result in restriction of movement due to muscular sclerosis. Other ocular findings may include normal visual acuity, diplopia, blepharoptosis, ocular proptosis, periorbital and eyelid edema, conjunctival injection, and chemosis. Inflammatory myositis due to infectious or immune etiology may present with reduced visual acuity and uveitis. The course of the disease may be acute with complete resolution after treatment, relapsing or chronic.

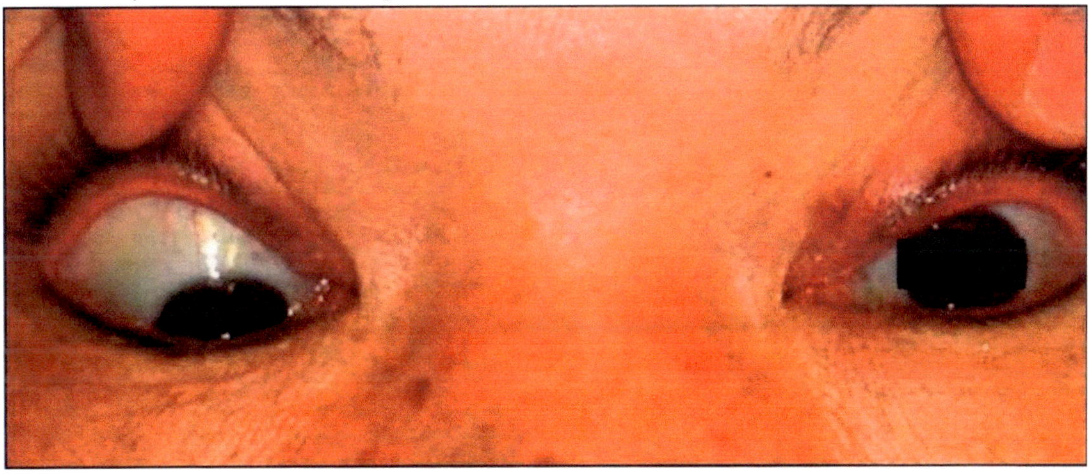

Figure 74: Orbital myositis with restriction of extraocular movements of the left eye in down gaze

Pathology/Pathogenesis: The etiology of idiopathic orbital myositis is suspected to be immune in nature. Histopathological studies of orbital myositis are characteristic for an inflammatory infiltrate composed mainly of small well-differentiated mature lymphocytes, mixed with plasma cells, in a diffuse or multifocal pattern. The muscle fibers are swollen and separated by edema and fibrosis, with loss of normal striations and degeneration of muscle fibers.

Diagnosis: The diagnosis of idiopathic orbital myositis (variant of idiopathic orbital pseudotumor) is confirmed only after all other possible etiologies have been excluded by appropriate testing. Orbital myositis may be the result of systemic or local etiologies including orbital infections, neoplasms, thyroid disease. Associations with orbital myositis include Rheumatoid arthritis, psoriatic arthropathy, Crohn's disease, Lyme disease, and granulomatosis with polyangiitis. Paraneoplastic syndromes may manifest as orbital myositis. The differential diagnosis includes thyroid orbitopathy, orbital cellulitis, neoplasms, metastasis, Tolosa-Hunt syndrome, trochleitis, and infectious myositis due to trichinosis. Diagnostic A-scan echography shows thickened extraocular muscles and tendons with low internal reflectivity and regular acoustic structure. CT scan or MRI imaging is characteristic for diffuse enlargement of the entire involved muscle.

Treatment: Idiopathic orbital myositis may be a self-limiting entity; it responds dramatically (24-48 hours) to treatment with corticosteroids given orally, IV or by sub-Tenon's injection. Other immunomodulating drugs have been used with variable success rates. Recurrent or refractory cases may respond to low-dose orbital irradiation (2500-3000 cGy). Chronic conditions with restriction or diplopia may be managed with surgery or botulinum injections.

References:

1) Weinstein GS, Dresner SC, Slamovits TL, Kennerdell JS. Acute and subacute orbital myositis. *Am J Ophthalmol.* 1983 Aug; 96(2): 209-17
2) Kennerdell JS, Dresner SC. The nonspecific orbital inflammatory syndromes. *Surv Ophthalmol.* 1984 Sep-Oct; 29(2): 93-103.
3) Mannor GE, Rose GE, Moseley IF, Wright JE. Outcome of orbital myositis: clinical features associated with recurrence. *Ophthalmology.* 1997; 104:409-13.
4) Nabili S, McCarey DW, Browne B, Capell HA. A case of orbital myositis associated rheumatoid. *Ann Rheum Dis* 2002;61:938-939.

Orbital Pseudotumor

Definition: Idiopathic orbital inflammation or orbital pseudotumor can be described as a non-specific inflammatory syndrome with a mass-like effect simulating a primary orbital neoplasm. Diagnostic criteria are: (1) orbital mass lesion, clinically manifesting with signs of mass effect, inflammation, or infiltration; (2) presence of focal or diffuse inflammatory lesion in neuroimaging; (3) fibroinflammatory findings in histopathologic speciments; and (4) lack of identifiable local or systemic diagnosis.

History: The first description of idiopathic orbital pseudotumor was published by Birch-Hirschfield in 1905. Garner divided non-neoplastic orbital masses into three classes based on the pathogenesis (known local, known systemic, unknown idiopathic).

Epidemiology: The peak incidence of orbital pseudotumor may be seen in the 4th and 5th decade of life. Males and females are equally affected and there is no racial predilection. Pediatric cases have been reported as early as in infancy. Bilaterality in adults is suggestive of a systemic disorder.

Clinical Features:

Systemic Manifestations: Rarely do systemic manifestations occur in adults. Constitutional symptoms, such as fever and malaise, can occur in children.

Ocular Manifestations: Orbital involvement may be diffuse or focal. Variants include myositis, dacryoadenitis, scleritis and optic perineuritis. Visual loss (due to compression, uveitis, retinal detachment, fibrosis of optic nerve, CRAO), diplopia, extraocular movement restriction, proptosis, moderate pain, lid swelling, chemosis, conjunctival vessel engorgement, palpable mass, and lacrimal gland enlargment can be seen. Uveitis and retinal detachment may be associated with scleritis. Bilateral involvement in children is more common than adults, Children with bilateral disease are more likely to have associated uveitis, disc edema and increased incidence of recurrence. Iritis may be the presenting symptom in children. Characteristics associated with recurrences include male gender, lack of proptosis, eyelid retraction, horizontal extraocular muscle involvement, multiple or bilateral extraocular muscle involvement, muscle tendon sparing on neuroimaging, and lack of response to corticosteroids or nonsteroidal anti-inflammatory agents.

Pathology/Pathogenesis: The exact pathogenesis of orbital pseudotumor has not been determined yet. Evidence suggests an autoimmune response directed against various orbital "target" tissues. Histopathological findings include a gray rubbery mass with polymorphous infiltrate of mature lympohocytes, plasma cells, macrophages and polymorphonuclear leukocytes and fibrosis.

Diagnosis: Orbital pseudotumor or idiopathic orbital inflammatory syndrome is a diagnosis of exclusion. Orbital inflammation may result from primary inflammatory conditions of the orbit or systemic disease. Serologic testing is crucial in determining the cause of orbital pseudotumor. Orbital imaging with CT scan or MM may show thickening and enhancement of the posterior Tenon's capsule, orbital mass or infiltrate which may mold to the globe or the optic nerve. Orbital biopsy may be performed for diagnostic purposes in unresponsive to treatment or diagnostically challenging cases. Dramatic response to oral systemic corticosteroid treatment should not be used a diagnostic criterion because many other orbital entities may respond similarly.

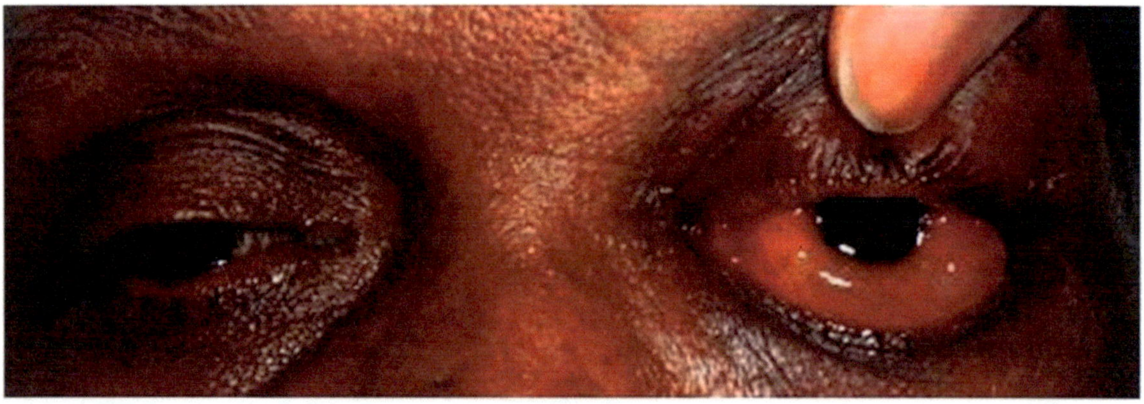

Figure 75: Chemosis and proptosis in a patient afflicted with orbital pseudotumor.

Treatment: Oral prednisone and an H2 blocker with a slow taper is initially the recommended treatment. Immunosuppressive and immunomodulatory agents such as monoclonal antibody treatments and inhibitors of the cytokine TNF-[alpha] have been used successfully for the treatment of orbital pseudotumor. Lesions that appear hyperintense compared with cerebral cortex on MM images may respond well to corticosteroid therapy. Lesions that are hypo- or iso- intense compared to extraocular muscle respond poorly. Radiation therapy may be used in refractory cases.

References:

1) Pendse S, Bilyk JR, Lee MS. The ticking time bomb. *Surv Ophthalmol.* 2006 May-Jun;51(3):274-9
2) Snebold NG. Orbital pseudotumor syndromes. *Curr Opin Ophthalmol.* 1997 Dec;8 (6):41-4.
3) Kapadia MK, Rubin PA. The emerging use of TNF-alpha inhibitors in orbital inflammatory disease. *Int Ophthalmol Clin.* 2006 Spring;46(2): 165-81.
4) Orbital inflammatory disease. RC DellaRocca, K. Schneider. In Hornblass, Albert, 1939-; Hanig, Carl J. *Oculoplastic, orbital, and reconstructive surgery* Baltimore : Williams & Wilkins, c1988.
5) Weinstein GS, Dresner SC, Slamovits TL, Kennerdell JS. Acute and subacute orbital myositis. *Am J Ophthalmol.* 1983 Aug;96(2):209-17.
6) Kennerdell JS, Dresner SC. The nonspecific orbital inflammatory syndromes. *Surv Ophthalmol.* 1984 Sep-Oct;29(2):93-103.

7) Manner GE, Rose GE, Moseley IF, Wright JE. Outcome of orbital myositis: clinical features associated with recurrence. *Ophthalmology*. 1997;104:409-413.
8) S Nabili, D W McCarey, B Browne, H A Capell. A case of orbital myositis associated with rheumatoid *Arthritis*. *Ann Rheum Dis* 2002;61:938-939
9) Mombaerts I, Goldschmeding R, Schlingemann RO, Koornneef L. What is orbital pseudotumor? *Surv Ophthalmol.* 1996;41:66-78.

Table 1: Differential Diagnosis of Orbital Inflammation

Amyloidosis
Bacterial
Carotid-cavernous fistula
Cystercercosis
Ehrlichiosis
Expanding lymphangioma
Foreign body reaction
Fungal (aspergillus or mucor)
Giant cell arteritis
Hematic cyst
Idiopathic
Infectious
Intraocular necrosis of choroidal melanoma
Lyme
Lymphoma
Metastasis
Myasis
Orbital ischemia
Paranasal sinus carcinoma
Polyarteritis nodosa
Primary or invasive tumor
Rhabdomyosarcoma
Rheumatoid arthritis
Ruptured dermoid cyst
Sarcoidosis
Syphilis
Systemic lupus erythematosis
Thyroid orbitopathy
Tuberculosis
Granulomatosis with polyangiitis

Ocular Rosacea

Introduction: Ocular rosacea is a dermatologic condition that affects the midfacial region with more than 50% of patients having associated ocular manifestations. Ocular symptoms may present prior to the cutaneous manifestations. There appears to be no correlation between the severity of the ocular disease and the severity of facial rosacea.

Epidemiology: Approximately 10% of the general population display dermatological manifestations of rosacea. Of these, up to 60% experience ocular involvement. The condition is much more common in fair-skinned white patients, and females are affected twice as commonly as males.

Clinical Features: Facial involvement may manifest in the form of telangiectasia, erythema, papules, pustules or rhinophyma. Ocular symptoms commonly include irritation, redness, itching, burning, photophobia, and foreign body sensation. Examination may demonstrate eyelid telangiectasia, blepharitis and meibomian gland dysfunction, often with thick viscous plugging of the meibomian gland orifices. Conjunctivitis may be chronic, and in rare cases may lead to cicatrization. The cornea may become secondarily involved with punctate epithelial keratopathy, marginal infiltrates, and frank neovascularization. Very rarely there may be corneal thinning, ulceration and perforation.

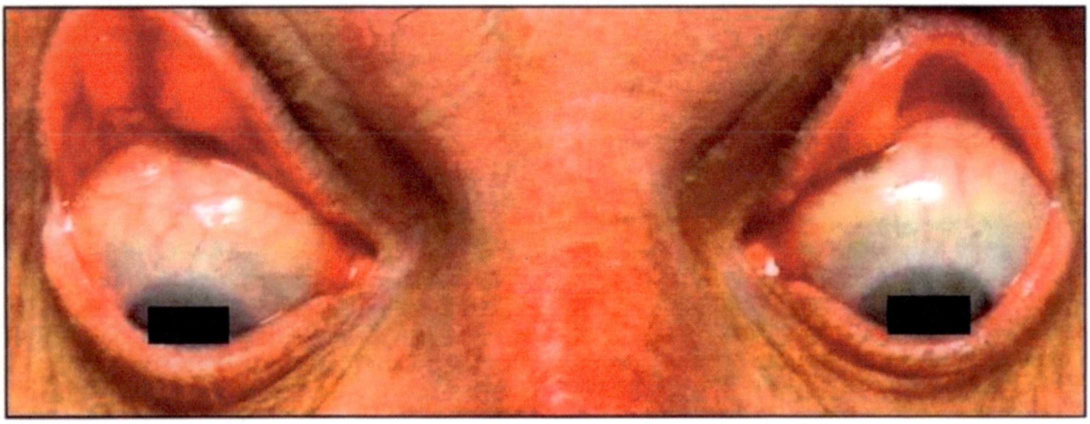

Figure 76: Floppy eyelid syndrome and blepharoconjunctivitis secondary to ocular rosacea

Pathogenesis: The pathogenesis remains unknown. Inflammatory changes are the hallmark of this condition which may be thought of as having both a vascular and inflammatory component. A type 4, cell mediated hypersensitivity reaction has been hypothesized as a possible mechanism. Other implicated stimuli include the possible involvement of demodex mites and Helicobacter pylori.

Diagnosis: The diagnosis of ocular rosacea is completely clinical. Laboratory or imaging studies are neither necessary nor useful in establishing the diagnosis.

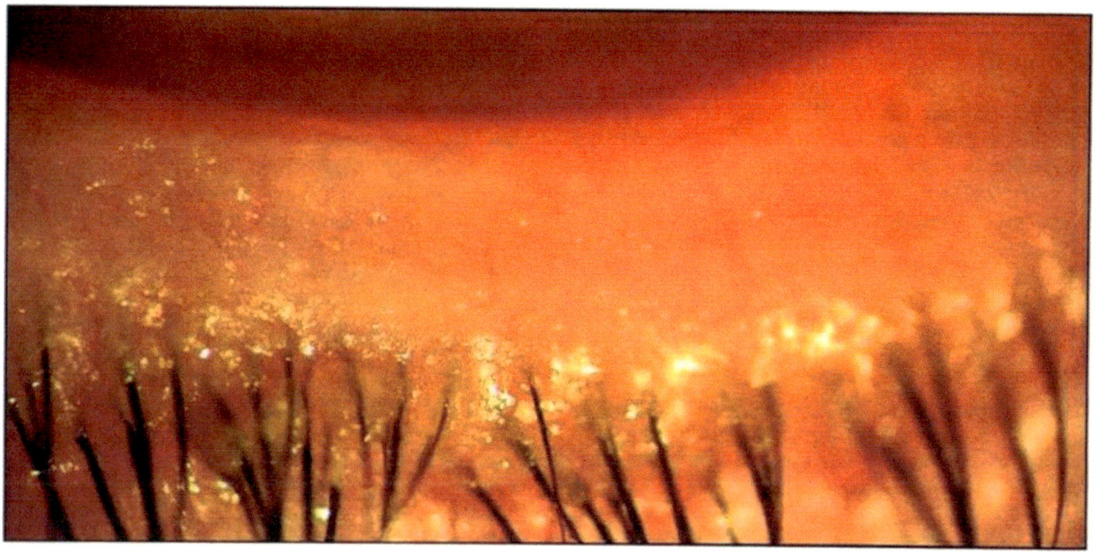

Figure 77: Meibomian gland dysfunction, lid crusting, and blepharitis in a patient with ocular rosacea

Treatment: Treatment of ocular rosacea is for symptomatic control rather than curative. No one therapeutic agent has found to be effective and most cases require a multi-treatment approach. Lid hygiene with hot compresses and digital massage, artificial tears, and systemic antibiotics (tetracyclines, erythromycin, azithromycin, clarithromycin, metronidazole), can be used to control symptoms. Topical steroids should be used judiciously but can prove useful for short term exacerbations. The use of retinoids is reserved for cases in which multiple agents have failed.

Reference:

Akpek EK, Merchant A, Pinar V, Foster CS. Ocular rosacea: patient characteristics and follow-up. *Ophthalmology*. Nov 1997; 104(11): 1863-7.

Scleritis

Definition: Scleritis is typically a painful and potentially sight-threatening inflammatory process centered in the sclera, but may also involve the cornea, adjacent episclera, and the underlying uvea. Careful clinical history taking, detailed ocular examination, appropriate investigation for ocular and systemic disease with timely intervention of immunosuppressant drugs when necessary, has improved the long-term outcome for patients with this disease.

History: Watson and Hayreh proposed a classification of scleritis and episcleritis in 1976, which is still used today.

Epidemiology: Patients presenting with scleritis are predominantly middle-aged and Caucasian. The mean age at onset is approximately 49 years with the majority of patients being female (71%). Systemic disease is associated in up to 50% of patients with scleritis. There is no known HLA association. Etiology can be classified as autoimmune, infectious, surgically induced, traumatic and drug induced. Scleritis may also present as a masquerade syndrome.

Etiology:

Autoimmune: The most common connective tissue disorder associated with scleral disease is rheumatoid arthritis, while granulomatosis with polyangiitis is the most commonly associated vasculitis. Other causative systemic diseases include relapsing polychondritis, inflammatory bowel disease, systemic lupus erythematosus and polyarteritis nodosa.

Infectious: Infectious scleritis is rare in the absence of infectious keratitis. The etiology may be viral, bacterial, fungal, and parasitic. Herpes zoster is the most common viral etiological agent while Pseudomonas aeruginosa is the most common pathogen reported.

Surgically-Induced Scleritis: Surgically-induced scleritis can occur after a variety of procedures but most commonly occurs in patients undergoing cataract surgery whereby a limbal incision was performed. Previous surgical procedures (two or more) represent an additional risk factor. It has been demonstrated that up to 90% of these patients present with an associated occult autoimmune systemic disease when investigated, emphasizing the importance of careful systemic evaluation.

Pathology: Studies of enucleated eyes with necrotizing scleritis demonstrate vasculitis with fibrinoid necrosis and neutrophil invasion of the vessel wall in 75% of cases, while vascular immunodeposits were found in the scleral tissue in 93% of cases. T cells and macrophages were the major inflammatory cells infiltrating the deep episcleral tissue with clusters of B cells in perivascular areas. Increased HLA-DR expression and increased IL-2 expression on T cells suggest an active cell-mediated immune response. Lack of antibody expression and complement further suggest that T cells represent the effector cells in Scleritis.

Clinical features: Scleritis may involve the anterior sclera, posterior sclera or both. Presentation may be unilateral or bilateral. Anterior scleritis, the most common form of the disease, may be diffuse, nodular, or necrotizing in presentation. Rarely, a necrotizing pattern of anterior scleritis may occur in the absence of pain and overt inflammation, and this is termed scleromalacia perforans. Posterior scleritis is defined as involvement of the sclera posterior to the insertion of the rectus muscles. Scleritic pain is characteristically dull and boring in nature, with a sub-acute onset that typically intensifies over several weeks. Patients with anterior scleritis may present with redness, and tenderness of the globe often in association with photophobia and lacrimation. Patients with posterior scleritis may present with reduced vision with or without pain. Up to 50% of patients with scleritis have evidence of an underlying systemic disease and therefore careful clinical examination is paramount.

Anterior Scleritis: This is the most common form of scleral inflammation and is characterized by diffuse involvement of the anterior sclera by edema and dilatation of the deep episcleral vascular plexus. Corneal infiltration, thinning and stromal keratitis may be present, as well as involvement of the underlying trabecular meshwork resulting in secondary raised intraocular pressure. Nodular anterior scleritis is characterized by distinct nodules, which are formed by localized areas of scleral edema and inflammation.

***Necrotizing Anterior Scleritis*:** This represents the most severe form of scleritis and is characterized by severe vasculitis and closure of the episcleral vascular bed. On examination there are visible areas of capillary non-perfusion with infarction and necrosis of the involved sclera. Inflammation commonly spreads to involve the cornea, ciliary body, and trabecular meshwork resulting in keratitis, anterior uveitis and elevated intraocular pressure.

Scleromalacia Perforans: This rare form of necrotizing anterior scleritis results from an obliterative arteritis that involves the deep episcleral vascular plexus. Clinically it is typically asymptomatic but may present with blurred vision from high astigmatism due to scleral thinning leading to loss of scleral rigidity. The sclera is parchment white, avascular and thinned. Corneal involvement is minimal except for limited peripheral thinning.

Posterior Scleritis: Posterior scleritis may occur in an isolated form or may be associated with anterior scleritis. B-scan ultrasonography and magnetic resonance imaging have delineated diffuse and nodular forms. Clinical presentation depends on the location, extent and severity of involvement of the posterior sclera. Patients older than fifty years of age, presenting with posterior scleritis have been shown to have a greater risk of an associated systemic disease and are more likely to require systemic immunosuppressive agents to achieve disease control. Ultrasound remains the gold standard for diagnosis with identification of a thickened posterior scleral coat (edema in Tenon's space greater than 2mm).

Diagnosis: A detailed history and careful systemic examination should be performed in all cases of scleritis. Serologic investigations should then be tailored to the clinical findings. An estimate to the extent of systemic involvement can be elucidated through assessment of the patient's blood pressure, renal function and acute phase reactants. Further core investigations should include complete blood count, urea and electrolytes, rheumatoid factor, anti-nuclear antibodies, anticytoplasmic antibodies and venereal disease research laboratory analysis. Ancillary imaging studies may be required in some cases for diagnostic confirmation.

Treatment: The principles of treatment in scleritis are to control the inflammation and to elucidate and treat any underlying associated local or systemic disease processes in order to prevent structural and functional damage to the eye and prevent systemic disease associated mortality. Patients presenting with posterior or necrotizing scleritis usually require more aggressive immunosuppressive therapy than those presenting with anterior non-necrotizing disease. Non-necrotizing scleritis is often responsive to non-steroidal anti-inflammatory drugs. Corticosteroids are reserved to those cases, which are non-responsive to cox-inhibitors and to cases of posterior and necrotizing scleritis. Second line agents used in the treatment of scleritis include cyclosporin, mycophenolate, methotrexate, and anti-TNF blockers. Cyclophosphamide may be required in patients with granulomatosis with polyangiitis, rheumatoid arthritis, polyarteritis nodosa, and relapsing polychondroitis.

Table 1 Clinical Classification of Scleral Inflammatory Disease

1. Episcleritis
    a. Simple
    b. Nodular
2. Scleritis
    a. Anterior
        i. Diffuse
        ii. Nodular
        iii. Necrotizing
            1. With inflammation
            2. Without inflammation (scleromalacia perforans)
    b. Posterior

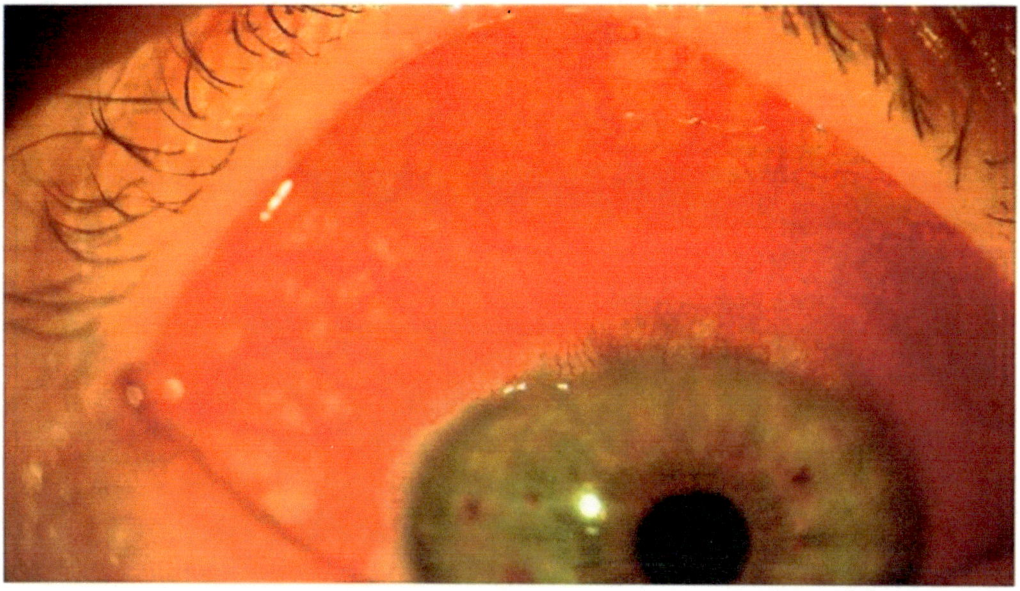

Figure 78: Peripheral keratouveitis in a patient with diffuse scleritis.

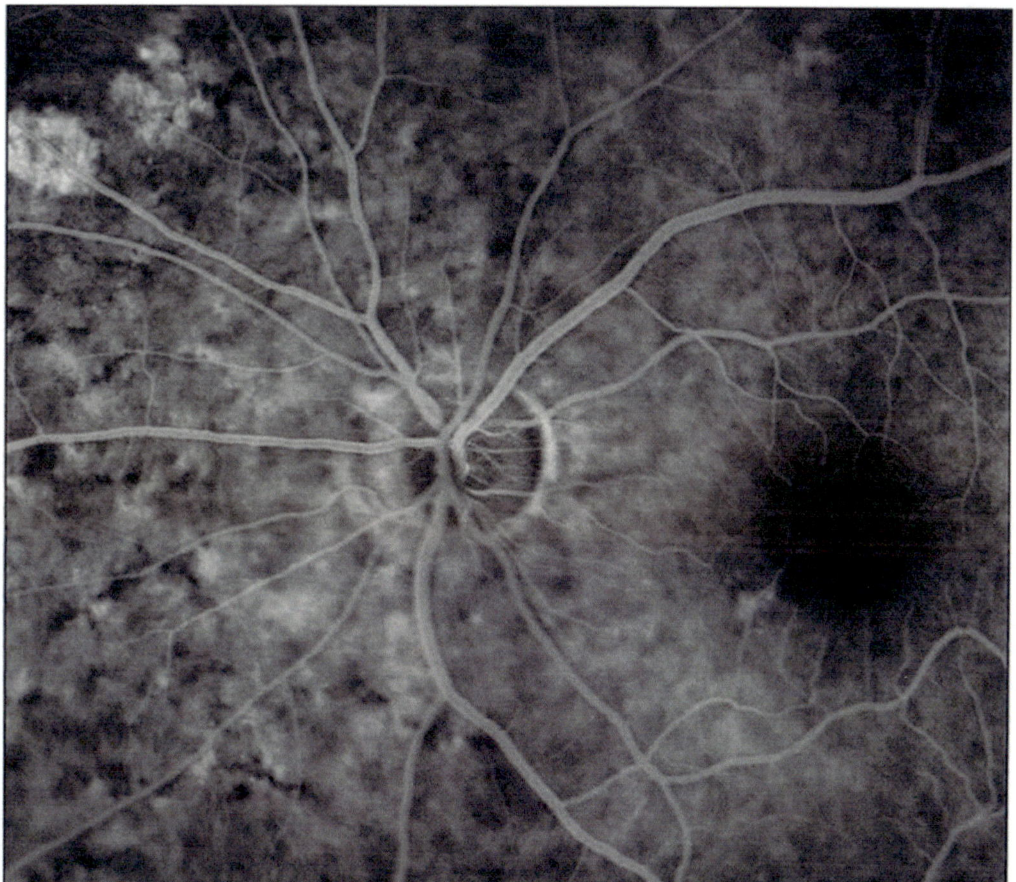

Figure 79: Note the leopard appearance in posterior scleritis.

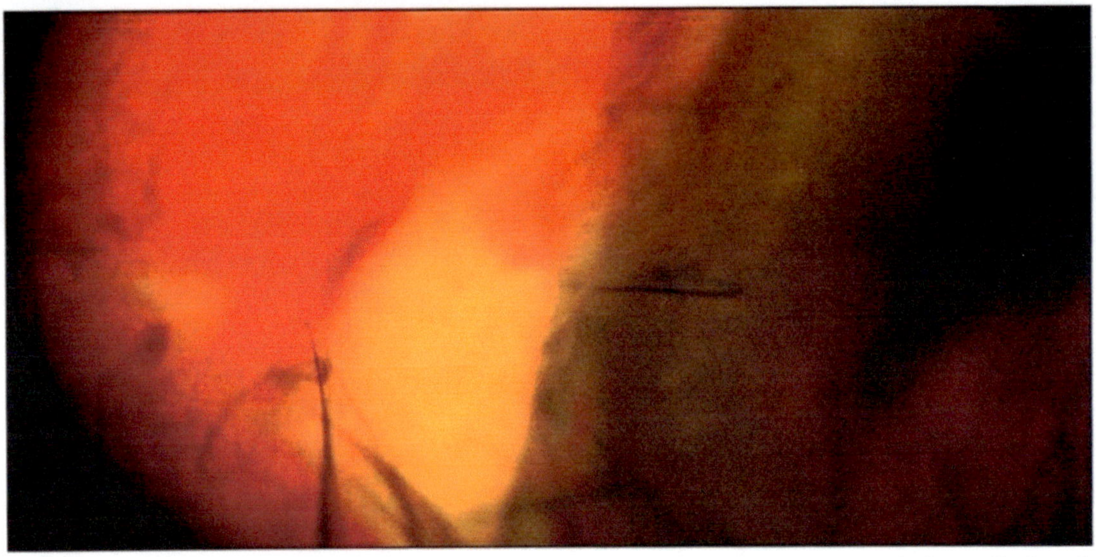

Figure 80: Scleral patch graft in a patient with necrotizing scleritis. Histopathology disclosed branching fungal hyphae.

Figure 81: Superior diffuse scleritis.

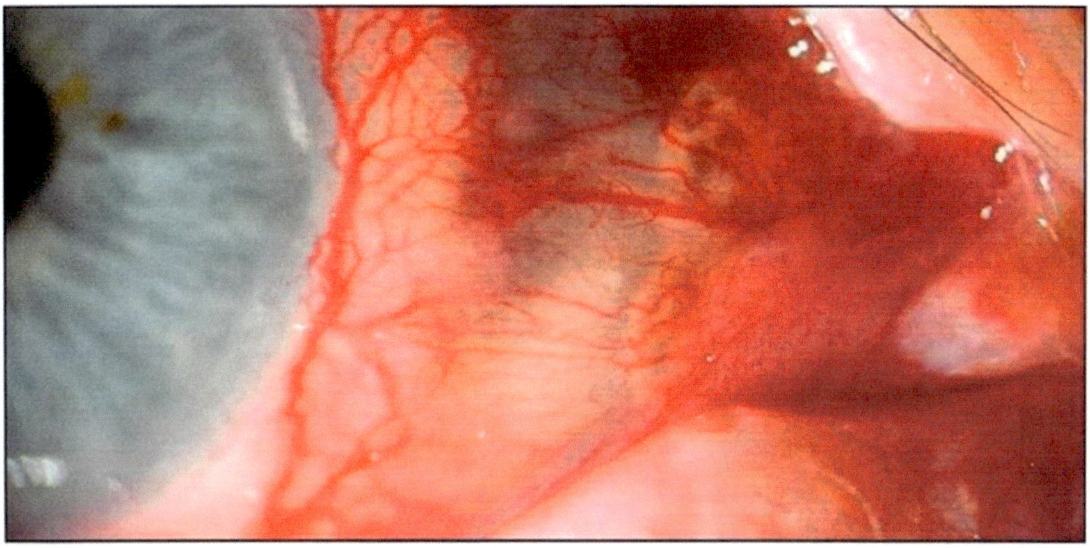

Figure 82: Nasal nodular and necrotizing scleritis

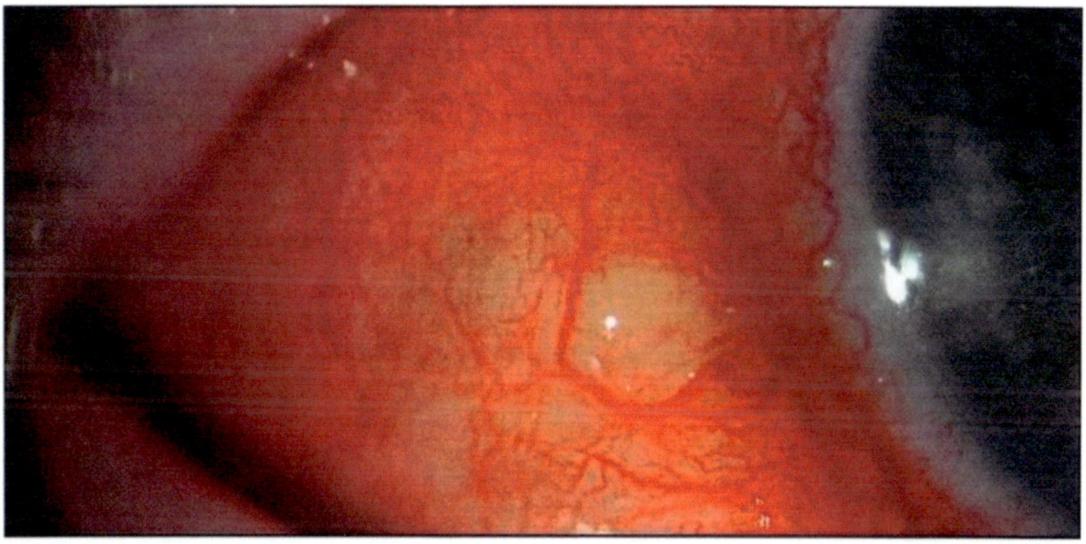

Figure 83: Elevated scleral nodule with diffuse scleritis

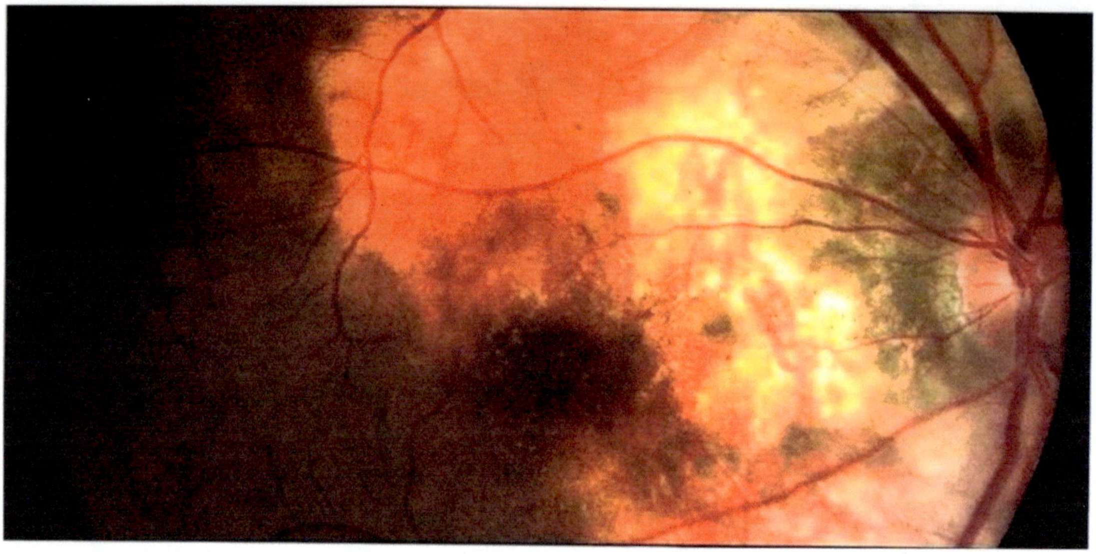

Figure 84: Healed posterior scleritis. Note the disseminated sclerochoroidal calcification.

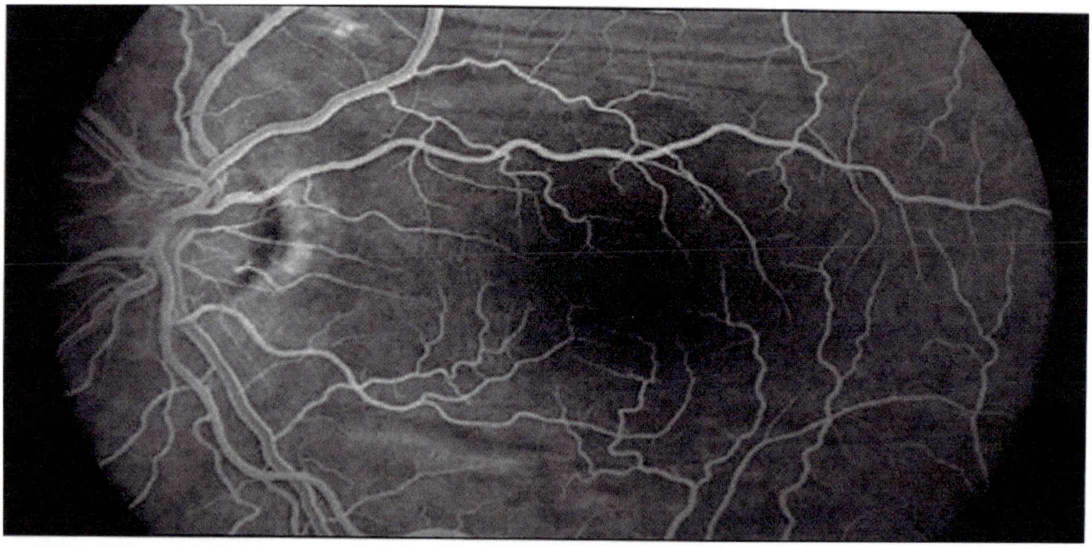

Figure 85: Early-phase fluorescein angiogram of a patient with posterior scleritis with prominent choroidal folds.

References:

Okhravi N, Odufawa B, McCluskey P, Lightman S. Scleritis; Major Review. *Surv Ophthalmol* 50:351-363, 2005

Stevens-Johnson Syndrome and Toxic Epidermal Necrolysis Syndrome

Definition/History: Stevens-Johnson Syndrome (SJS) and TENS (Toxic Epidermal Necrolysis Syndrome) are severe mucocutaneous adverse drug reactions with prolonged courses. SJS was first described in 1922 by pediatricians A.M. Stevens and S.C. Johnson after observing two children with severe ocular and oral mucosal reactions to unknown causes. Erythema multiforme (EM), its milder counterpart, was originally described by von Hebra in 1866. Thomas divided EM into 2 categories: erythema multiforme minor and erythema multiforme major (EMM), in 1950. EMM also became known as Stevens-Johnson syndrome. Since 1983, the eponym of Stevens-Johnson syndrome had been used as a synonym for EMM. Ten years later, Bastuji and Roujeau proposed that EMM and SJS are 2 distinct disorders, stating that both had similar mucosal erosions, but different patterns of cutaneous lesions. TEN, also called Lyell's syndrome was first described by the Scottish dermatologist Alan Lyell in 1956. He coined the term "necrolysis," by combining the key clinical feature "epidermolysis" with the characteristic histopathological feature "necrosis." Based on clinical manifestations and pathology results, SJS and TENS appear to be variants of the same disease, the latter being more severe.

Epidemiology: Stevens-Johnson syndrome (SJS) is part of a spectrum of adverse cutaneous and mucous membrane reactions to an inciting drug or infection that most commonly occurs in children and young adults. The incidence of SJS is approximately 6 cases per million persons per year, and that of TEN is approximately 2 cases per million persons per year. TEN affects women more frequently than men with a ratio of 1.5:1, and the incidence increases with age. Both diseases are characterized by having a low incidence but high mortality rates. Erythema and erosions of the buccal, ocular, and genital mucosa are present in more than 90% of patients. Approximately 50% of patients with SJS have acute ophthalmic manifestations. Chronic ocular involvement leading to permanent loss of vision may occur in up to 35% of affected individuals. The most frequently incriminated drugs are antibiotics (especially sulfonamides), non-steroidal anti-inflammatory drugs and anti-convulsants. The risk of developing SJS-TEN is reported to be highest during the initial week(s) of therapy.

Pathology/Pathogenesis: Delayed hypersensitivity reaction to drugs has been described in patients with SJS. The lack of lymphocyte response to native drug and positive patch test suggests that the immune response may be directed at drug-modified epidermal cells. This is associated with an impaired capacity to detoxify reactive intermediate drug metabolites. Genetic susceptibility may play a role, as evidenced by the increased incidence of HLA-B12 in individuals affected by TEN. We found HLA-DQB1*0601 in a significantly disproportionate number of white patients with SJS and ocular complications. Recently, it has been shown that the tissue damage is due to massive Fas-mediated keratinocyte cell death by apoptosis. Both PA and psoriasis are associated with human leukocyte antigen (HLA) A2, B17, B38, B39, Cw6, and DR7a. genes.

Clinical Features:

Systemic manifestations: Both SJS and TEN are characterized by epidermal detachment ranging from mild (1-10%) of total body surface area (TBSA) in SJS, to moderate (10-30% TBSA) in the SJS-TEN overlap, and severe (>30% TBSA) in TENS. Mortality rates correlate with the degree of epidermal detachment. Initial symptoms of both TEN and SJS can be fever, stinging eyes, and pain upon swallowing, any of which can precede cutaneous manifestations by 1 to 3 days. Skin lesions tend to appear first on the trunk, spreading to the neck, face, and proximal upper extremities.

Ocular manifestations: Ocular symptoms include red eye, tearing, dry eye, pain, blepharospasm, and itching. Keratinization of the eyelid margin with variable degrees of meibomian gland dysfunction are common. Aberrant conjunctival and corneal cicatrizations are important ocular findings in both entities. DiPascuale and colleagues found a strong correlation between the severity of eyelid margin and tarsal pathology and the extent of corneal complications. External examination reveals conjunctival hyperemia and entropion. Trichiasis, conjunctival subepithelial fibrosis, foreshortening of fornices, and symblepharon formation are evident upon slit-lamp examination. Madarosis, or loss of eyelashes, is common. Corneal keratinization, conjunctivalization, and perforation may also occur.

Diagnosis: The diagnosis is most often clinical, based upon exposure to new medication, history of aprodrome, and evolution of a mucocutaneous rash. Skin biopsy is the only diagnostically helpful laboratory study, revealing interleukin 6 (IL-6), tumor necrosis factor-alpha, interferon gamma, interleukin 18 (IL-18), and Fas ligand (FasL) in the lesional epidermis and/or blister fluid of some patients. Conjunctival biopsies from patients with active ocular disease show subepithelial plasma cells and lymphocyte infiltration.

Treatment: Optimal medical management of SJS and TEN requires early diagnosis, immediate discontinuation of the causative drug (s), supportive care, and specific therapy. The use of systemic corticosteroids remains controversial. Some advocate short-term use during the acute phase, while others discourage using steroids believing they may increase the individual's susceptibility to sepsis and gastrointestinal hemorrhage.

Most recently, the use of intravenous immunoglobulin (WIG) has been reported to improve outcomes, by inhibiting Fas-FasL interactions and cell death. Cyclosporine, cyclophosphamide, plasmapheresis, and low-dose N-acetylcysteine have shown promising results.

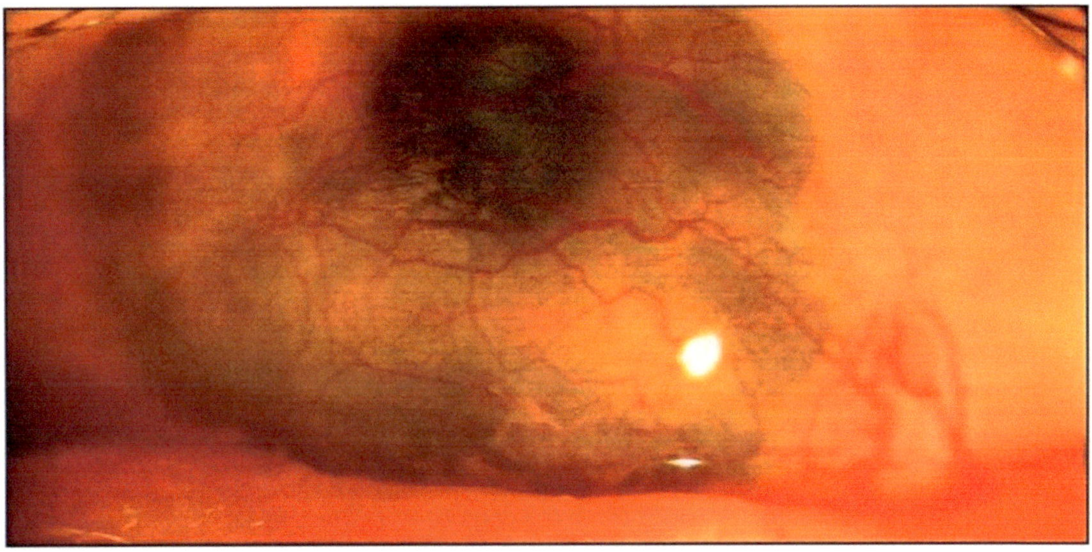

Figure 86: Widespread branches of neovascularization spanning the corneal surface in SJS. Note the madarosis of the lower eyelid (a common sequela).

Ocular care involves aggressive lubrication of the ocular surface along with mucolytic agents. If untreated, lid margin keratinization and tarsal scarring, together with lipid tear deficiency, contribute to corneal complications because of blink-related microtrauma. Attempts to suppress inflammation and scarring by amniotic membrane transplantation at the acute stage and to prevent microtrauma at the chronic stage may help to avoid sight-threatening complications.

As inflammation and cicatricial changes ensue, most ophthalmologists use topical steroids, antibiotics, and symblepharon lyses. In case of exposure keratopathy, tarsorrhaphy and/or amniotic membrane grafting may be required. Ocular surface reconstruction can be achieved through the use of adhesive glues, lamellar grafts, and penetrating keratoplasty. Attempted visual rehabilitation in patients with visual impairment can be considered once the eye has been quiet for at least 3 months. Removal of keratinized plaques, along with mucous membrane grafting, is important for the future success of corneal surgeries. Limbal stem cell transplantation may be employed and is useful in certain cases. Keratoprosthesis is ultimately performed on end-stage cases that failed at least one of the previously mentioned procedures.

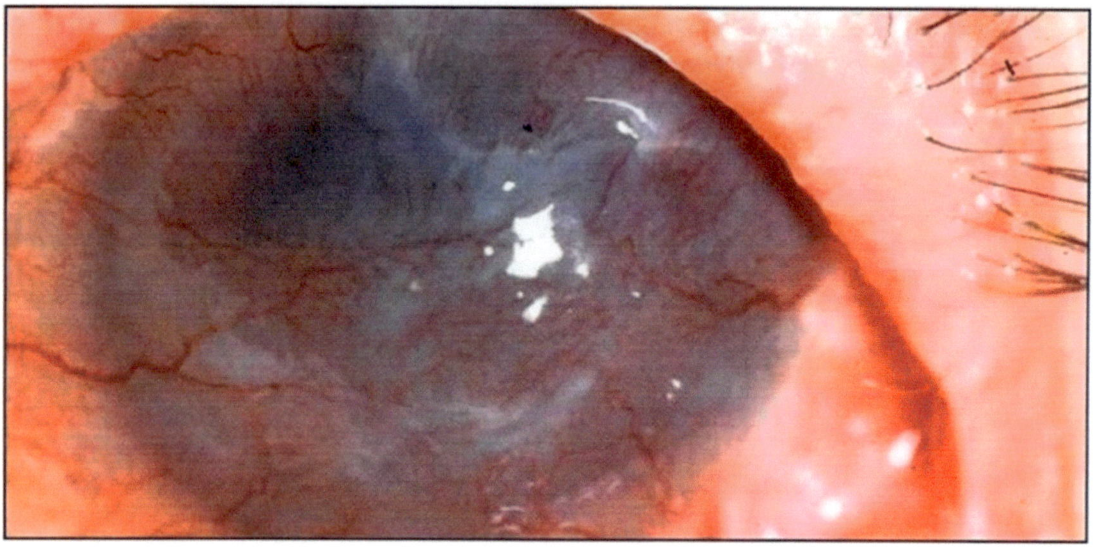

Figure 87: Extensive corneal neovascularization in Stevens-Johnson syndrome.

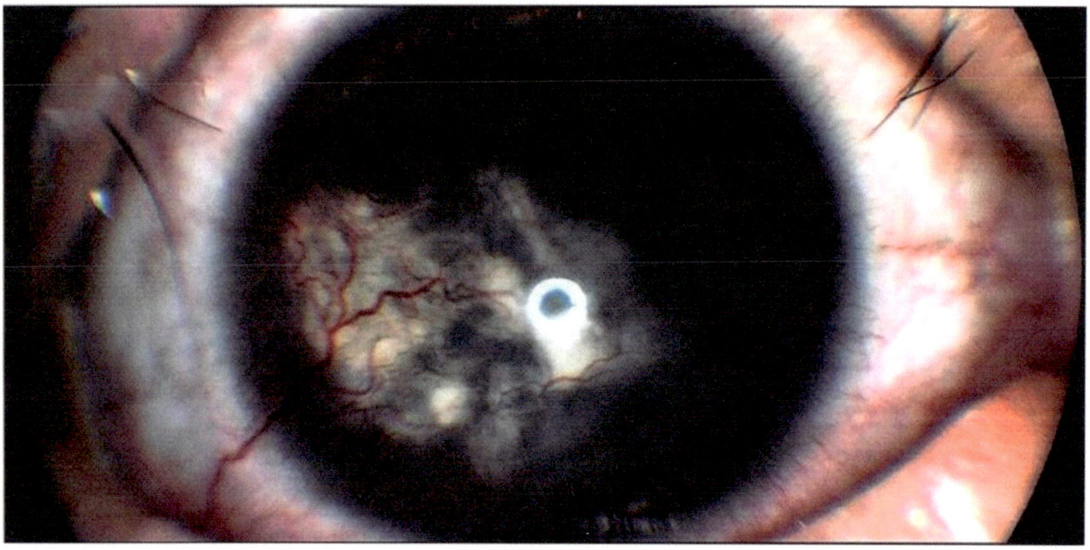

Figure 88: Corneal neovascularization with white deposits in a patient with SJS.

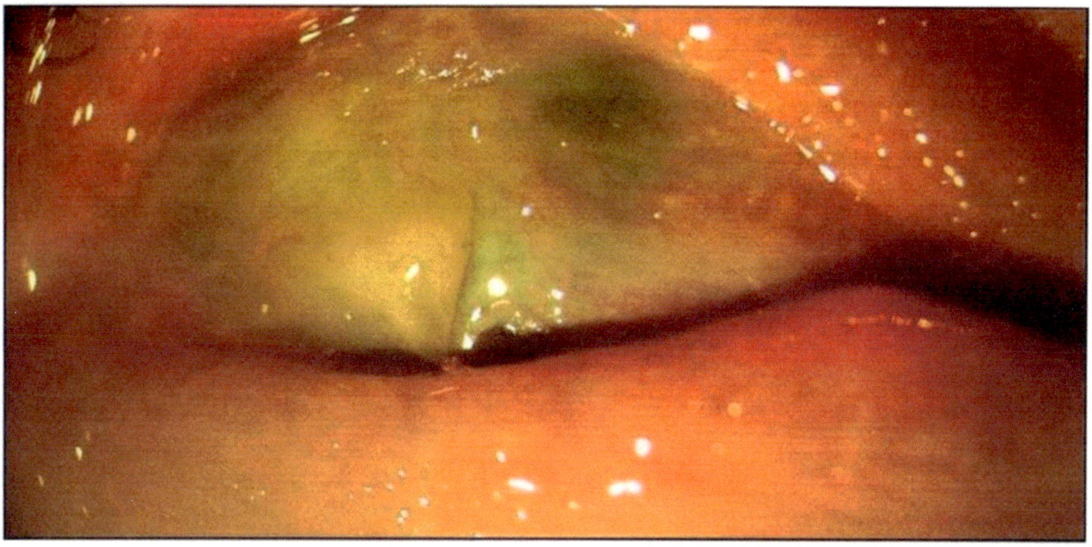

Figure 89: Complete vascularization, opacification, and keratinization in a 12 year-old patient with SJS.

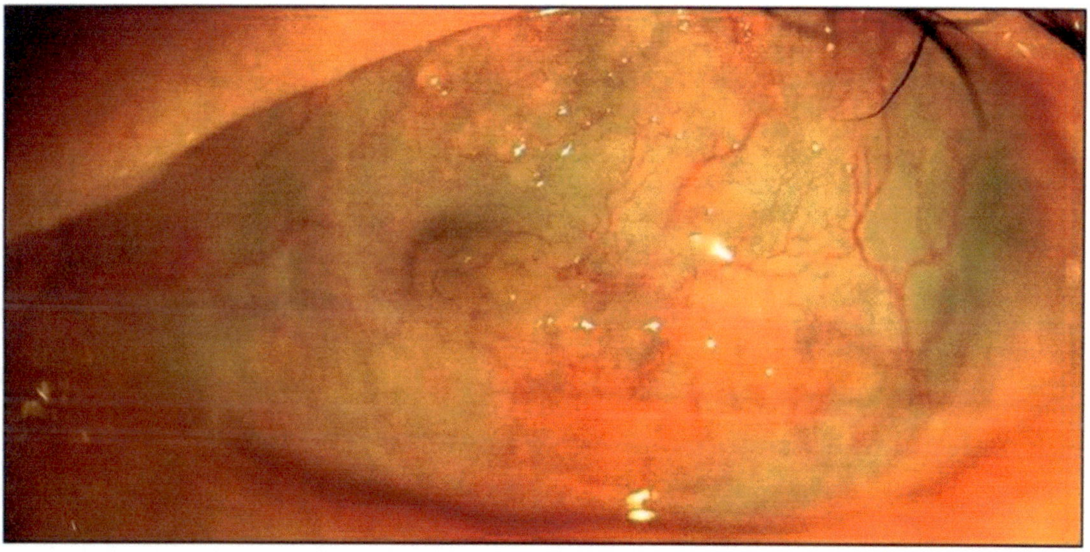

Figure 90: Madarosis, symblepharon, and total corneal opacification with neovascularization in the other eye of the same patient as in Figure 89.

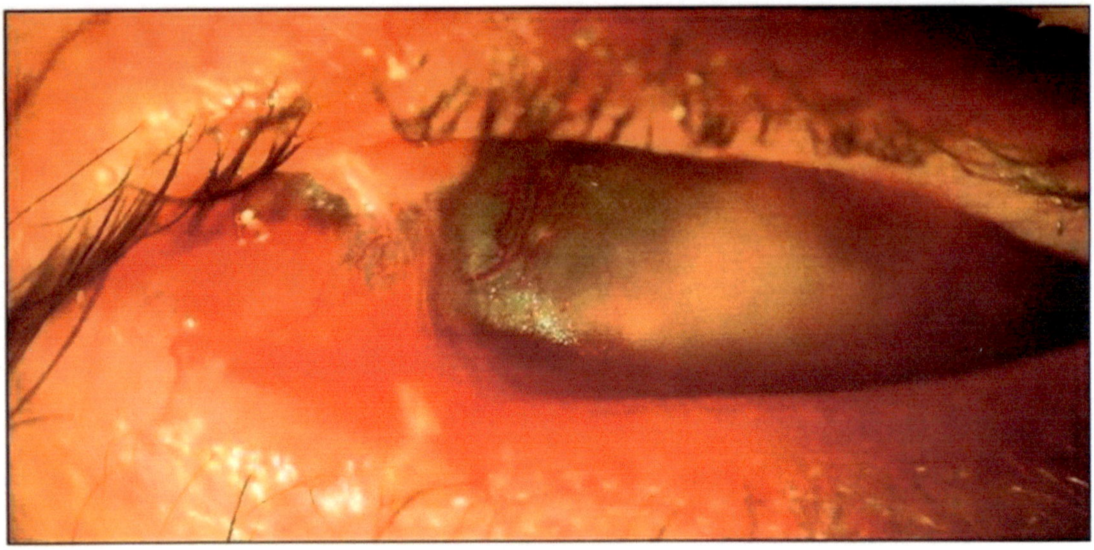

Figure 91: Extensive symblepharon secondary to SJS.

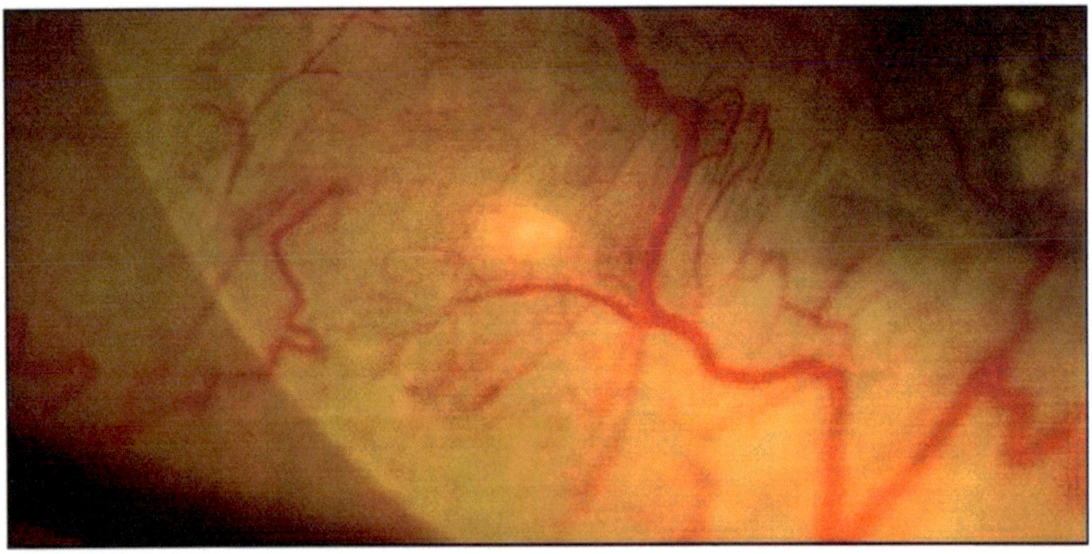

Figure 92: Bandage contact lens used to protect eyes affected by SJS from further migration of neovascularization into the cornea.

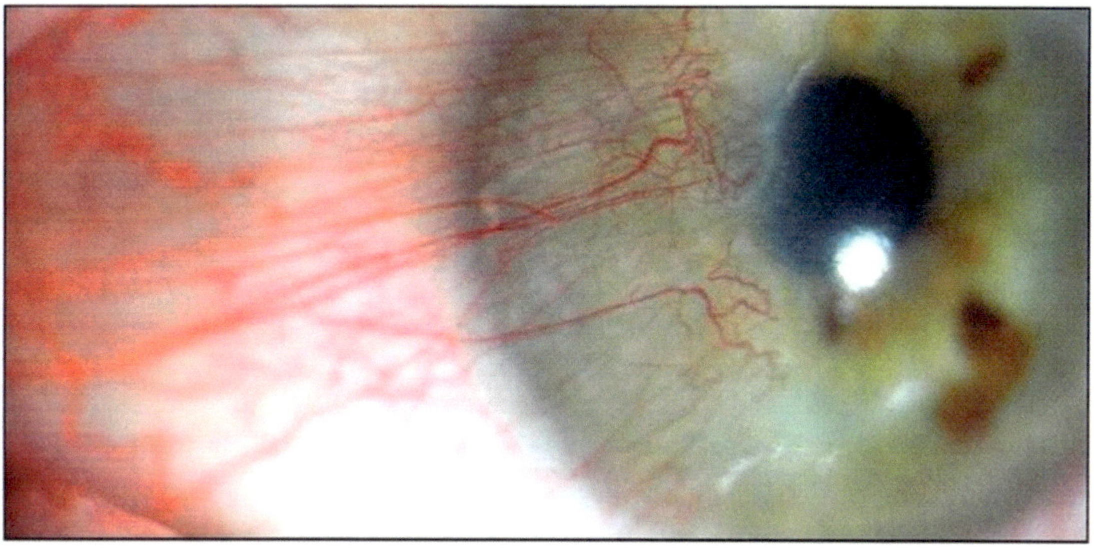

Figure 93: Limbal stem cell deficiency: A common feature of Stevens-Johnson syndome. Note the encroaching nasal neovascularization upon the central corneal surface.

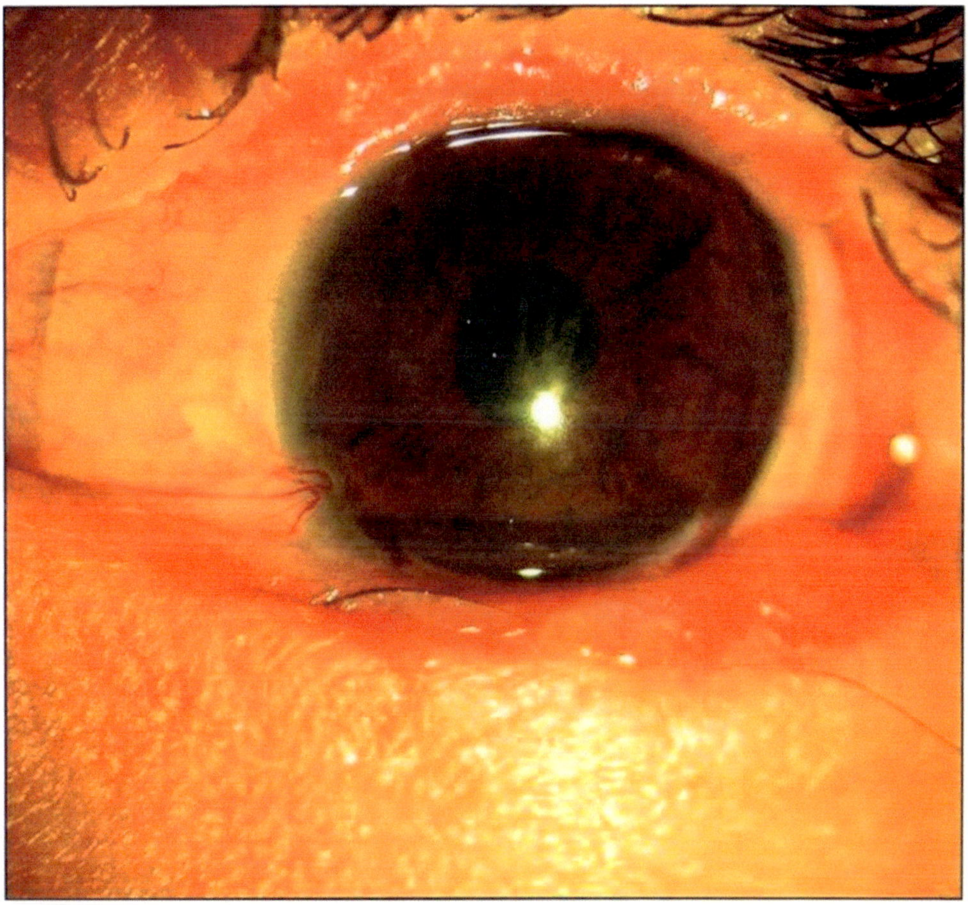

Figure 94: Bandage contact lens in SJS patient status-post amniotic membrane graft transplantation. Note the madarosis and trichiasis of the inferior eyelid.

References:

1) Lyell A. Toxic epidermal necrolysis: an eruption resembling scalding of the skin. *Br. J. Dermatol.* 1956;68:355-61.

2) Roujeau JC, Stern RS. Severe adverse cutaneous reactions to drugs. *N. Engl. J. Med.* 1994;331:1272-1285.

3) Power WJ, Ghoraishi M, Merayo-Lloves JM, et al Analysis of the acute ophthalmic manifestations of the erythema multiforme/Stevens Johnson syndrome/toxic epidermal necrolysis disease spectrum. *Ophthalmology* 1995; 102: 1669-76.

4) Howard GM. The Stevens—Johnson syndrome. Ocular prognosis and treatment. *Am J Ophthalmol* 1963; 55: 893-900.

5) Power WJ, Saidman SL, Zhang DS, Vamvakas EC, Merayo-Lloves JM, Kaufman AH, Foster CS. HLA typing in patients with ocular manifestations of Stevens-Johnson syndrome. *Ophthalmology* 1996;103:1406-9.

6) French LE. Toxic epidermal necrolysis and Stevens Johnson syndrome: our current understanding. *Allergol Int* 2006;1:9-16.

7) Di Pascuale MA, Espana EM, Liu DT, Kawakita T, Li W, Gao YY, Baradaran-Rafii A, Elizondo A, Raju VK, Tseng SC. Correlation of corneal complications with eyelid cicatricial pathologies in patients with Stevens-Johnson syndrome and toxic epidermal necrolysis syndrome. *Ophthalmology* 2005;5:904-12.

8) Patterson R, Miller M, Kaplan M, et al. Effectiveness of early therapy with corticosteroids in Stevens-Johnson syndrome: experience with 21 cases and a hypothesis regarding pathogenesis. *Ann Allergy*. 1994;73: 27-34

Part Three:

Autoimmune Diseases

Fuchs' Heterochromic Iridocyclitis

Definition: Fuchs' heterochromic iridocyclitis (FHI, or Fuchs' uveitis syndrome) is a chronic, non-granulomatous uveitis of unknown origin. Often asymptomatic, it is characterized by a classic clinical spectrum of small stellate keratic precipitates, iris atrophy (with or without heterochromia), abnormal angle vessels, and absence of posterior synechiae. However, clinical features in FHI are probably more variable.

History: The first report of FHI was made in 1904 by Weill. Years later Fuchs described both the clinical and histopathological features of this entity.

Epidemiology: The prevalence of FHI in uveitis populations ranges from 1.2 to 4.5%. True prevalence is probably higher because the syndrome is diverse, often presenting with variations, resulting in its being one of the most under-diagnosed uveitic syndromes. It does not have any sexual or racial predilections, is mostly unilateral, and usually affects young to middle-aged individuals.

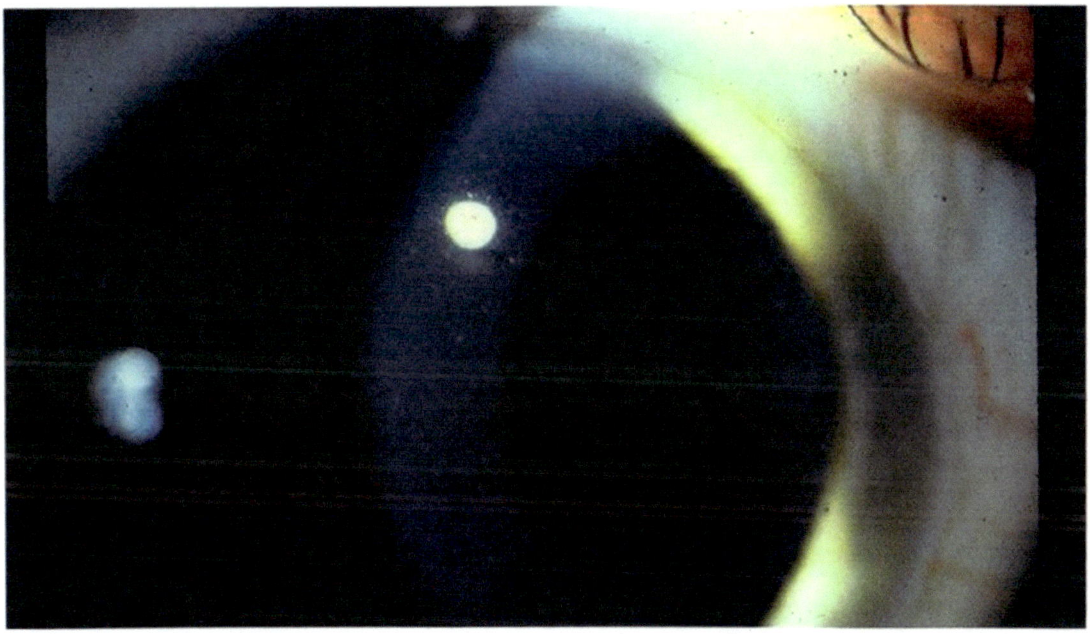

Figure 95: Fuchs Heterochromic Iridocyclitis - note the fine stellate keratic precipitates.

Clinical Features: FHI is considered an unusual form of uveitis with a variable clinical appearance. Many patients are unaware of their disease, which is often recognized during a routine ophthalmologic examination.

Anterior segment: Anterior chamber inflammation is mild. Keratic precipitates, usually small and stellate, are diffusely scattered over the cornea. Iris changes often precede obvious heterochromia and are a more sensitive and reliable sign. They include iris stromal smoothing (with loss of the normal corrugated texture), iris nodules (which can lead to misdiagnosis as granulomatous uveitis), small refractile iris crystals (Russell bodies), and, heterochromia. Heterochromia is not a universal feature: hypochromia is often subtle or absent (especially in darker irides). In pale blue eyes, loss of the paler anterior iris stroma can result in a darker iris (inverse heterochromia). Abnormal iris and anterior chamber (AC) angle vessels are common, and may be responsible for the occurrence of bleeding after AC paracentesis (Amsler's sign). Cataract formation and secondary glaucoma are common complications, and the latter is the most common cause of visual loss in patients with FHI.

Posterior segment: Vitritis is a common finding. In general, this is mild and not associated with macular edema or retinal vasculitis. Peripheral inflammatory chorioretinal scars resembling those of Toxoplasma retinochoroiditis may be seen.

Pathogenesis: Cellular phenotype (high levels of CD8+ T cells) and cytokine profile in aqueous humor of FHI patients is different from that observed in other chronic uveitides. Specific intraocular antibody production against rubella virus and non-identified antigens have been reported and many pathogenetic mechanisms considering these particular features have been proposed. There is inadequate evidence at present to formulate a common pathophysiologic mechanism.

Diagnosis: The diagnosis is clinical, though the formal criteria have not yet been internationally accepted. The differential diagnosis includes conditions with hypopigmentary heterochromia and a raised IOP, such as glaucomatocyclitic crisis, syphilis, and herpetic uveitis.

Treatment: No anti-inflammatory treatment is known to change the course of the disease. Treatment is mostly reserved for sight-threatening complications: cataract, glaucoma, and vitreous opacification. Long term steroids are not indicated. However, a short trial of topical steroids may be helpful in differentiating FHI from conditions such as glaucomatocyclitic crisis or idiopathic anterior uveitis with trabecular damage, Cataract surgery may be necessary. Glaucoma is the most damaging complication of FHI, and requires prompt and aggressive therapy. This is a result of steroid-responsive trabeculitis. A high proportion of patients fail to respond to maximal medical therapy, and require surgery. Vitrectomy may be necessary in selected cases.

1) Liesegang reported 66% of patients with secondary glaucoma requiring surgery
2) Le Hey reported failed medical therapy in 73% of cases with secondary glaucoma
3) Jones reported that only 63% of the patients with Fuchs and Glaucoma remained controlled on topical medication.

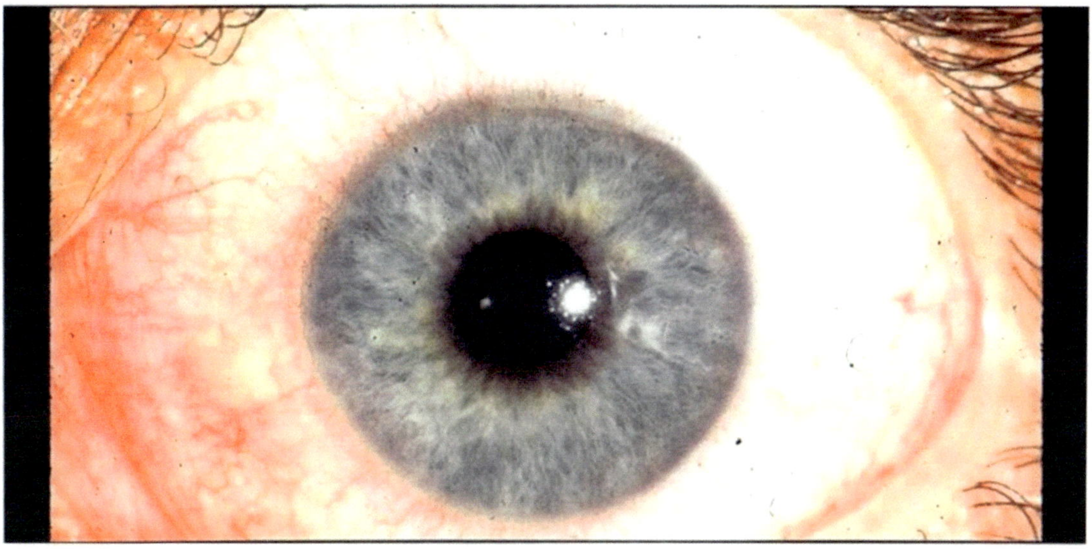

<u>Figure 96:</u> Note the heterochromia in the left eye.

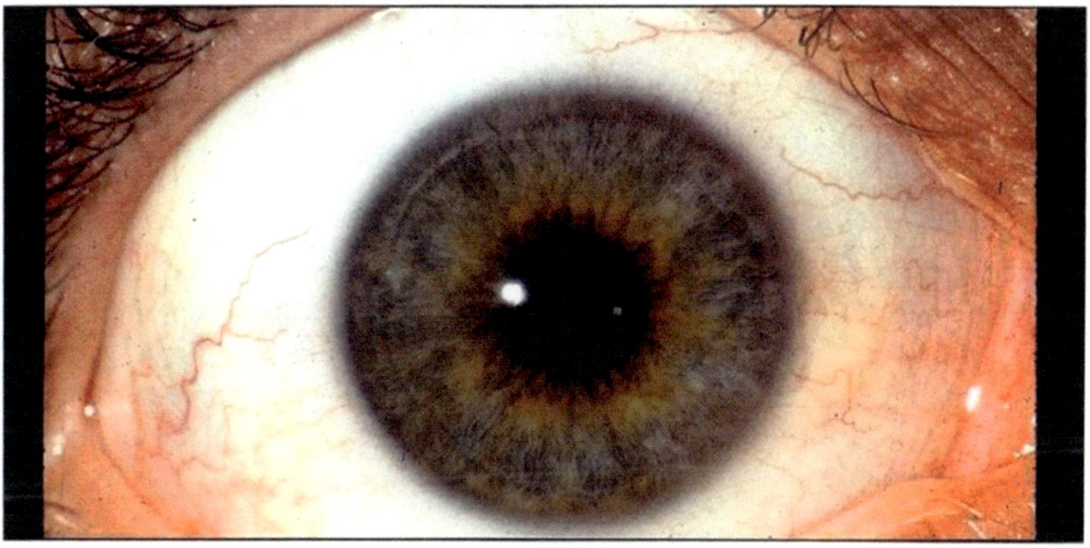

<u>Figure 97:</u> The uninvolved eye.

References:

1) Mohamed Q, Zamir E. Update on Fuchs' uveitis syndrome. *Curr Opin Ophthalmol* 2005; 16:356-63.
2) Livir-Rallatos C. Fuchs' heterochromic iridocyclitis; in: Foster CS, Vitale AT. *Diagnosis and treatment of uveitis.* Saunders. Philadelphia 2002:693-700.
3) Muhaya M, Calder V, Towler HM, et al. Characterization of T-cells and cytokines in the aqueous humor (AH) in patients with Fuchs' heterochromic cyclitis (FHC) and idiopathic anterior uveitis (IAU). *Clin Exp Immunol* 1998; 111:123-8.
4) De Groot-Mijnes, de Visser L, Rothova A, et al. Rubella virus is associated with Fuchs' heterochromic iridocyclitis. *Am J Ophthalmol* 2006; 141:212-4.

Human leukocyte antigen testing

Human leukocyte antigen testing

Uveitic syndromes are sometimes associated with certain human leukocyte antigen (HLA) types[1]. HLA is the human major histocompatibility complex (MHC) in humans and is located on the short arm of chromosome 6. HLA genes subtypes are defined as HLA class I molecules and HLA class II molecules—according to their molecular structure. HLA class I molecules are expressed on almost all somatic cells, although the levels of expression varies from tissue to tissue and can be modulated by several cytokines, especially the interferons (IFN).

Class I molecules bind peptides derived from endogenously synthesized proteins (e.g., viral proteins in virus-infected cells) and present them to CD8 T cells. Normal human corneal endothelium does not express HLA class I molecules, which is thought to promote ocular immune privilege and the survival of corneal grafts[2.] Albeit Human uveal cells, with the exception of vascular endothelium, do not normally express[3,4] or express in low concentration.

Class II molecules are found on relatively few cell types, such as macrophages, B lymphocytes, and dendritic cells. The expression of HLA class II molecules can also be induced by various pro-inflammatory stimuli. Retinal pigment epithelial (RPE) cells do not normally express HLA class II molecules[4]. However, expression of these HLA molecules has been detected on RPE cells in patients with uveitis[5], proliferative vitreoretinopathy[6], and retinitis pigmentosa[7]. Furthermore, the induction of these molecules by IFN-y has been demonstrated[8]. Class II molecules bind peptides derived from exogenous proteins that have been internalized by antigen presenting cells and present them to CD4 T cells. Thus, HLA plays an important role in the immune system to recognize self from non-self, to present foreign antigens, and ultimately to stimulate T cells.

Association between HLA antigen and disease were published since 1967 and showed that Hodgkin's lymphoma was related to a specific group of HLA antigens[10]. The association between some uveitic entities and HLA antigens has been acknowledged since 1970s.

There are several associations between HLA molecules and eye inflammation, one of the strongest is the association with birdshot choroidoretinopathy and the HLA A29. Up to 90-99% [11,12,13] of the patients with an HLA A29 positive test have birdshot. HLA A29 is subdivided into HLA A29.1 and HLA A29.2. Both of these subtypes are associated with this distinctive ocular inflammatory disease. B27 molecule has also a strong correlation with ocular disease. Patients with acute anterior uveitis are positive in the 50% of the cases. This particular molecule has certain mimicry with some bacterial antigens such as *Klebsiella, Salmonella, Shigella*, and *Yersinia*, which somehow triggers autoimmunity in these patients. But molecular mimicry does not explain by itself all the immunologic events and other pathways have to be studied. In Behcet's disease the HLA B51 subtype HLA-B*5101 is strongly associated in many different ethnic groups from the Middle East to the Far East[15,16]. The presence of this HLA molecule can increase the risk of developing the disease by a 6t to 11 fold[17-20]. In spite of this fact there is not substantial number of cases of Behcet's disease in family members, so maybe also some environmental factors are also associated in the pathogenesis.

In patients with Vogt-Koyanagi-Harada syndrome is found some association with HLA DR4 molecules among Japanese, Chinese and Hispanics. There are 27 subtypes of this particular molecule, but HLA DRB1*4 is the one which confers susceptibility to get the disease. Apparently this HLA molecule facilitates CD4+ lymphocytes to selective infiltrate melanocytes which explain such selective pigmented cell destruction in the course of the disease. Sympathetic Ophthalmia shares the same susceptibility as patients with Vogt-Koyanagi-Harada syndrome to HLA DR4 molecules but also HLA DR53 [21] confers an elevated risk for this entity. In Sarcoid patients there is a clear association with HLA molecules HLA-B8-DR3, -DR5, and -DR6 haplotypes among Caucasian patients, and in Japanese population HLA-DR52 was significant higher than in Caucasian. The presence of these molecules can increase the risk of having the disease by 2-7 fold. On the other side HLA DRB1*1302 seems to be protective, this related to a glutamic acid residue at position 71 (unique to DRB1*1302) which interferes with the interaction of T helper cell receptor[22] . In patients with juvenile idiopathic arthritis HLA DR8 and its associated HLA-D specificity (Dw8) are described to be present in patients with pauciarticular form (which is the most frequent among uveitic patients). In male patients and with an older onset there is a strong association with HLA B27 molecule. Patients with pars planitis have increased association with HLA DR2 molecules[23-25]. Multiple sclerosis is frequently found in patients with pars planitis and they share this occurrence of HLA molecules, particularly the subtype DR15 (which is exclusively found in patients with both pars planitis and multiple sclerosis).

Nevertheless, there are strong associations of HLA molecules in different uveitic syndromes, other mechanism must be considered, since most of them are currently unknown.

References

1) Yabuki K, Inoko H, Ohno S. HLA testing in patients with uveitis. *Int Ophthalmol Clin.* 2000 Spring;40(2):19-35.
2) Treseler PA, Foulks GN, Sanfilippo F: The expression of HLA antigens by cells in the human cornea. *Am J Ophthalmol* 98:763-72, 1984-
3) Abi-Hanna D, Wakefield D: Expression of HLA antigens on the human uvea. *Br J Rheumatol* 27:68-71, 1988.

4) Abi-Hanna D, Wakefield D, Watkins S: HLA antigens in ocular tissues. I. In vivo expression in human eyes. *Transplantation* 45:610-3, 1988.
5) Chan CC, Detrick B, Nussenblatt RB, et al: HLA-DR antigens on retinal pigment epithelial cells from patients with uveitis. *Arch Ophthalmol* 104:725-9, 1986.
6) Jerdan JA, Pepose JS, Michels RG, et al: Proliferative vitreoretinopathy membranes. An immunohistochemical study. *Ophthalmology* 96:801-10, 1989
7) Detrick B, Rodrigues M, Chan CC, et al: Expression of HLADR antigen on retinal pigment epithelial cells in retinitis pigmentosa. *Am J Ophthalmol* 101:584 90, 1986.
8) Abi-Hanna D, McCluskey P, Wakefield D: HLA antigens in the iris and aqueous humor gamma interferon levels in anterior uveitis. *Invest Ophthalmol Vis Sci* 30:990-4,1989.
10) Yabuki K, Inoko H, Ohno S. HLA testing in patients with uveitis. *Int Ophthalmol Clin.* 2000 Spring;40(2):19-35.
11) Baarsma GS, Kijlstra A, Oosterhuis JA, Kruit PJ, Rothova A. Association of birdshot retinochoroidopathy and HLA-A29 antigen. *Doc Ophthalmol* 1986;61:267
12) Tabary T, LeHoang P, Betuel H, et al. Susceptibility to birdshot chorioretinopathy is restricted to the HLA-A29.2 subtype. *Tissue Antigens* 1990;36:177-179.
13) Priem HA, Kijlstra A, Noens L, Baarsma GS, De Laey JJ, Oosterhuis JA. HLA typing in birdshot chorioretinopathy. *Am J Ophthalmol* 1988;105:182-185.
14) Be' atrice Donvito et al. Different HLA Class IA Region Complotypes for HLA-A29.2 and A29.1 Antigens, Identical in Birdshot Retinochoroidopathy Patients or Healthy Individuals. *Invest Ophthalmol Vis Sci.* 2005;46:3227-3232.
15) Yazici H, Chamberlain MA, Schreuder I, et al. HLA antigens in Behc, et's disease: a reappraisal by a comparative study of Turkish and British patients. *Ann Rheum Dis* 1980;39:344-348.
16) Yabuki K, Mizuki N, Ota M, et al. Association of MICA gene and HLA-B*5101 with Behget's disease in Greece. *Invest Ophthalmol Vis Sci* 1999;40:1921-1926.
17) Mizuki N, Inoko H, Tanaka H, et al. Human leukocyte antigen serologic and DNA typing of Behget's disease and its primary association with B51. *Invest Ophthalmol Vis Sci* 1992;33:3332-3340.
18) Mizuki N, Ohno S, Ando H, et al. A strong association between HLA-B*5101 and Behget's disease in Greek patients. *Tissue Antigens* 1997; 50:57-60.
19) Mizuki N, Ota M, Kimura M, et al. Triplet repeat polymorphism in the transmembrane region of the MICA gene: a strong association of six GCT repetitions with Behget's disease. *Proc Natl Acad Sci U S A* 1997;94:1298-1303.
20) Yabuki K, Mizuki N, Ota M, et al. Association of MICA gene and HLA-B*5101 with Behget's disease in Greece. *Invest Ophthalmol Vis Sci* 1999;40:1921-1926.
21) Davis JL, Mittal KK, Freidlin V, et al. HLA associations and ancestry in Vogt-Koyanagi- Harada disease and sympathetic ophthalmia. *Ophthalmology* 1990;97:1137-1142.
22) Brown JH, Jardetzky T, Saper MA, et al. A hypothetical model of the foreign antigen binding site of class II histocompatibility molecules. *Nature* 1988;332:845-850.
23) Malinowski SM, Pulido JS, Goeken NE, et al. The association of HLA-B8, B51, DR2, and multiple sclerosis in pars planitis. *Ophthalmology* 1993;100:1199-1205.
24) Tang WM, Pulido JS, Eckels DD, et al. The association of HLA-DR15 and intermediate uveitis. *Am J Ophthalmol* 1997;123:70-75.
25) Raja SC, Jabs DA, Dunn JP, et al. Pars planitis: clinical features and class II HLA associations. *Ophthalmology* 1999;106:594-599

Disease	**HLA association**
Acute Posterior Multifocal Placoid Pigment Epitheliopathy	HLA-B7
	HLA-D R2
Adamantiades-Behcet Disease	HLA-B51
	HLA-B*5101
Ankylosing Spondylitis	HLA-B27
Birdshot Retinochoroidopathy	HLA-A29
Giant Cell Arteritis	HLA-DR3
	HLA-DR4
	HLA-B8
	HLA-DRBi
	HLA-Cw3
Inflammatory Bowel Disease	HLA-B27
Juvenile Idiopathic Arthritis	HLA-DQA1*0101
	HLA-DRB1*0101
	HLA-DRB1*0102
	HLA-DRB1*1104
Multiple Sclerosis	HLA-DQ6
	HLA-DR15
Pars Planitis	HLA-DR2
	HLA-DR15
Presumed Ocular Histoplasmosis Syndrome	HLA-B7
	HLA-DRw2
Psoriatic Arthritis	HLA-A2
	HLA-B17
	HLA-B38
	HLA-B39
	HLA-Cw6
	HLA-DR7a
Reiter's Syndrome	HLA-B27
Rheumatoid Arthitis	HLA-DR1.
	HLA-DR2
	HLA-DR3
	HLA-DR4
	HLA-DR5
	HLA-DR7
Serpiginous Choroiditis	HLA-B7
Sympathetic Ophthalmia	HLA-DR4
	HLA-DR53
	HLA-DQB1*0401
	HLA-DRB1*0405
Tubulointerstitial Nephritis and Uveitis Syndrome	HLA-DQA1*01
	HLA-DQB1*05
	HLA-DRB1*01
Vogt-Koyanagi-Harada Disease	HLA-DR1
	HLA-DR4
	HLA-DQB1*0401
	HLA-DRB1*0405
Whipple's Disease	HLA-B27

HLA-B27 Associated Uveitis

Definition: The association between the human major histocompatibility complex (MHC), HLA (human leukocyte antigen)-B27, and its spectrum of HLA-B27-associated inflammatory diseases and uveitis remains one of the strongest HLA-disease associations. However, HLA-B27 acute anterior uveitis (AAU) and its related systemic inflammatory conditions is by far the most common association. The presence of the HLA-B27 antigen has been shown to be a predictor of disease severity.

History: Brewerton was the first to describe the association between HLA-B27 and acute anterior uveitis in 1973. They also described a strong association between this genotype and other systemic conditions, such as Reactive arthritis and ankylosing spondylitis.

Epidemiology: HLA-B27 AAU is the most common identifiable cause of anterior uveitis, accounting for between 18-32% of all anterior uveitis cases in Western countries and a lower frequency in Asia (at least in part by the lower frequency of HLA-B27 in these populations). HLA-B27+ AAU is characterized by a clear male preponderance, occurring between the ages of 20 and 40. The association between HLA-B27 and other types of uveitis is much less frequent. Posterior segment involvement has been reported in 25% of all HLA-B27 associated uveitis. Patients with HLA-B27 have an approximately 2% lifetime risk of developing uveitis.

Clinical Features:

Systemic manifestations: HLA-B27 related conditions are ankylosing spondylitis, reactive arthritis (formally known as Reiter's syndrome), psoriatic arthritis, enteropathic arthropathy, and inflammatory bowel disease. These entities are often grouped together as the 'seronegative spondyloarthropathies'. The most frequent extraocular symptom is lumbar or buttock pain.

Ocular manifestations: Anterior uveitis has been reported to become chronic in up to 5% of the patients. Other common findings are posterior synechiae, vitritis, and hypopyon. (Figure 96). Intermediate uveitis and elevated intraocular pressure are less common. Cystoid macular edema is by far the most frequent finding. Papillitis may also appear. (Figures 97 and 98)

Pathology/Pathogenesis: The exact mechanisms by which HLA-B27 predisposes individuals to disease remains elusive. It is likely that in individuals who express HLA-B27, a change in the intracellular peptide pool (which may result from infection with an intracellular pathogen), could potentially alter the normal balance of HLA-B27 cell surface molecules. A perturbation of this balance may result in a more potent trigger of an immune activation of prolonged inflammatory responses.

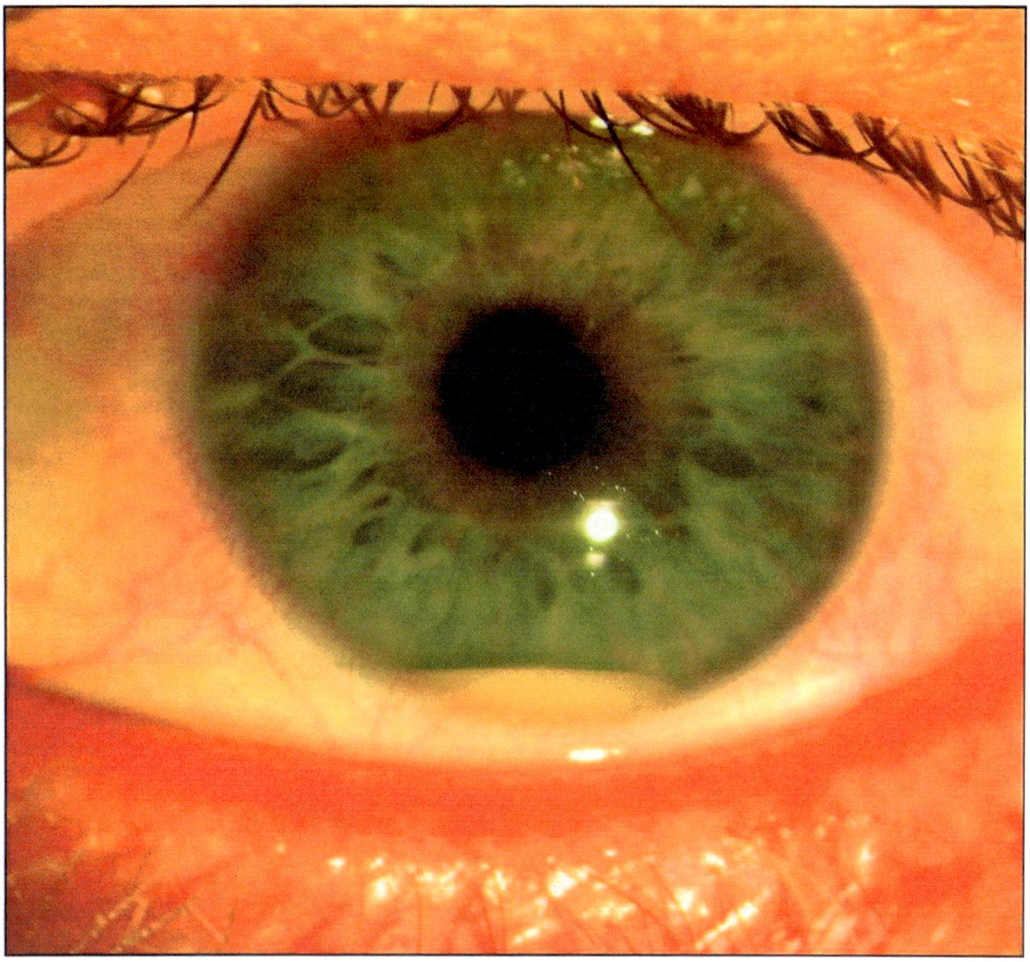

Figure 98: Hypopyon in a patient with HLA-B27 uveitis.

Diagnosis: Diagnosis is mainly based on clinical examination. We emphasize that HLA-B27 associated uveitis may appear independently as the sole or inflammatory manifestation associated with this genotype, although careful questioning of patients with seemingly isolated ocular disease may uncover subtle or early manifestations of a seronegative spondyloarthropathy.

Serologic testing of patients with recurrent episodes of uveitis (especially acute anterior uveitis) should include HLA haplotype determination because of its value as a predictor of disease severity and its profound relationship with other systemic inflammatory conditions, which may coexist or emerge with ocular involvement.

Treatment: First-line therapy for acute uveitis is corticosteroids. The route of administration corresponds with the severity of inflammatory reaction. In mild cases, topical steroids should suffice, whereas in moderate and severe cases, sub-Tenon injections and/or oral corticosteroids may be necessary. Cycloplegic/mydriatic drops reduces pain from ciliary spasm and may break/prevent posterior synechia if used early. Systemic immunomodulatory agents may be required in refractory cases.

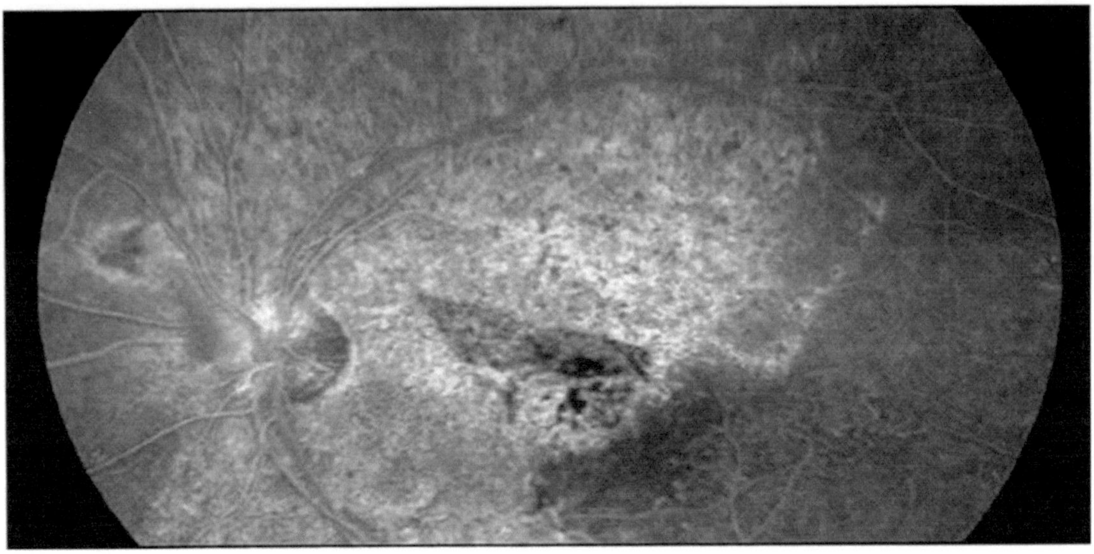

Figure 99: Early-phase FA of HLA-B27 positive patient with retinal vasculitis. Note the staining of the RPE and window defects.

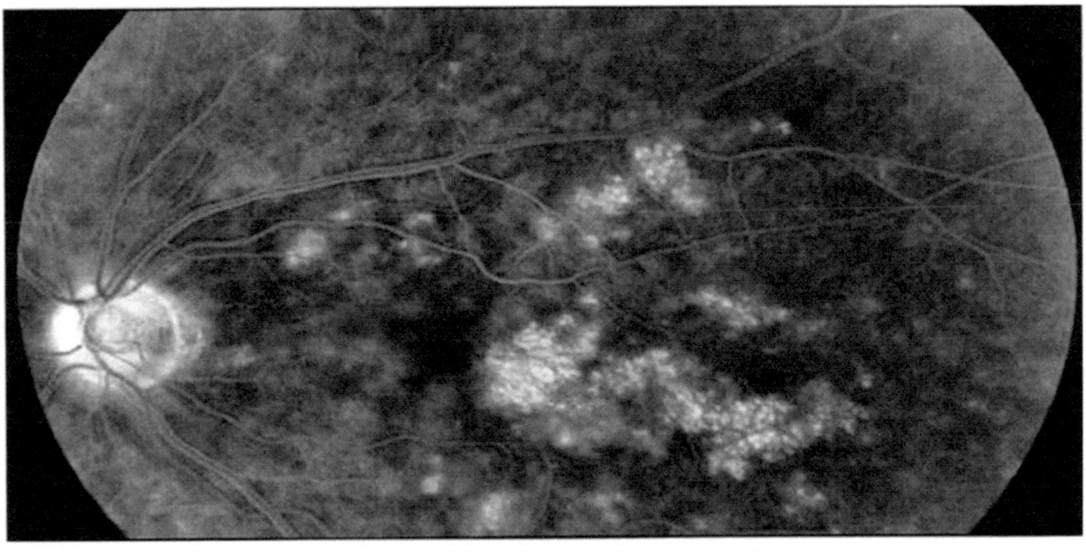

Figure 100: HLA B-27 positive panuveitis with cystoid macular edema.

References:

1) Chang JH, McCluskey PJ, Wakefield D. Acute anterior uveitis and HLA-B27. *Surv Ophthalmol.* 2005;50(4):364-88.
2) Suhler EB, Martin TM, Rosenbaum JT. HLA- B27-associated uveitis: overview and current perspectives. *Curr Opin Ophthalmol.* 2003;14 (6)378-83

Intermediate Uveitis

Definition: The term intermediate Uveitis (IU) refers to an intraocular inflammatory syndrome mainly involving the anterior vitreous, peripheral retina, and pars plana. It does not designate a single disease entity; it is a category of uveitides based on an anatomic classification system that can include diseases of various etiologies and clinical manifestations. The term pars planitis is often used to describe a subset of IU syndromes which are present on the pars plana. The syndrome is bilateral in 80% of the patients and chronic with periods of exacerbation and remission.

History: This entity was described by Fuchs in 1908, who named it chronic cyclitis. However, it was Schepens, decades later, who gave the first complete description of the disease entity capturing most of the classic clinical characteristics.

Epidemiology: IU has been reported in 8% to 22% of uveitis patient populations. It usually affects patients from 5 to 30 years old, without a gender or racial predilection.

Clinical Features: The etiology of IU is unknown but there are several associated systemic diseases, including multiple sclerosis (MS), idiopathic optic neuritis, sarcoidosis, thyroid diseases, and inflammatory bowel diseases.

Ocular manifestations:

Anterior segment: Clinical signs of inflammation may be present or absent. Anterior chamber cellularity, keratic precipitates, and (less frequently) posterior synechia may be seen. Complications may include ocular hypertension (corticosteroid-induced in most cases) and cataract formation.

Posterior segment: Vitreous cells are the most typical finding. Vitreal yellowish white aggregates (called "snowballs") may form and are mostly found in the inferior periphery. In addition, frank exudates on the pars plana may be seen varying from yellowish white and confluent ("snowbanks") in the acute stage, to a white sharp-edged collagen band (pars plana fibrosis) seen chronically in some patients, during inactive disease periods.

Signs of vasculitis including venous sheathing and/or retinal neovascularization are also common. Optic nerve involvement causing disc edema, and less frequently disc atrophy, and neovascularization may also be seen. Optic neuritis (with or without associated MS) has been reported in a substantial number of patients with IU.

Complications involving posterior segment include macular edema (which is the most common cause of severe visual loss in these patients), vitreous hemorrhage, cyclitic membrane formation, and retinal detachment.

Diagnosis: Diagnosis is based on clinical examination:

- A thorough peripheral retinal examination with scleral depression is imperative in the evaluation of all patients with IU.
- Laboratory and ancillary tests together with a careful review of systems may search for an associated disorder including Lyme disease, tuberculosis, syphilis, cat-scratch disease, multiple sclerosis, and sarcoidosis.
- Serologic tests should include angiotensin-converting enzyme (ACE), and lysozyme levels.
- Chest X-ray, Gallium scan, and spiral chest-CT scan are appropriate. Magnetic resonance imaging may also be helpful to rule out associated demyelinating diseases.
- Ophthalmologic tests should include fluorescein angiography (which can illustrate findings such as vasculitis and/or macular edema), echography, and electroretinogram. A vitrectomy may be necessary, therapeutically or diagnostically.

Figure 101: View of the posterior segment in an eye affected by immediate uveitis. Observe the vitreal yellowish white aggregates, the so-called "snowballs," and the obscured view of the retina due to dense cellular infiltration of the vitreous humor.

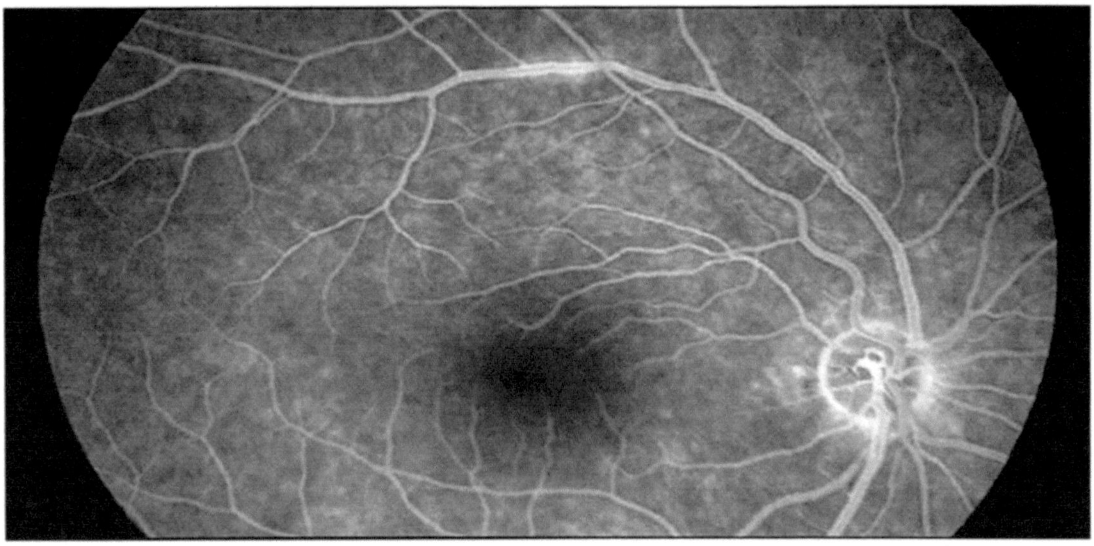

Figure 102: Angiographic view of an eye affected by idiopathic intermediate uveitis. Note the focal active vasculitis along the superior vein.

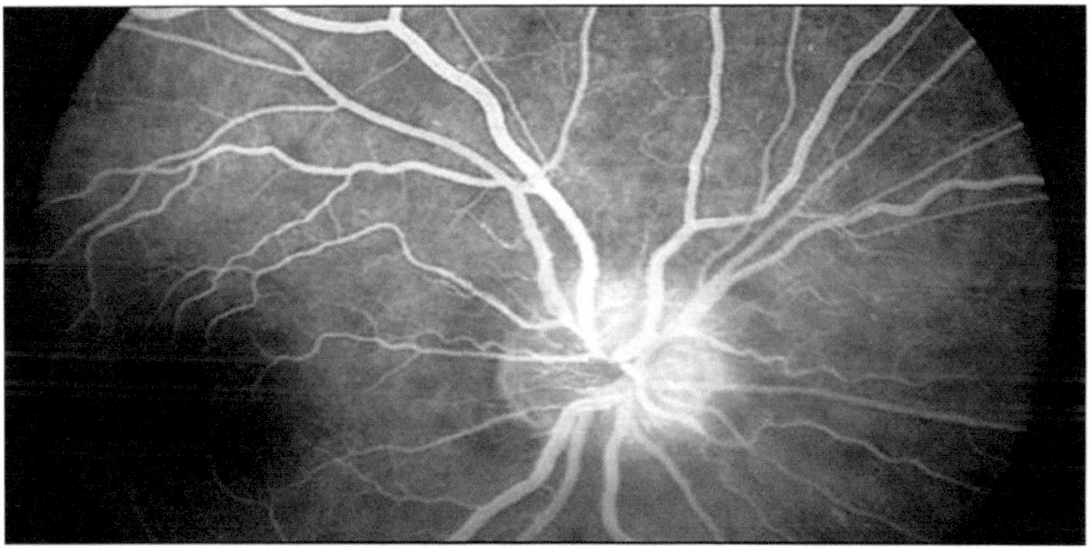

Figure 103: Papillitis in a patient with immediate uveitis.

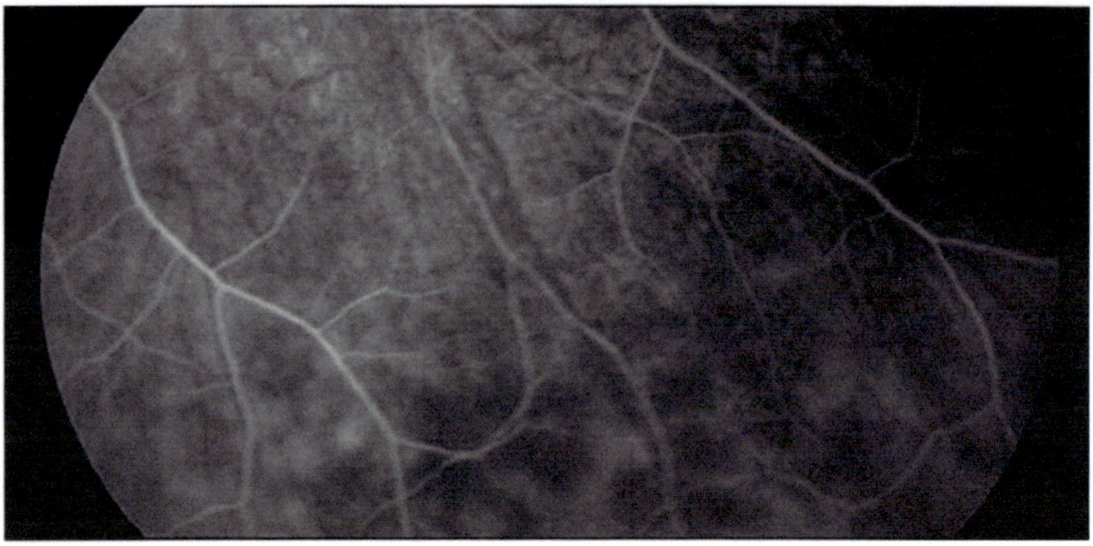

Figure 104: Late-phase FA of an eye affected by pars planitis. Note the pars plana infiltration located inferiorly.

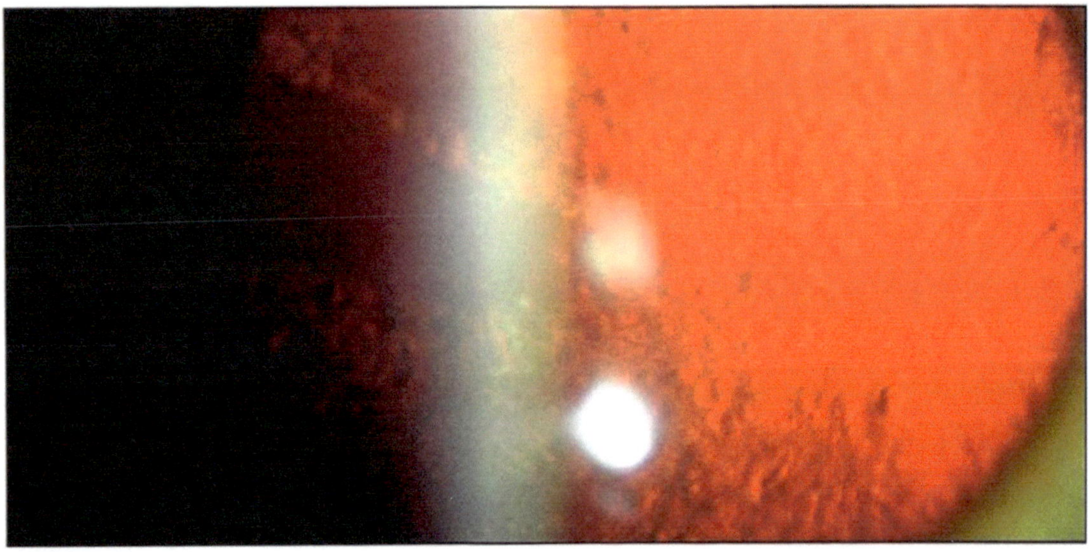

Figure 105: Transillumination view of an advanced (4+) posterior subcapsular cataract in a patient affected by pars planitis.

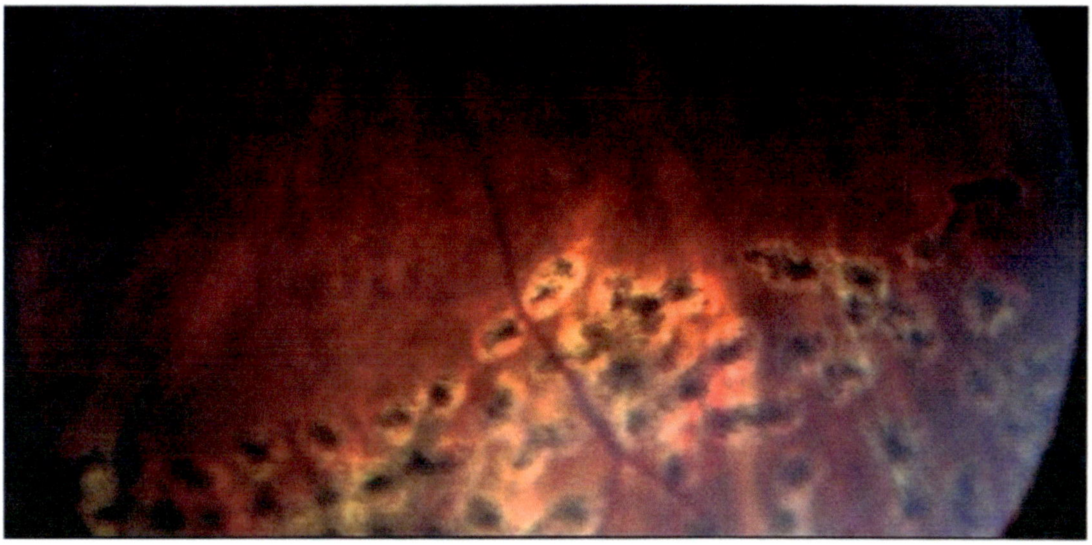

Figure 106: View of the inferior peripheral retina of an eye affected by intermediate uveitis. Note the pigmented chorioretinal scars secondary to laser photocoagulation following vitrectomy and endolaser therapy in an attempt to successfully control persistent inflammation.

Treatment: Whether acute IU should be treated depends on the presence of inflammation, the extent of vasculitis, coexisting macular edema, and the degree of pars plana infiltration. Having excluded treatable infectious and non-infectious entities that may simulate or present a clinical picture of IU, a five-step program (quite similar to that treatment approach initially described by Kaplan) approach is recommended as follows: (1) topical corticosteroids in the presence of anterior chamber inflammation, together with regional corticosteroid injections; (2) oral NSAIDs, if inflammation persists following the third injection, and topical NSAIDs in the presence of macular edema; (3) Systemic corticosteroids (short course) if inflammation persists or recurs despite previous interventions; (4) Peripheral retinal cryopexy or indirect laser photocoagulation if inflammation recurs after a sixth regional steroid injection; (5) Offer therapeutic pars plana vitrectomy versus immunomodulatory therapy if inflammation is recalcitrant to the previous treatment modalities.

References:

1) Vitale AT, Zierhut M, Foster CS. Intemediate uveitis; in: Foster CS, Vitale AT. *Diagnosis and treatment of uveitis*. Saunders. Philadelphia 2002:844-57.
2) Bonfioli AA, Damico FM, Curi AL et al. Intermediate uveitis. *Semin Ophthalmol.* 2005; 20 (3)147-54

Lens-Induced Uveitis

Definition: Lens-induced uveitis (LIU) results from an inflammatory reaction to protein leaking from an injured lens or hypermature cataract.

History: Straub is credited with first recognizing the clinical entity in 1919.

Epidemiology: The incidence is unknown. LIU is more common in developing nations where eye trauma is frequently neglected.

Clinical Features: Anterior capsule phimosis is often present, lens opacity is universal. Phacolytic glaucoma is frequently found. The anterior chamber reaction consists of both white cells and lens particles. Intermediate uveitis is frequently masked by lens opacity.

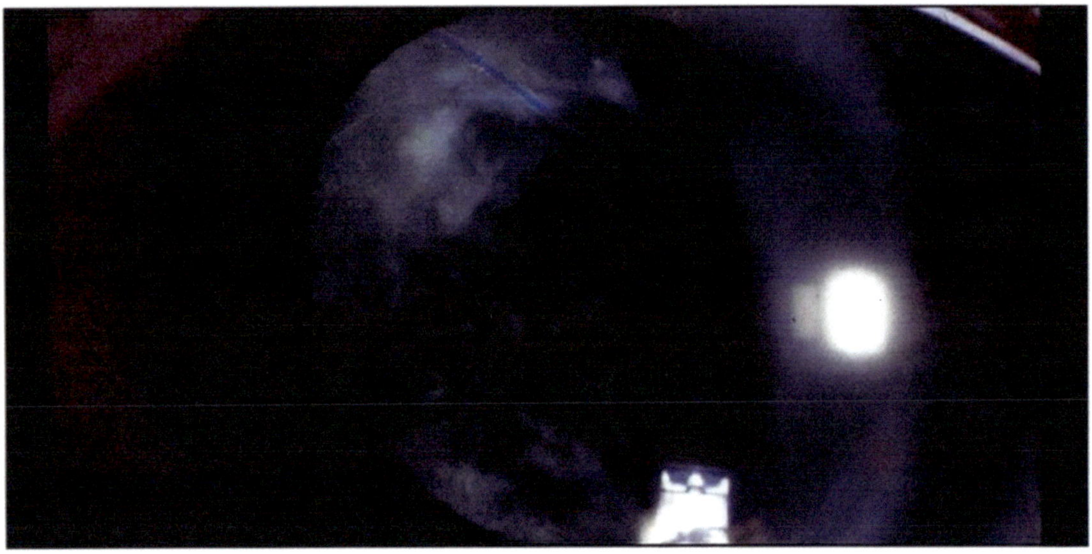

Figure 107: Lens Induced Uveitis - note the cortical lens material remaining in the anterior segment.

Pathology/Pathogenesis:. Lens protein is normally sequestered from the immune system. Lens material present in the anterior chamber induces a granulomatous inflammatory response characterized by autoreactive T lymphocytes and macrophages.

Diagnosis: Histopathologic examination of ocular specimens discloses zonal granulomatous inflammation and lens protein-laden macrophages.

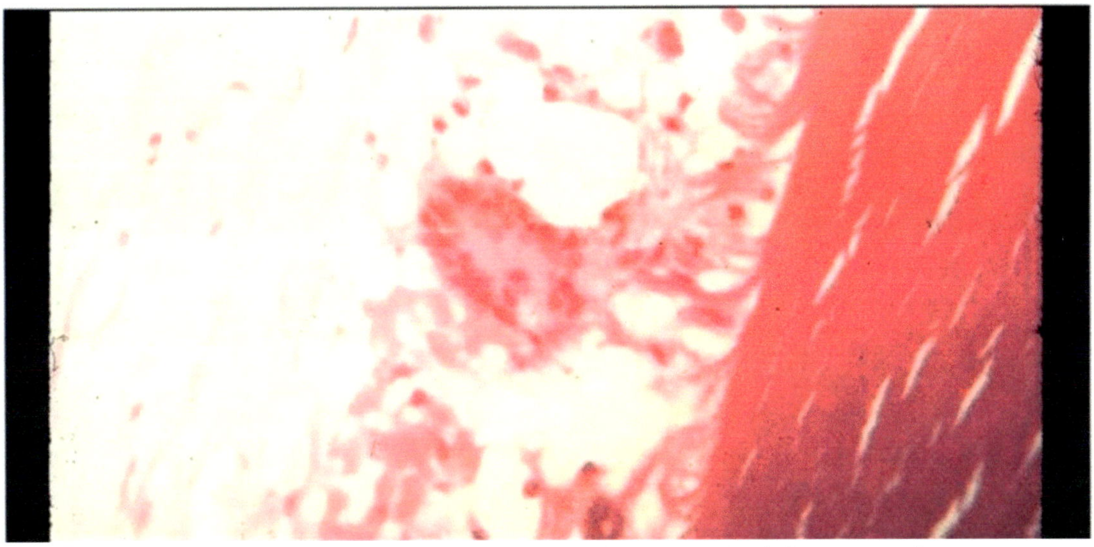

Figure 108: Zonal Granulomatous inflammation and lens protein-laden macrophages.

Treatment: Removal of all lens material is curative. If a small amount of lens material is present following extracapsular cataract extraction, corticosteroid therapy may temporize until resorption occurs. When pars plana vitrectomy is indicated for removal of posteriorly located lens fragments, vitreous specimens should be submitted for culture.

Reference

Michel SS, Foster CS. Lens-Induced Uveitis; in: Foster CS, Vitale AT. *Diagnosis and treatment of uveitis.* Saunders. Philadelphia 2002:817-821

Multiple Sclerosis

Definition: Multiple sclerosis (MS) is a chronic demyelinating central nervous system disease characterized by exacerbations and remissions.

History: Sir Augustus d'Esti first described MS in 1822. Charcot first reported ophthalmic manifestations in 1835. Central nervous system plaques and sclerosis were separately reported in London and Paris in the mid 1800s.

Epidemiology: The incidence varies from 5 to 30 cases per 100,000 and increases with increasing latitude on both sides of the equator. Uveitis occurs in up to 25% of cases. Onset is most common in early to mid-adulthood. Females are affected more often than males.

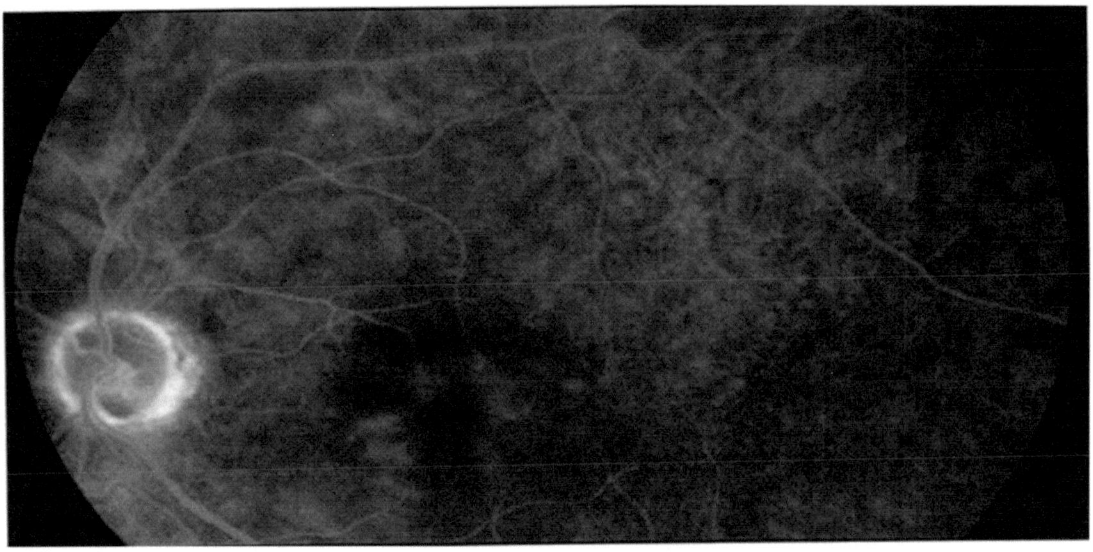

Figure 109: Cystoid macular edema in a patient with multiple sclerosis. Note the ring of optic disc hyperfluorescence, a mark of optic atrophy.

Clinical Features: Demyelination can affect any central nervous system tract. MS is associated with intermediate uveitis and posterior uveitis.(Figure 110). Neurophthalmologic manifestations are common and include optic neuritis (Figure 109), oculomotor nerve palsies, and internuclear ophthalmoplegia.

Pathology/Pathogenesis: The etiology is unknown. As yet unidentified infectious agents, environmental factors, and Vitamin D deficiency may be contributing factors.

Diagnosis: MS is associated with HLA-DR2. MRI demonstrates periventricular white matter changes which do not correlate with clinical symptomatology. Oligoclonal bands are frequently present in cerebrospinal fluid.

Treatment: The Optic Neuritis Treatment Trial delineated the most effective steroid regimen for acute retrobulbar optic neuritis. Interferon beta-1-a therapy delays progression to clinically definite multiple sclerosis following an initial demyelinating event such as optic neuritis. Glatiramer acetate reduces relapse rates

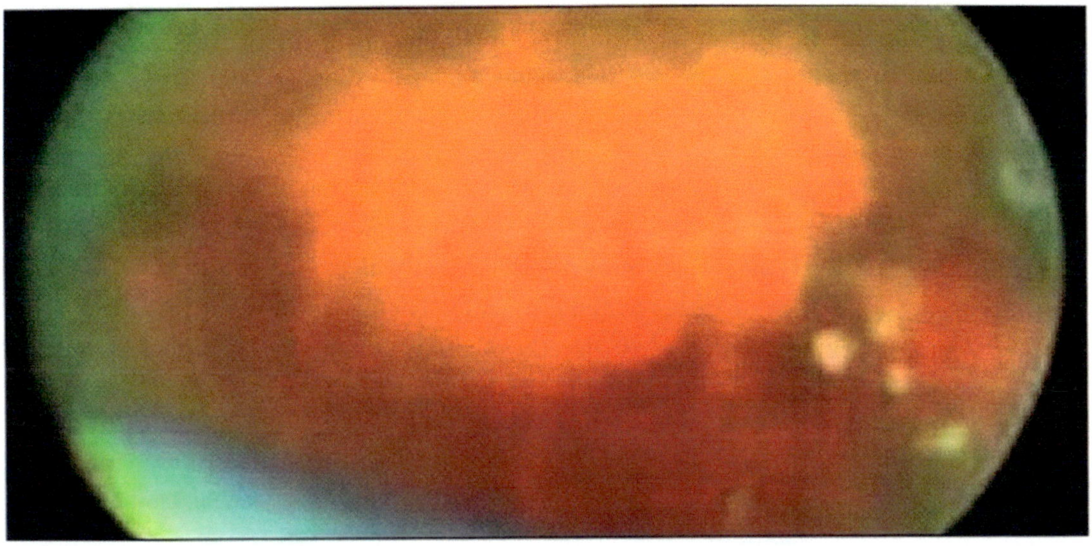

Figure 110: View of the inferior vitreous with the presence of clumped cells in a patient with multiple sclerosis.

Reference:

Markomichelakis N. Multiple Sclerosis; in: Foster CS, Bitale AT. *Diagnosis and treatment of uveitis* Saunders. Philadelphia 2002:701-709

Polyarteritis Nodosa

Definition: Polyarteritis nodosa (PAN), the prototype of systemic vasculitis, is a rare condition characterized by necrotizing inflammation of medium-sized muscular arteries and small vessels.

History: PAN was described by Kussmaul and Maier in 1866, who termed it periarteritis nodosa in attempt to reflect the nodular appearance of the affected vessels. In 1903, Ferrari renamed it polyarteritis, emphasizing the transmural and multifocal nature of the inflammation.

Epidemiology: PAN is an uncommon disease, mostly affecting 40-60 year old-adults. There is a preponderance of males to females (2:1). The exact incidence varies between 5 and 10 patients per million, and is directly related with the incidence of hepatitis B infection (much higher rates in hepatitis B hyperendemic populations).

Clinical Features: Virtually any organ, with the exception of the lungs, may be affected with peripheral neuropathy and symptoms from osteoarticular, renal artery, and gastrointestinal tract involvement are the most frequent clinical manifestations. Significant potential exists for end organ injury resulting from ischemia, infarcts, and hemorrhage.

Ocular manifestations This can be the first manifestation of the disease in 10-20% of patients. PAN can involve almost every tissue of the eye.

External involvement: Orbital vessel involvement may produce exophthalmos or a pseudotumor condition. Cranial nerve palsies may appear as a consequence of vasculitic involvement of the nervous system.

Anterior segment: The conjunctiva may be hyperemic and/or edematous, and sometimes present pale yellow, raised, and friable lesions due to infarcts.

Vasculitis affecting scleral, episcleral, and limbal vessels may lead to scleritis, episcleritis and keatitis. Necrotizing anterior scleritis (the most frequent type) is often associated with peripheral ulcerative keratitis (PUK), which progresses both circumferentially and centrally, requiring prompt diagnosis and systemic and aggressive therapy.

Acute non-granulomatous iritis may be seen.

Posterior segment: The most common ocular findings in PAN are choroidal and retinal vasculitis. Involvement of the posterior ciliary arteries and choroidal vessels may manifest as choroidal infarcts and exudative retinal detachments. Vitreous, subhyaloid, and retinal hemorrhages and other findings such as macular edema, cotton-wool spots, distortion of retinal vasculature, and lipid exudates may also be seen. (Figure 111). Vascular occlusion is less frequent. Papillitis due to optic nerve vasculitis may occur.

Pathology/Pathogenesis: The cause of the arteritis is unknown. It is likely that various antigens may trigger a circulating immune complex-mediated vasculitis. Viruses may contribute to the pathogenesis of arteritis (between 30% and 70% of patients have hepatitis B antibodies). Other known associated factors are drug abuse, hyposensitization treatment, B-cell neoplasm, and acute otitis media.

Superficial biopsies of cutaneous lesions will not show the characteristic segmental necrotizing vasculitis; these diagnostic changes are seen in muscular arteries taken from muscle, kidney, testes, or deep incisional skin biopsies.

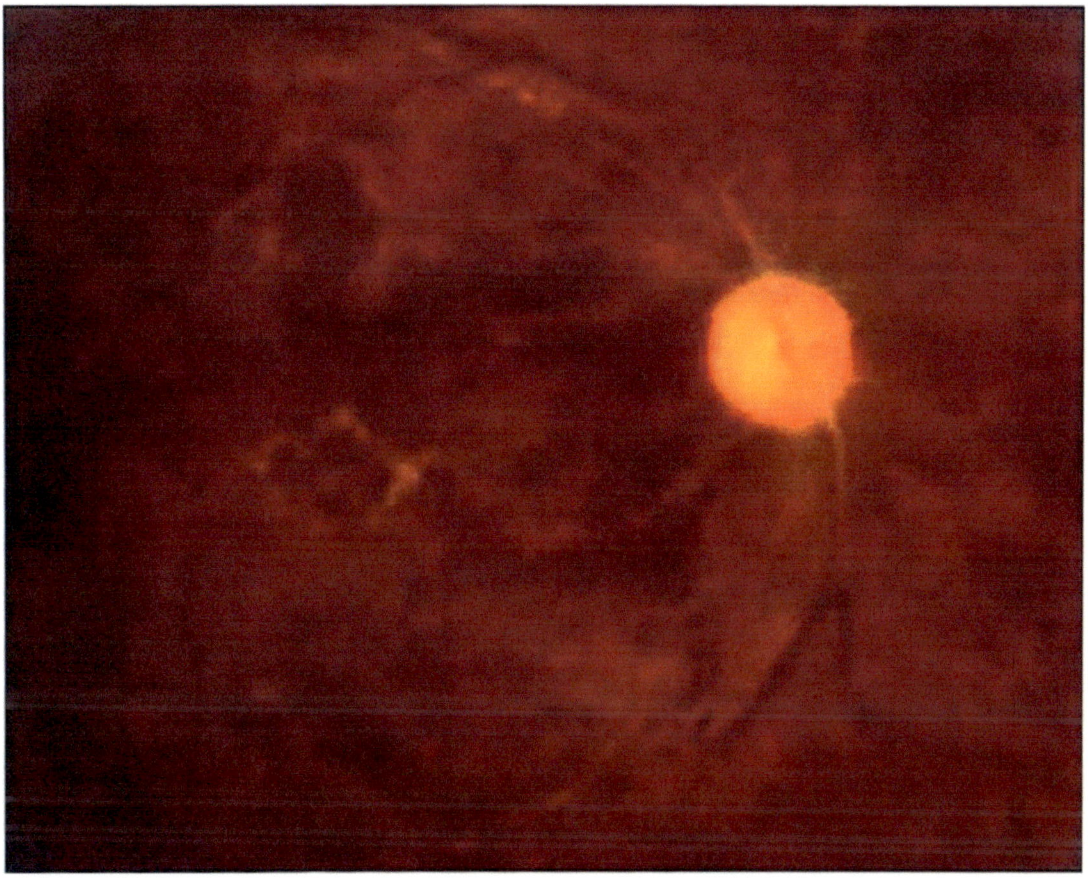

Figure 111: Right eye affected by polyarteritis nodosa-related vasculitis. Extensive areas of retinal hemorrhages with edema and lipid exudation, cotton-wool spots, and hyalinosis of the retinal vessels. Note the severe optic disc pallor.

Diagnosis: Establishing a definitive diagnosis of polyarteritis nodosa is challenging, and mandates dialogue between the pathologist and the clinician A tissue diagnosis is usually necessary for confirmation. Most laboratory tests are non-specific. It is important to note the following:

- Eosinophilia is relatively frequent.
- Hypocomplementemia may reflect more active disease.

- A high percentage (between 30% and 70%) of PAN patients have hepatitis B antigenemia.
- Cryoglobulins may be present and circulating immune complexes may be detected.
- Anti-neutrophil cytoplasmic antibody testing is typically negative

Fluorescein angiography (FA): Frequently shows arteritis with staining of involved arterial segments, dilated and tortuous capillaries, and leakage through diseased vessels. Thrombosis of the retinal veins (usually without evident periphlebitis) or delayed choroidal filling can also be seen.

Treatment: A clear distinction between limited versus systemic disease and idiopathic versus hepatitis B related PAN should be made because there are differences in their treatment and prognosis. Currently, systemic corticosteroids plus cyclophosphamide is the standard of care for idiopathic PAN, in particular for patients with adverse prognostic factors in whom this combination prolongs survival. In contrast, for hepatitis B-related PAN, treatment consists of schemes that include plasmapheresis and antiviral agents. The use of antiplatelet drugs concomitantly with the initiation of treatment might modify the potential vasospastic and platelet-aggregation effects of the disease.

References:

1) Soheilian M. Polyarteritis nodosa; in: Foster CS, Vitale AT. *Diagnosis and treatment of uveitis*. Saunders. Philadelphia 2002:653-60.
2) Colmegna I, Maldonado-Cocco JA. Polyarteritis nodosa revisited. *Curr Rheumatol* Rep. 2005;7(4):288-96.

Relapsing Polychondritis

Definition: Relapsing Polychondritis (RP) is a rare autoimmune disease which commonly affects the eye, causing episcleritis, scleritis, uveitis, or vasculitis.

The most distinctive characteristics of this condition are episodes of auricular, nasal, and laryngotracheal cartilage inflammation and inflammatory arthritis.

History: RP was first described by Jaksch-Wartenhorst in 1923 who called it polychondropathia. It was later named relapsing polychondritis by Pearson in 1960. Verity first reported ocular histological findings in an episcleritis specimen, which included a decrease in basophilia, fragmentation of elastic tissue with accumulation of mast cells, plasma cells, and lymphocytes around episcleral vessels.

Epidemiology: Most series have reported an equal male to female ratio and preponderance for white persons. The average age of onset is in the fourth decade with multisystemic involvement at presentation.

Clinical Features:

Systemic involvement: Auricular and nasal chondritis is painful, and patients can develop epistaxis. Auricular chondritis occurs initially in about half of the patients and later develops in about 80-90%. Saddle nose deformity can affect 30-60% of RP patients (Figure 113) Laryngotracheal involvement, with inflammation of cartilage, edema and narrowing of the airway, can present with hoarseness or aphonia, and local tenderness. Bronchitis or pneumonia can occur secondary to impaired lower airway mucocilliary function and poor cough reflex. Airway lesions cause about 50% of RP related deaths. Constitutional signs and symptoms are common, such as fever, weight loss, fatigue, night sweats, and enlarged lymph nodes. Nonerosive, rheumatoid factor-negative arthritis involving any joint can occur periodically. Cardiovascular disease such as aortic or mitral regurgitation, aortic aneurysms, myocarditis, pericarditis, and myocardial infarction are the second leading cause of death in patients with RP. Skin lesions such as dermatitis or leukocytoclastic vasculitis and renal complications (glomerulonephritis) may occur.

Ocular involvement: About 50% of RP patients develop ocular symptoms during the course of the disease, and 20-30% of these patients have ocular findings on presentation. Conjunctivitis, episcleritis, and scleritis are common. The scleritis can be diffuse, nodular, or necrotizing. (Figure 112) Posterior scleritis is uncommon. Iridocyclitis is another common finding. Peripheral corneal thinning with infiltrates or ulceration and keratitis sicca may be seen. Posterior segment findings include exudative retinal detachment, retinal infiltrates and chorioretinitis.

Other less common manifestations include extraocular muscle paresis with diplopia, lid ptosis, optic neuritis and papilledema. Orbital manifestations can include proptosis, chemosis, and lid edema, which can mimic pseudotumor or cellulitis.

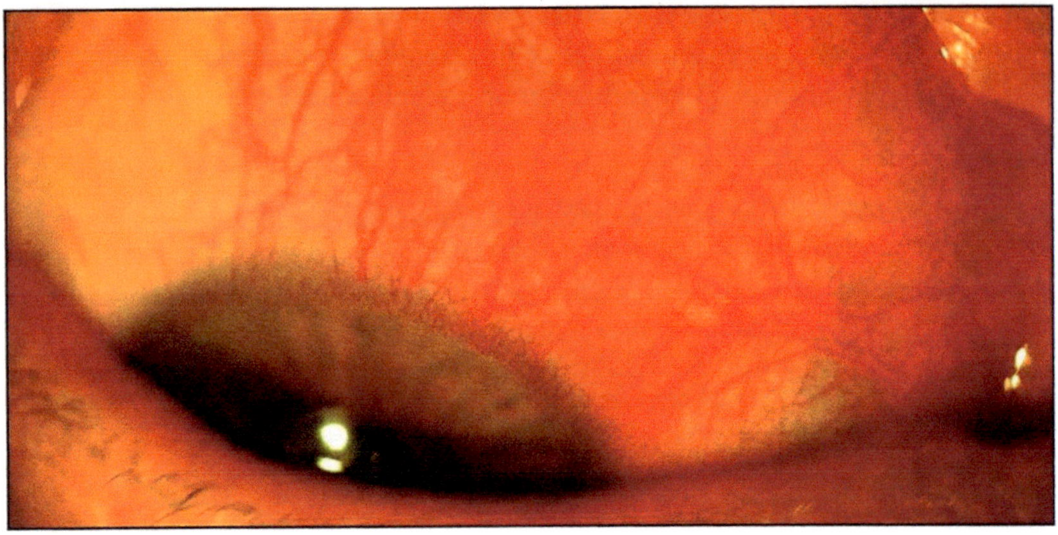

Figure 112: Diffuse scleritis in a patient with relapsing polychondritis

Pathology/Pathogenesis: Autoantibodies to collagen type II and IX and XI have been reported. The presence of immune complexes is suggested by immunofluorescence microassays that show granular deposits of IgG, IgA, IgM and complement at the junction of cartilaginous and fibrous tissue. A cell-mediated immune response to collagen has been reported. A significant association between RP and HLA-DR4 has been found. Histologic examination reveals loss of basophilic staining of cartilage matrix, perichondral inflammation at the cartilage-soft tissue interface, perivascular mononuclear and neutrophil infiltrates. Necrotic, vacuolated chondrocytes are replaced by fibrous tissue. Biopsy in a patient with RP and scleritis shows mast cells, plasma cells, and lymphocytes in the substantia propria and vasculitis with vessel wall infiltration with neutrophils and deposition of IgG, IgM and complement C3 in the vessel walls. There is strong evidence to support the hypothesis that RP is an autoimmune disease with vasculitis as the cause of the ocular, cardiovascular, dermatologic, neurologic, and audiovestibular manifestations.

Diagnosis: The diagnosis of RP is made clinically. The basis for diagnosis is the presentation of three or more of the following six signs: recurrent chondritis of both auricles, chondritis of nasal cartilage, nonerosive inflammatory polyarthritis, inflammation of ocular structures, chondritis of the respiratory tract, or cochlear/vestibular damage. Any of these signs and a positive biopsy is diagnostic. The diagnosis can also be made based on chondritis in two or more separate anatomic locations that responds to corticosteroids or dapsone. There are no diagnostic laboratory tests for RP, but most patients with RP show nonspecific inflammation, with elevated erythrocyte sedimentation rate (ESR), and C reactive protein. Patients with RP can have associated diseases, such as SLE, rheumatoid arthritis, or Sjogren's syndrome.

Treatment: Dapsone is often effective in treating the extraocular manifestations of RP. Topical steroids are not effective in controlling eye disease, and systemic steroids are usually required. Immunosuppressive therapy with azathioprine, methotrexate, and cyclosporine has also been used. Cyclophosphamide is usually reserved for severe refractory RP.

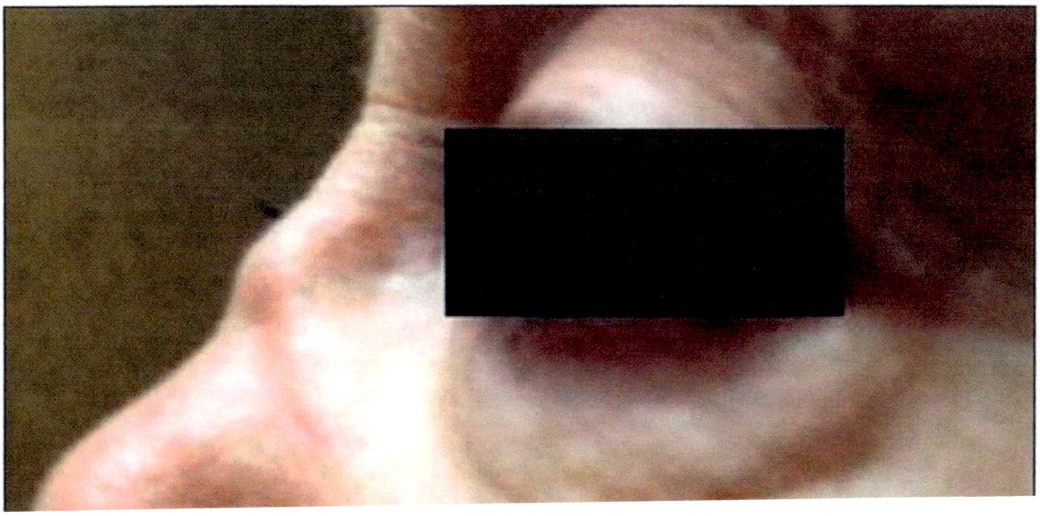

Figure 113: Saddle-nose deformity as seen in a patient with relapsing polychondritis.

Reference:

Wetzig RP. Eye Disease and Systemic Correlates in Relapsing Polychondritis; in: Foster CS, Vitale AT. *Diagnosis and treatment of uveitis*. Saunders. Philadelphia 2002:676-682.

Retinal Vasculitis

Definition: Retinal vasculitis (RV) represents a group of diseases causing retinal vasculature inflammation. The retinal veins are most frequently involved (retinal phlebitis).

History: RV was first described during the 19th century by van Trigt. H. Eales studied the association between recurrent vitreous hemorrhages and systemic symptoms, such as constipation. The clinical picture of retinal phlebitis was first described by Wadsworth in 1887. The association of RV with systemic diseases became recognized in the middle of the 20th century.

Epidemiology: Primary RV (also termed idiopathic RV) is a rare condition, with an estimated incidence of 2 cases per 100,000 per year, predominantly affecting adult females. However, RV is seen more frequently as a manifestation of ocular infections or systemic disorders, and the incidence of these pathologies varies worldwide.

Clinical Features: RV typically occurs in association with an underlying systemic or ocular disease. The list of associated diseases is extensive.

Systemic: Systemic symptoms and signs may be present and suggest an underlying etiology. Important systemic manifestations include oral and genital ulcers, skin ulceration, arthritis, rash, neurologic disease, and evidence of embolic disease. Therefore, a comprehensive review of systems is crucial to the evaluation of the patient with RV.

Ocular manifestations:

Anterior segment: Anterior uveitis may be seen in about one third of cases.

Posterior segment: Retinal vascular sheathing is the most characteristic feature of RV. Focal areas of fluffy-white cuffing as well as "skip areas" are commonly seen. The sheathing is most often seen around retinal veins, but can also affect arteries. Inferior vitreous snowballs and posterior vitreous detachments are also common. Additional findings include retinal hemorrhages, cystoid macular edema, optic disc edema, or optic atrophy. Chronic complications are associated with a poor visual prognosis and include branch vein occlusion, central vessel occlusion, macular ischemia, persistent neovascularization, vitreous hemorrhage, and tractional retinal detachment.

Pathology/Pathogenesis: Numerous studies have demonstrated the presence of CD4+ T cells within and surrounding the retinal vessels in patients with RV. Thus, cell-mediated immunity appears to play a major role in the pathogenesis of the disorder. However, humoral immunity and immune complex formation may also participate in the immunopathogenesis.

Diagnosis: A diagnostic evaluation should be performed on all patients with RV to search for an underlying cause of the disease and to guide the choice of therapy. Infectious causes of RV should be differentiated from non-infectious etiologies. Evaluation of suspected infectious RV may include ocular and/or systemic cultures, serologic tests, polymerase chain reaction (PCR), and tuberculin skin testing among others. In patients with suspected noninfectious systemic diseases, the diagnostic evaluation typically focuses on the collagen vascular diseases and systemic vasculitis syndromes. Human leukocyte antigen (HLA) testing is another useful technique for diseases such as birdshot retinochoroidopathy or Adamantiades-Behcet's disease. Imaging studies (CT and /or MRI scans) may also be beneficial in selected patients.

Fluorescein angiogram (FA): FA is especially helpful in cases of RV. Diffuse capillary leakage is a common finding in these patients. Macular ischemia is important to recognize, particularly in patients whose visual acuity fails to improve despite aggressive therapy. Late staining of vessels may be seen in two-thirds of patients. Neovascularization, secondary to inflammatory mediators rather than of retinal ischemia, develops in 15% of patients with idiopathic RV.

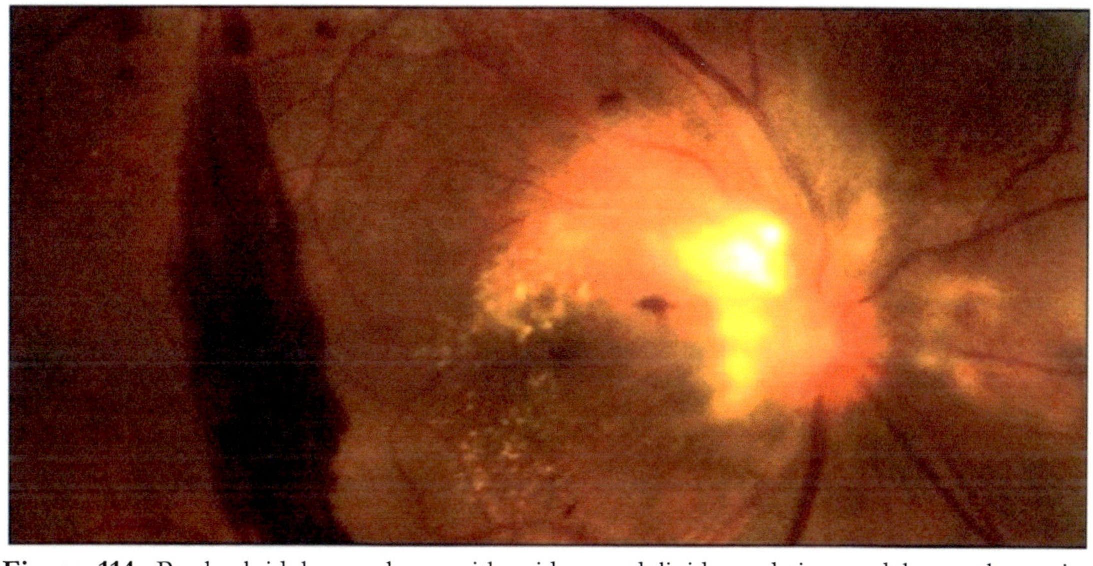

Figure 114: Pre-hyaloid hemorrhage with widespread lipid exudation and hemorrhages in patient with retinal vasculitis.

Treatment: Identification of any underlying systemic condition is crucial to control life-threatening complications of systemic diseases. Therapy may not be required for some patients with mild RV and good visual acuity. For most patients with non-infectious RV, initial therapy consists of systemic corticosteroids. However, some cases of RV may be unresponsive or inadequately controlled by these drugs. Additionally, some patients may experience intolerable side effects associated with systemic corticosteroids. Cyclosporine A, tacrolimus, methotrexate, azathioprine, mycophenolate mofetil, cyclophosphamide, or chlorambucil have all been used as steroid-sparing therapy. More recent medical options include tumor necrosis factor-alpha blockers and other biologic response modifiers. Laser photocoagulation is mainly indicated for neovascularization secondary to retinal ischemia. Pars plana vitrectomy may be beneficial in cases of recurrent vitreous hemorrhage, which often lead to proliferative vitreoretinopathy.

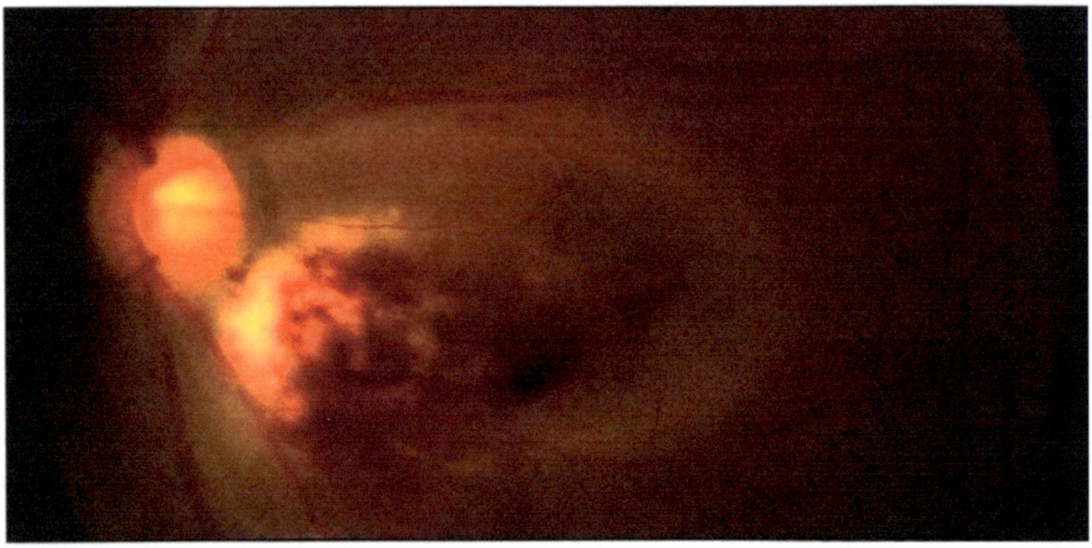

Figure 115: Idiopathic retinal vasculitis with retinal hemorrhaging and edema in papillomacular bundle. Improvement of visual acuity was attained with chlorambucil therapy.

References:

1) Ayliffe W. Retinal vasculitis; in: Foster CS, Vitale AT. *Diagnosis and treatment of uveitis*. Saunders. Philadelphia 2002:822-43.
2) Abu El-Asrar AM, Herbort CP, Tabbara KF. Retinal vasculitis.*Ocul Immunol Inflamm.* 2005 Dec;13(6):415-33.

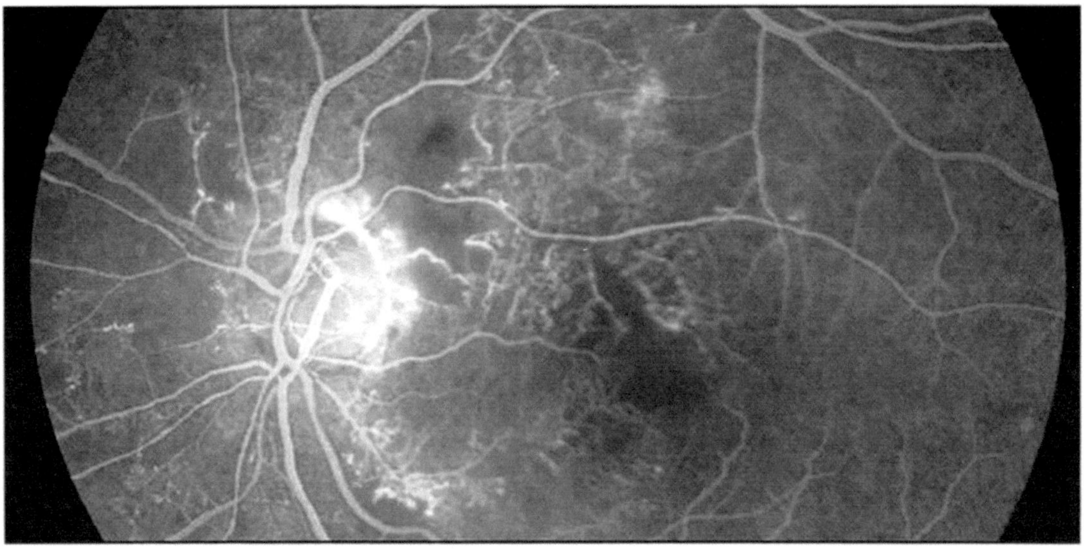

Figure 116: Retinal vasculitis and extensive capillary dropout secondary to radiation retinopathy.

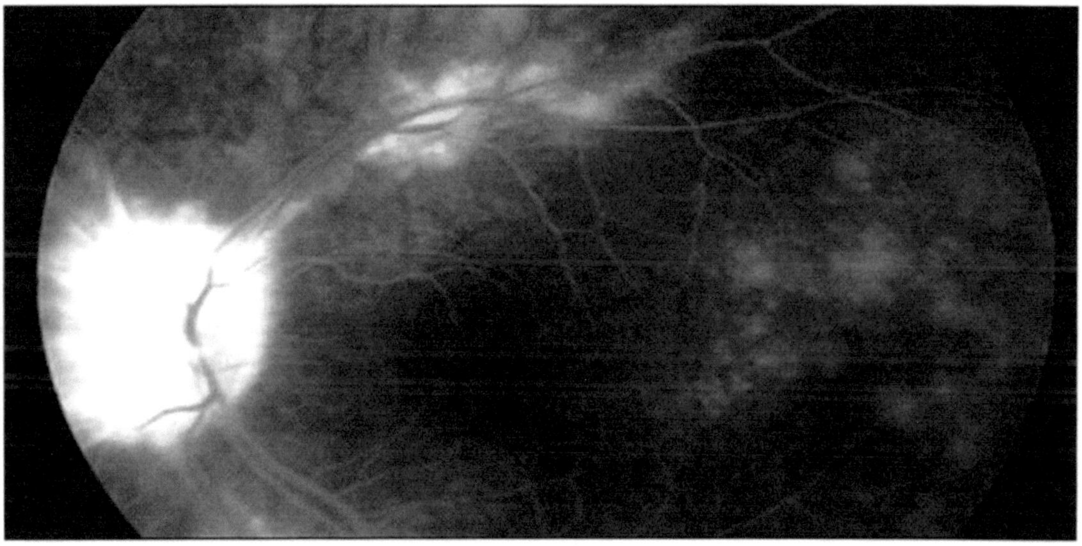

Figure 117: Papillitis in a patient with diffuse retinal vasculitis.

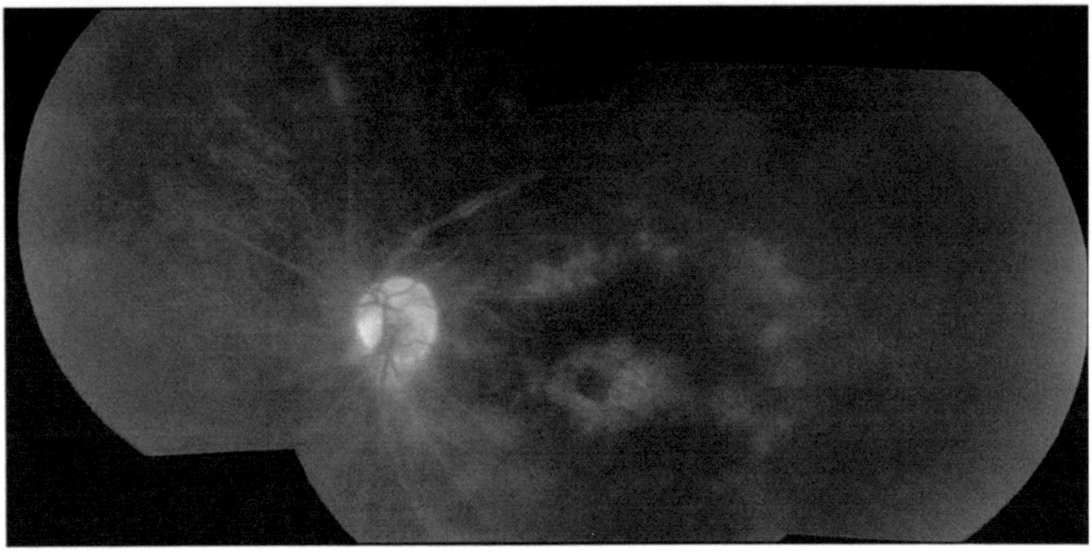

Figure 118: Retinal Vasculitis with diffuse cystoid macular edema. Note the focal phlebitis along the superior arcade.

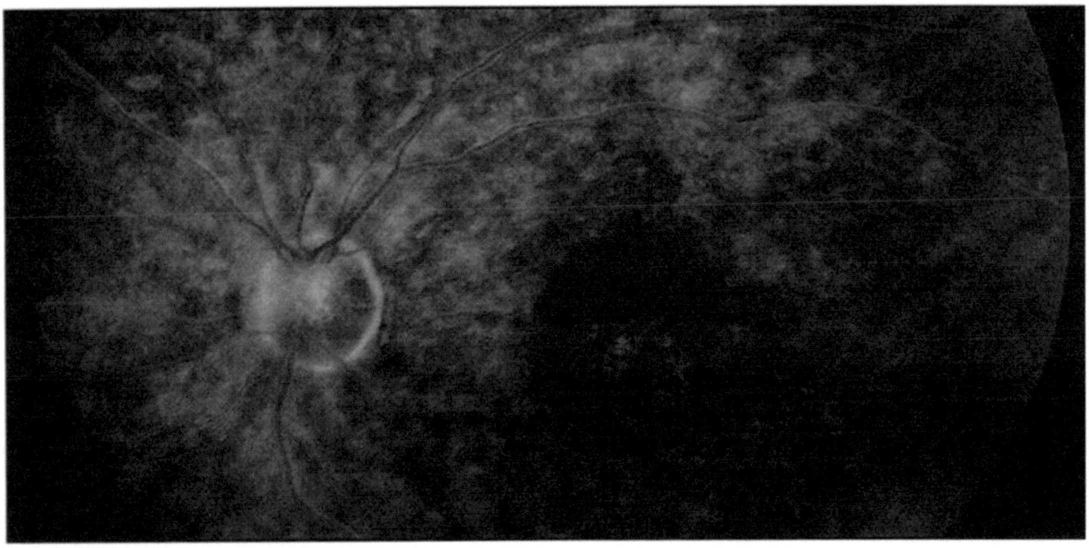

Figure 119: Ischemic maculopathy in a patient with retinal vasculitis.

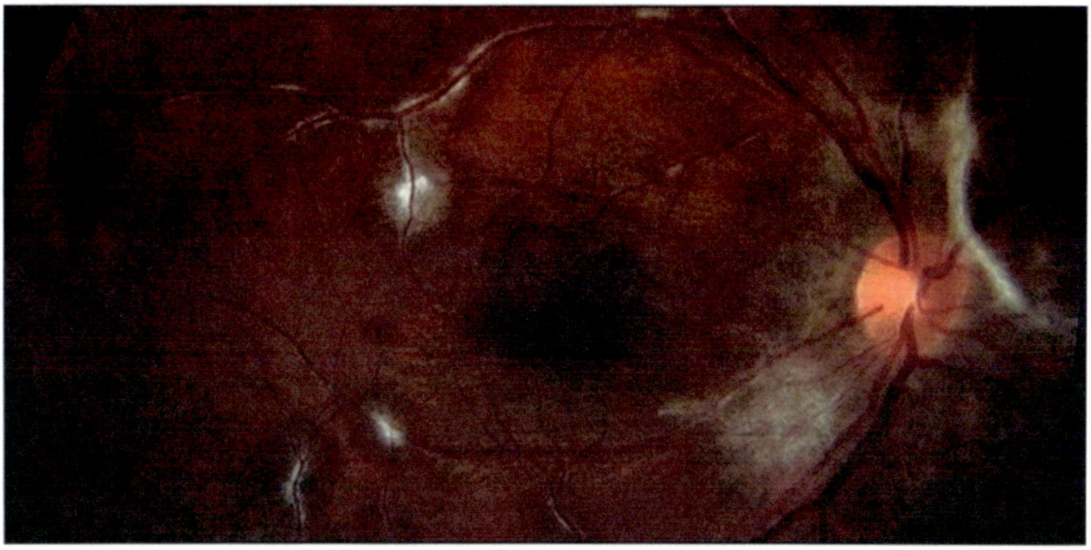

Figure 120: Sheathing of the retinal vessels seen as fluffy white cuffing in an eye affected by idiopathic retinal vasculitis. Note the abundant fibrotic tissue formation around the optic disc, and the epiretinal membrane affecting the macula.

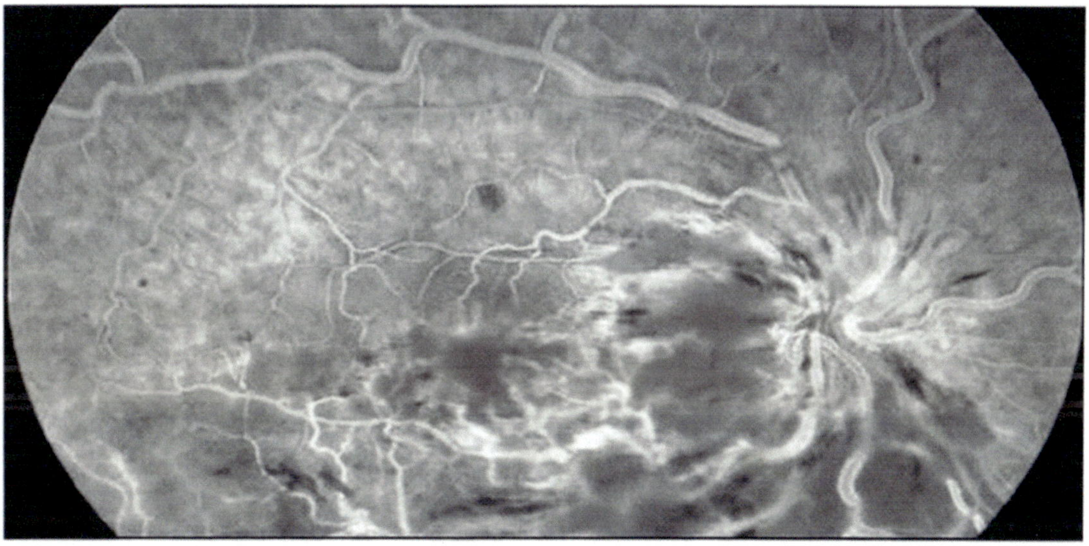

Figure 121: Retinal vasculitis with splinter hemorrhages and diffuse exudates as seen on fluorescein angiography.

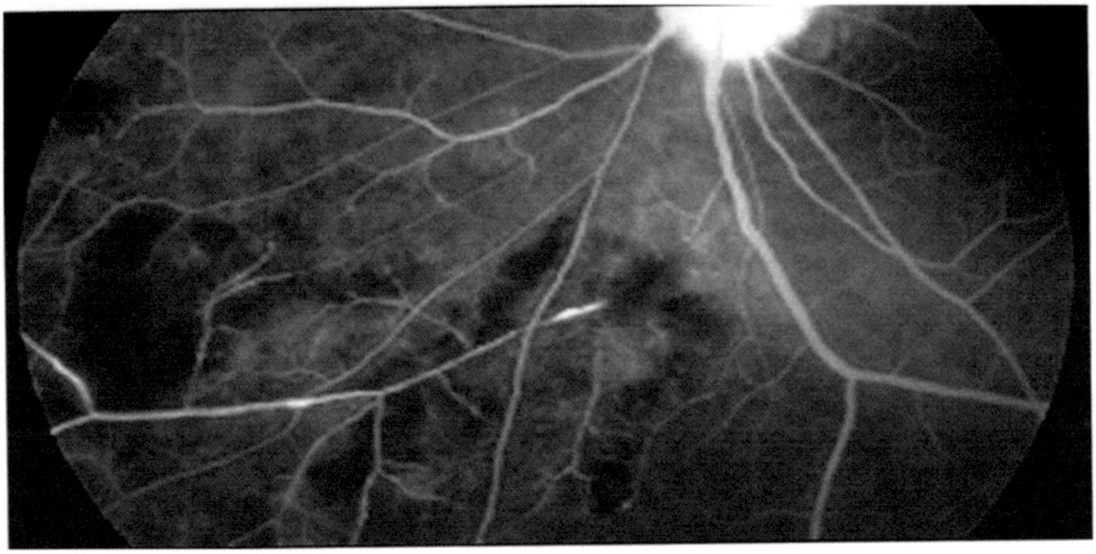

Figure 122: Hypofluorescencent areas due to blockage (secondary to retinal hemorrhages) in an eye affected by retinal vasculitis. Note the "skip lesions" of the retinal vessel in the affected area.

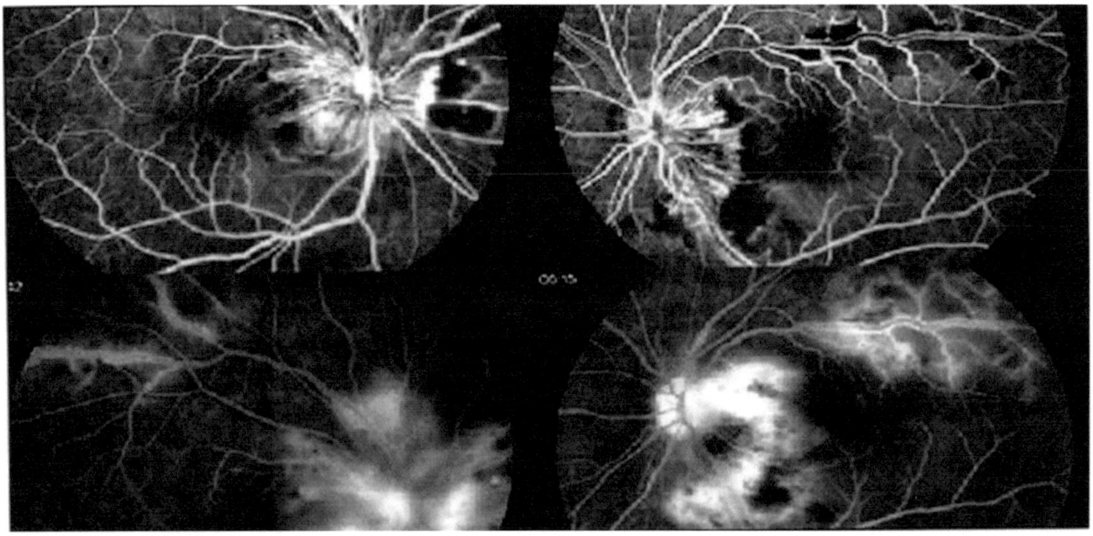

Figure 123: Vasculitis along the superior vein and stemming from the optic nerve with fluorescein blockage by hemorrhages in both eyes. Note the increased leakage in the later phases of the fluorescein angiogram.

Rheumatoid Arthritis

Definition: Rheumatoid arthritis (RA) is a chronic multisystemic disease of unknown etiology. The characteristic feature of RA is persistent inflammatory synovitis, usually involving peripheral joints with symmetric distribution. The subsequent changes in joint integrity are the hallmark of the disease.

Epidemiology: The prevalence of RA is approximately 1% of the population, with a female: male ratio of 3:1. The prevalence increases with age. RA is seen throughout the world and affects all races. Seventy-percent of the patients with classic or definite RA express the HLA DR4 or HLA DR1 antigen or both. Additional HLA-DR alleles may convey susceptibility to RA, including DR5, DR2, DR3, and DR7.

Pathogenesis: It has been suggested that RA might be a manifestation of the response to an infectious agent in a genetically susceptible host. Another possibility is that the infecting microorganism might prime the host to cross-reactive determinants expressed within the joint as a result of "molecular mimicry." Of all the potential environmental triggers, the only one clearly associated with the development of RA is cigarette smoking.

Clinical Features:

Systemic Manifestations: The onset of RA is insidious; only 10% experience an abrupt onset. The arthritis is classically a symmetric, deforming polyarthritis. Typically, the small joints of hands, especially proximal interphalangeal joints and feet are involved. The arthritis is characterized by morning stiffness that improves with exercise during the day. X-ray shows erosions of bone at the joint margin. Joint destruction appears as a consequence of uncontrolled disease. The most common extra-articular lesions are rheumatoid nodules. The main pulmonary manifestations are: pleurisy, pulmonary effusions, pleural nodules, pulmonary nodules, and interstitial fibrosis. Cardiac involvement includes pericarditis, which may be detected in as many as 50% of patients with RA at autopsy. Vascular complication can also be also present. The common presentation of RA arteritis is a polyneuropathy, particularly with lower extremity anesthesia or hypoesthesia, or as poorly healing leg ulcers. Visceral ischemia may also be manifestations of rheumatoid vasculitis. Chronic leg ulcers with recurrent infection and hyperpigmentation of the skin are also characteristic features.

Ocular Manifestations: Ocular complications occur less frequently. Keratoconjunctivitis sicca (secondary Sjogren's syndrome), scleritis, and corneal melts are the most frequent. Sclera' inflammation can be classified as episcleritis or scleritis. Scleromalacia perforans may be seen with long-standing RA. Anterior scleritis is most common. A large cohort showed that approximately 1% of patients with RA had scleral disease. Of patients with scleritis, 10% to 33% have RA. Scleritis is associated with rheumatoid vasculitis and systemic (often occult) mild disease activity; 14% of patients with rheumatoid vasculitis have scleritis. Necrotizing scleritis is a poor systemic prognosis sign due to its association with vasculitis. Patients with RA can develop peripheral ulcerative keratitis associated with corneal melting; this may be necrotizing in nature. Peripheral ulcerative keratitis requires prompt aggressive medical therapy with systemic corticosteroids and immunomodulatory therapy.

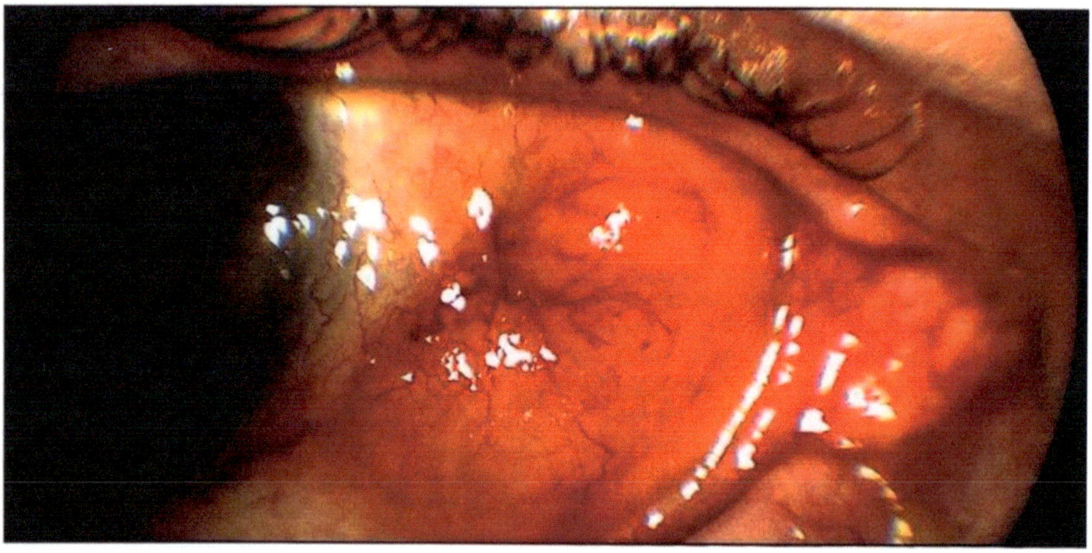

Figure 124: Vascularized and elevated scleral nodule in a patient with rheumatoid arthritis-associated scleritis.

Diagnosis: The diagnosis of RA is clinical. Serologic testing of rheumatoid factors, which are autoantibodies reactive with the Fc portion of IgG, are found in more than two-thirds of adults with the disease, may help in the diagnosis.

Treatment: The old paradigm of the base down pyramid treatment approach for RA beginning with nonsteroidal anti-inflammatory drugs (NSAID) followed by antimalarials (hydroxychloroquine), and gold has been turned upside down after evidence-based medicine evaluations outcomes disclosed, quite clearly, that aggressive immunomodulatory therapy early in the course of the disease results in considerably less damage, less overall morbidity, and superior quality of life assessments. Immunomodulatory therapy is also useful in the treatment of rheumatoid vasculitis. Low-dose prednisone, at approximately 5 to 10 mg daily or its alternate-day equivalent, is sometimes used in conjunction to increase the patient's mobility and functional capacity.

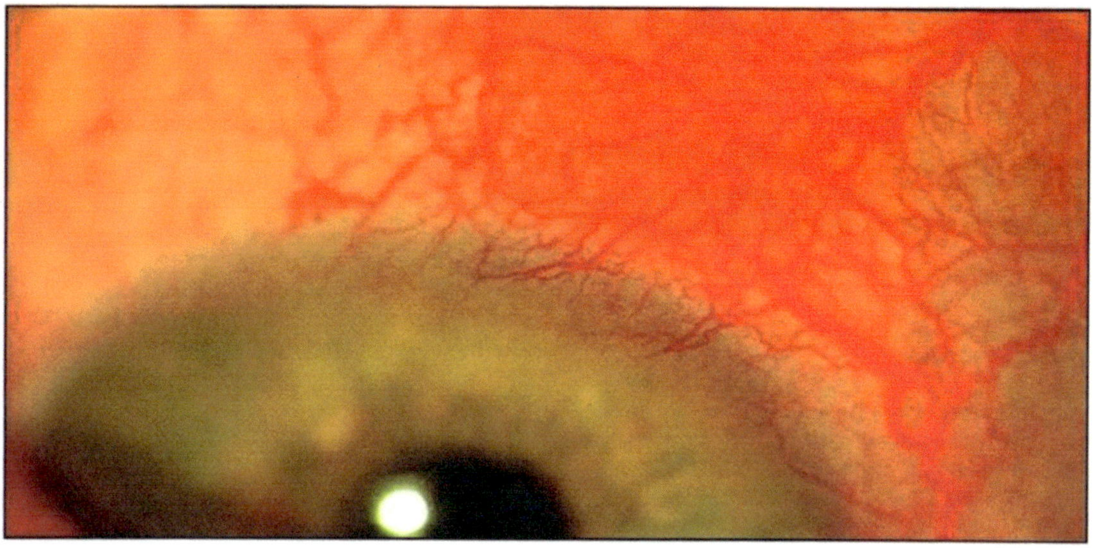

Figure 125: Sectoral scleritis secondary to rheumatoid arthritis.

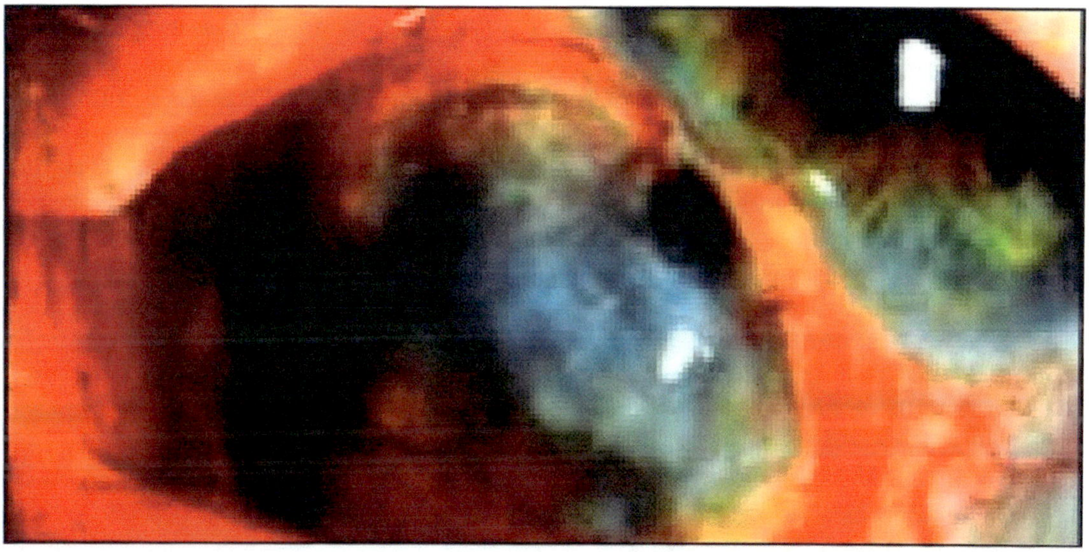

Figure 126: Active necrotizing scleritis in a patient with rheumatoid arthritis.

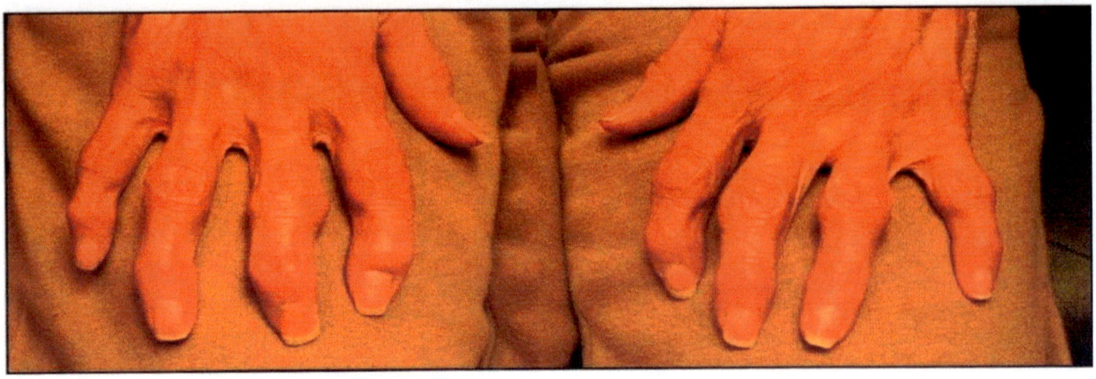

Figure 127: Hands afflicted by rheumatoid arthritis.

References:

1) Wolfe AM: The epidemiology of rheumatoid arthritis: A review. Parts I and 1I, *Bull Rheum Dis* 19:518, 1968.
2) McDermot EM, McDevitt H: The immunogenetics of rheumatic diseases. *Bull Rheum Dis* 38: 1, 1988.
3) Decker JL, Malone DG, Haraqui B et al: Rheumatoid arthritis: Evolving concepts of pathogenesis and treatment. *An Intern Med* 101: 810, 1984.
4) Harris ED: Rheumatoid arthritis: The clinical spectrum. In Kelly WN, Harris ED, Ruddy S et al (eds): *Textbook of Rheumatology*, 2nd ed, pp 915-950. Philadelphia, WB Saunders, 1985.
5) Williamson J: Incidence of eye disease in cases of connective tissue disease. *Trans Ophthalmol Soc* UK 94:742, 1974.
6) Watson PG, Hazelman BL: *The Sclera and Systemic Disorders*. Philadelphia, WB Saunders, 1976.
7) Sevel D: Necrogranulomatous keratitis. *Am J Ophthalmol* 63:250, 1967.
8) Hurd ER, Snyder WB, Ziff M: Choroidal nodules and retinal detachments in rheumatoid arthritis: Improvement in immunoglobulin levels following prednisolone and cyclophosphamide therapy. *Am J Med* 48:273, 1970.
9) Foster CS, Forstot SL, Wilson LA: Mortality rate in rheumatoid arthritis patients developing necrotizing scleritis or peripheral ulcerative keratitis. *Ophthalmology* 91:1253, 1984.
10) Williamson J: Incidence of eye disease in cases of connective tissue disease. *Trans Ophthalmol Soc* UK 94:742, 1974.
11) Scott DGI, Bacon PA, Tribe CR: Systemic rheumatoid vasculitis: A clinical and laboratory study of 50 cases. *Medicine* 60:288, 1981.
12) Sainz de la Maza M, Foster CS, Jabbur NS, Baltatzis S. Ocular characteristics and disease associations in scleritis-associated peripheral keratopathy. *Arch Ophthalmol.* 2002 Jan;120 (1):15-9.
13) Clewes AR, Dawson JK, Kaye S, Bucknall RC. Peripheral ulcerative keratitis in rheumatoid arthritis: successful use of intravenous cyclophosphamide and comparison of clinical and serological characteristics. *Ann Rheum Dis.* 2005 Jun;64(6):961-2.
14) Ducoulombier V, Solau E, Coquerelle P, Houvenagel E, Siame JL, Desprez X, Fauquert P, Guyot MH, Delcambre B, Flipo RM. Long-term results of infliximab therapy in rheumatoid arthritis: Experience acquired by the North-Pas-de-Calais hospital network. *Joint Bone Spine.* 2006 Nov 13.
15) Genta MS, Genta RM, Gabay C. Systemic rheumatoid vasculitis: a review. *Semin Arthritis Rheum.* 2006 Oct;36(2):88-98.
16) Ruddy S: The management of rheumatoid arthritis. In Kelly WN, Harris ED, Ruddy S et al (eds): *Textbook of Rheumatology*, 2nd ed, pp 950-966. Philadelphia, WB Saunders, 1985.

Sarcoidosis

Definition: Sarcoidosis is a multisystem granulomatous disease of unknown etiology characterized by non-caseating granulomas in the involved organs. The clinical manifestations are variable and its course (which may be acute or chronic) is unpredictable.

History: This entity was first described by Hutchinson in 1878. In 1899, Boeck reported the non-caseating granulomatous inflammation as the pathological hallmark. Schaumann, in 1914, recognized the multisystemic nature of the disease.

Epidemiology: It has a worldwide prevalence, but variable incidence among different geographical regions. The disease usually affects adults between 20 and 40 years of age, and is slightly more common in women than men. It is 3 to 4 times more prevalent in US blacks than whites. Several cases of familial sarcoidosis have been described. Sarcoidosis favors non-smokers.

Clinical Features: The lung is the most frequently affected organ in patients with sarcoidosis. Lymph nodes are involved in almost all cases, especially hilar and mediastinal nodes. The majority of patients are asymptomatic. Other frequently affected organs and/or tissues are the spleen, skin and heart.

Ophthalmic involvement occurs in approximately 30% of the patients and could be the first manifestation of the disease and precede pulmonary involvement for many years.

External involvement: The lacrimal gland is frequently affected. Dry eye can occur with or without palpable lacrimal gland enlargement. The nasolacrimal drainage system may also become involved. Orbital, lid and extraocular muscle involvement may also occur.

Anterior segment: Anterior segment involvement is the most common ocular manifestation. It is usually granulomatous and chronic in nature. Conjunctivitis (with the classic solitary, yellow, "millet-seed" nodules which may be difficult to differentiate from the classic lymphoid follicles) is also common. Iris nodules are frequently associated with anterior uveitis (especially with exacerbations). Other findings are posterior synechiae, cataract, band keratopathy, and scleritis.

Posterior segment: Vitritis is the most common manifestation of ocular sarcoidosis involving the posterior segment. Uveitis, when related to sarcoidosis, may be anterior (the most common), intermediate, panuveitis, and posterior uveitis (the least common). Retinal vasculitis and optic nerve involvement are also common. Periphlebitis is a hallmark of sarcoidosis (although not pathognomonic), and may be associated with yellow perivenous exudates ("taches de bougie" or candle wax drippings). Other manifestations include choroidal nodules, cystoid macular edema, and exudative retinal detachment.

Pathology/Pathogenesis: Non-necrotizing (non-caseating) granulomas (with histiocytes, epithelioid cells, and multinucleated giant cells making up the center of the granuloma, surrounded by lymphocytes, plasma cells, and fibroblasts in the periphery) are the hallmark. Sarcoidosis represents a unique type of autoimmune disease, in which a monocyte-associated autoantigen is attacked by cell-mediated immune mechanisms, with CD4+ lymphocytes as the main supporters of the inflammatory reaction.

Diagnosis: Definitive diagnosis requires histologic confirmation. The evaluation is as follows:

- Chest radiograph, serum angiotensin converting enzyme (ACE) determination, lysozyme, serum and urine calcium, and liver enzymes. Biopsy of clinically suspicious, easily accessible tissue (for example, conjunctiva), may be helpful.
- If these are negative, but suspicion persists, chest CT and whole body 67Ga scans, and pulmonary function tests should be done. If they support the diagnosis, bronchoalveolar lavage and transbronchial lung biopsy can be pursued. Open lung biopsy is indicated if there is clinical and radiographic evidence with no histological confirmation.

Treatment: Given the severity of ocular complications in many patients with ocular sarcoidosis when inflammation persists and/or recurs, prompt and aggressive therapeutic intervention is mandatory. Anterior uveitis should be initially managed with topical steroids and mydriatics. Systemic steroids are indicated in anterior uveitis that does not respond to topical therapy, and in patients with posterior uveitis, neovascularization, or orbital disease with visual symptoms or optic nerve involvement. If inflammation persists, other immunomodulatory agents may be required. Successful results have been reported with azathioprine, cyclosporine, methotrexate, and cyclophosphamide. Cataract formation due to persisting inflammation and/or steroids treatment is common, and, surgery is frequently needed. Secondary glaucoma not responding to medical treatment often requires drainage devices or trabeculectomy using topical antimetabolites.

References:

1) Stavrou P, Foster CS. Sarcoidosis; in: *Diagnosis and treatment of uveitis*. Saunders. Philadelphia 2002:710-25.
2) Bonfioli AA, Orefice F. Sarcoidosis. *Semin Ophthalmol.* 2005;20(3):177-82.
3) Baughman RP, Lower EE. Novel therapies for sarcoidosis. *Semin Respir Crit Care Med.* 2007 Feb;28(1):128-33.

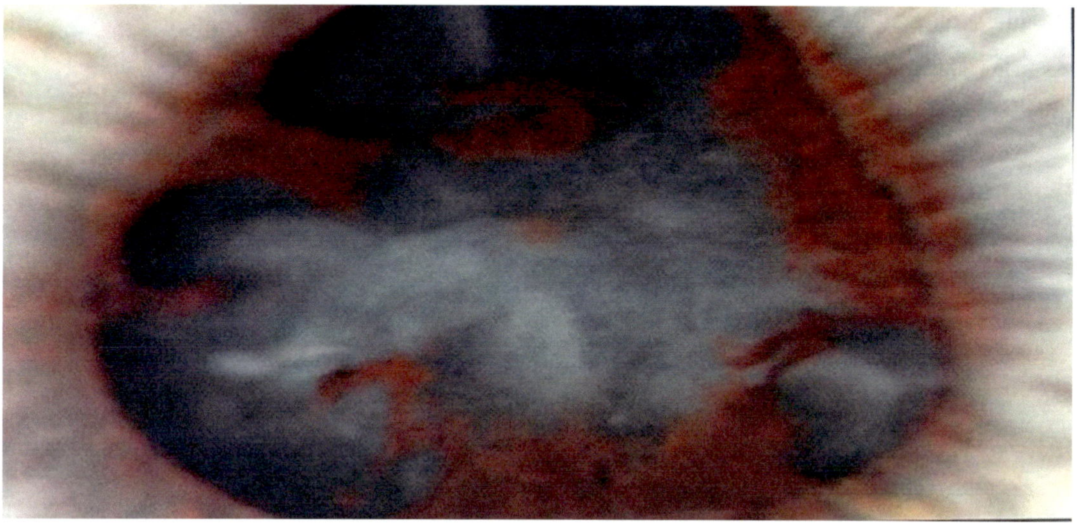

Figure 128: Pigment on anterior lens and affected by sarcoidosis.

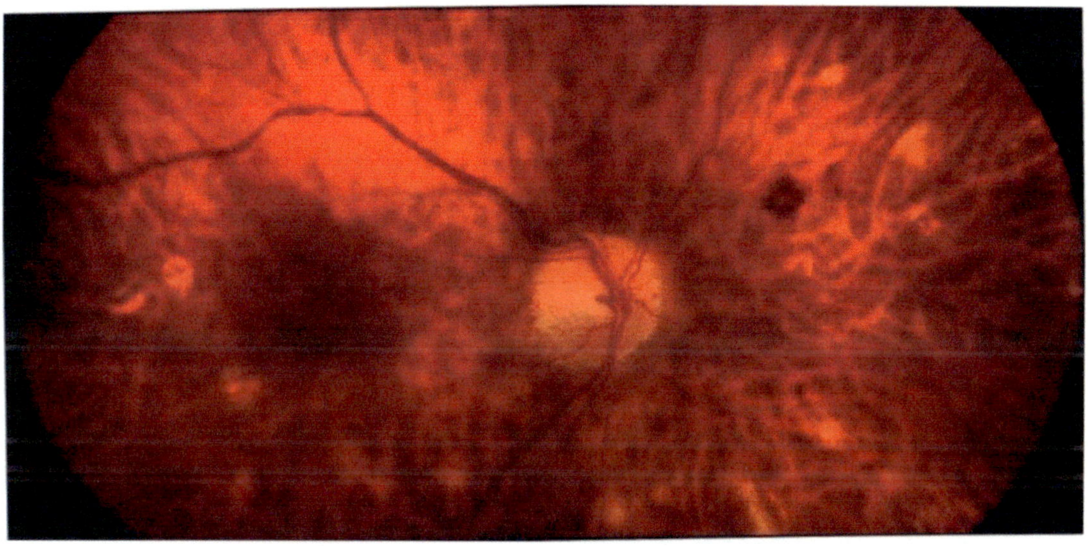

Figure 129: Fundus photograph of the right eye reveals the existence of multifocal chorioretinal scars in a "punched-out" appearance.

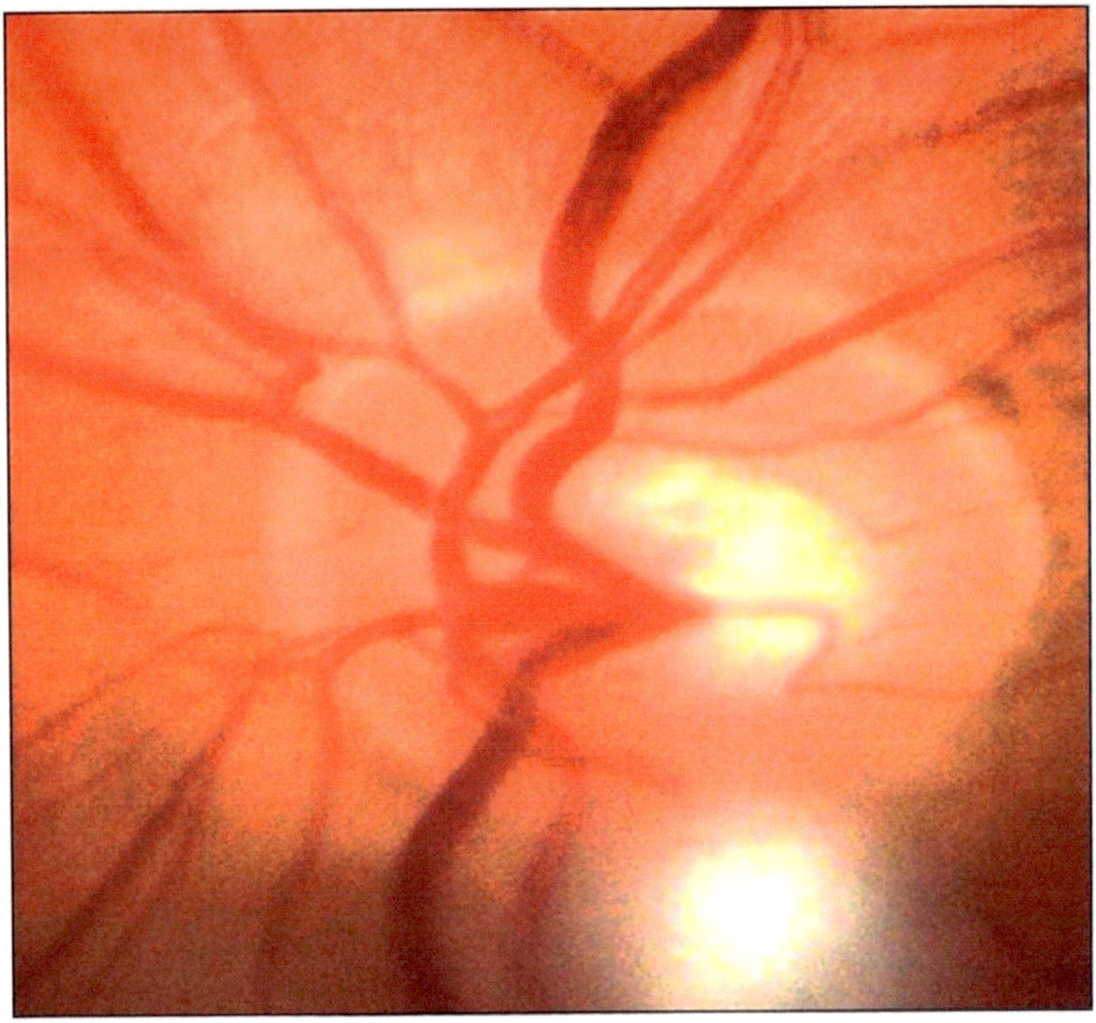

Figure 150: Juxtapapillary granuloma in a patient with ocular sarcoidosis.

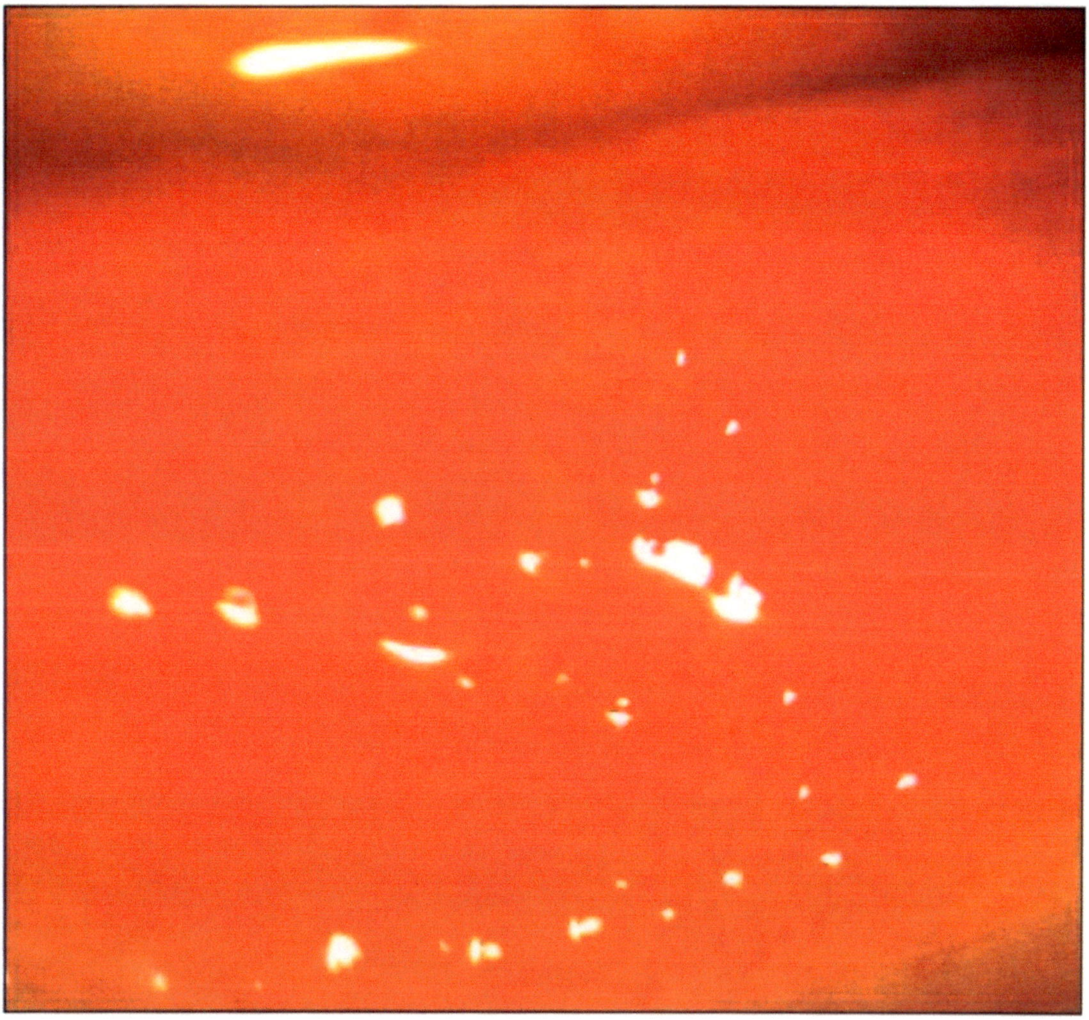

Figure 131: Follicular conjunctivitis in a patient with ocular sarcoidosis.

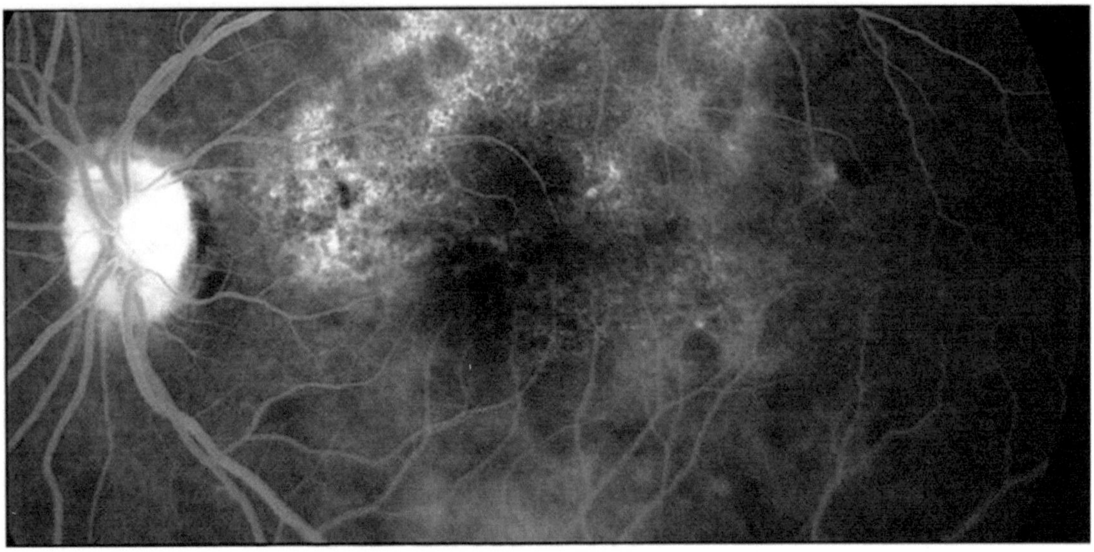

Figure 132: During the mid-phase of the FA, note the diffuse RPE scarring and cellophane maculopathy in an African-American female affected by ocular sarcoidosis.

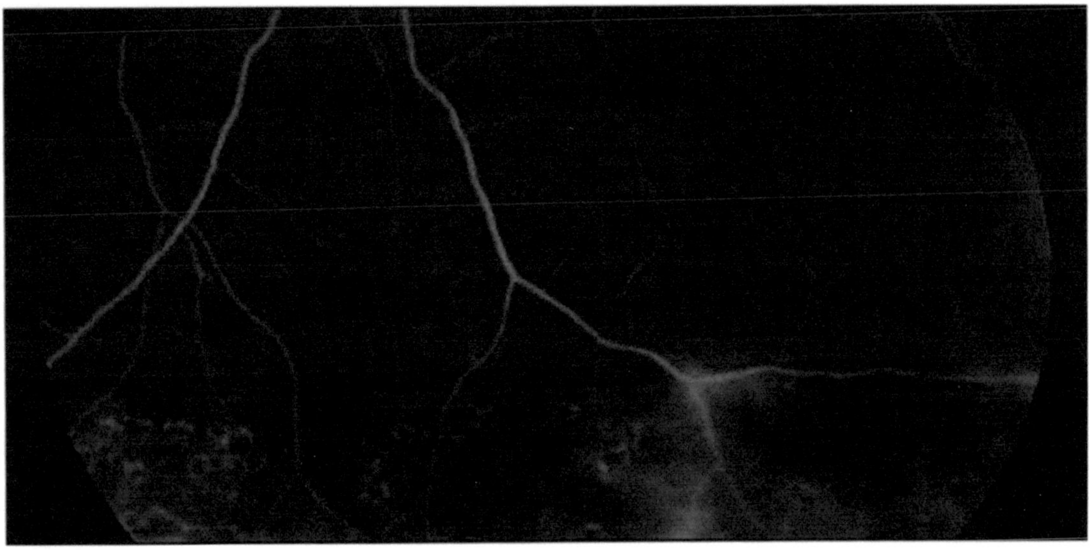

Figure 133: Fluorescein angiography of a 27 year-old African-American female affected by ocular sarcoidosis. This photo demonstrates signs of focal active vasculitis with dye leakage at the edge of the panretinal photocoagulation.

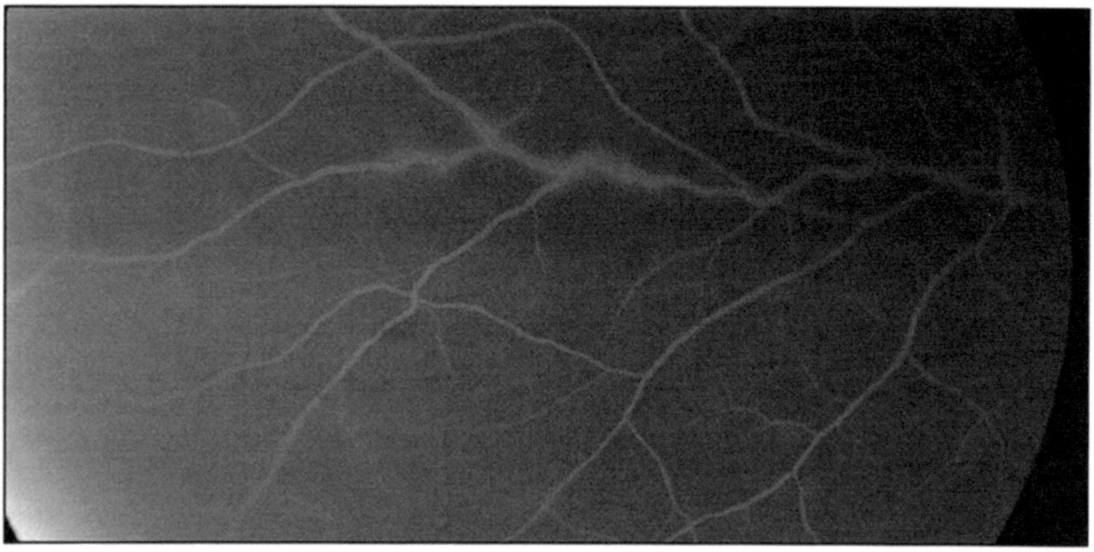

Figure 134: FA showing retinal vascular staining and deformation of a retinal vessel secondary to inflammation in the temporal periphery.

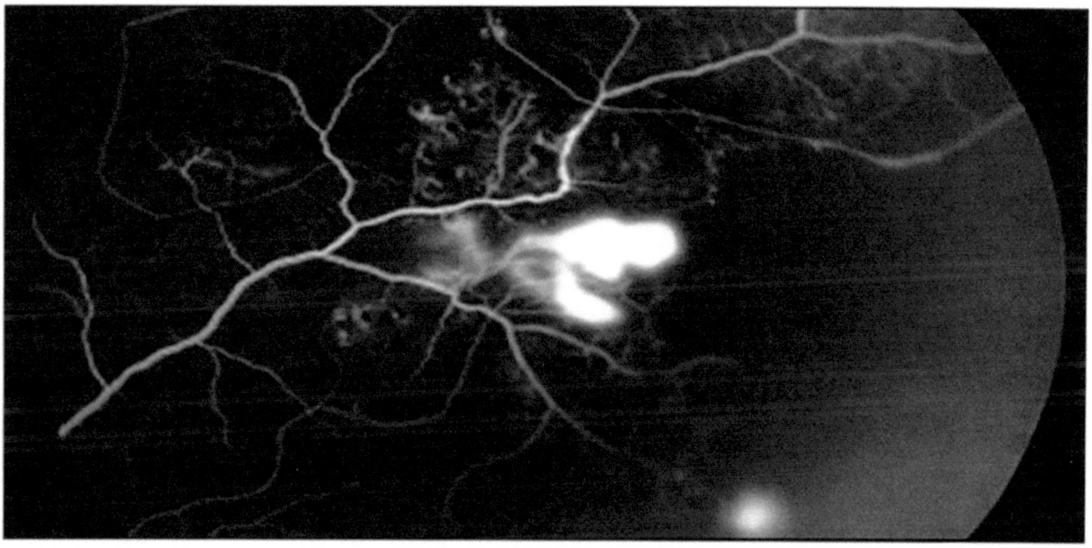

Figure 135: Peripheral retinal neovascularization and capillary dropout secondary to recalcitrant sarcoidosis-related inflammation during the early phase of the angiographic study.

Sclerodema

Definition: Scleroderma is a multisystem connective tissue disease characterized by disturbances in the microvasculature, prominent inflammatory and immunologic alterations, and excessive deposition of intracellular matrices (including collagen) in the skin and internal organs (lungs, kidneys, and gastrointestinal tract.) Scleroderma exists in two forms: (1) Localized scleroderma (morphea) which comprises a group of distinct conditions that involve the skin and subcutaneous tissue, characterized by thickening and fibrosis with a variety of extracutaneous features, and (2) Systemic sclerosis, with visceral involvement.

History: Gintrac introduced the term scleroderma in 1847 (skleros-hard, derma-skin), emphasizing that the skin was the most obvious organ involved. Raynaud documented the association between scleroderma and abnormal vasoconstriction years later, and subsequently, other associations were observed and reported. Mayes introduced the current classification of the disease at the end of the last century.

Epidemiology: Scleroderma is a rare disease with a prevalence of 240 cases per million and an incidence of approximately 19 cases per million. Disease onset is higher between ages 30 and 50 years, and more women than men are affected. Diffuse disease is more frequent than the limited form in black patients. The disease has a worldwide distribution, although it is less frequent in Asia.

Clinical Features:

Systemic manifestations: Preliminary criteria for the diagnosis of scleroderma (One major or two minor criteria) are:

Major criterion: Sclerodermatous skin changes proximal to the metacarpophalangeal or metatarsophalangeal joints.

Minor criteria (In the absence of proximal scleroderma): Sclerodactyly; sclerodermatous skin changes of finger or toes, digital pitting scars of fingertips or loss of substance of the distal finger pad, bibasilar pulmonary fibrosis not attributable to primary lung disease, Raynaud's phenomenon (sequential development of pallor, cyanosis, and rubor of the digits on cold exposure, emotional stress, or both) is the initial symptom in most patients. Visceral involvement may affect (in order, of frequency) gastrointestinal tract, lungs, heart, kidneys, and nervous system.

Ocular manifestations:

External involvement: Eyelids and periorbital tissue are frequently affected. Fibrotic changes involving the eyelids may lead to difficult lid eversion and blepharophimosis.

Periorbital edema is also relatively common in both forms. Reduced tear secretion is a frequent feature. Orbital involvement with subsequent ocular myopathy, most notably affecting the superior rectus muscle, may also be seen.

Anterior segment: The vast majority of corneal findings result from keratoconjunctivitis sicca (KCS). Subepithelial fibrosis with associated conjunctival fornix foreshortening is common.

Posterior segment: Abnormalities of the choroidal vasculature are the most common finding affecting the posterior segment. These are areas of nonperfusion with damage to the choriocapillaris, microaneurysmal dilatation of the terminal venules, and atrophy of the overlying retinal pigment epithelium. Retinal vasculature is usually unaffected.

Pathology/Pathophysiology: Histopathologic features of scleroderma are influenced by the stage of the disease. In the early phase there is lymphocytic and monocytic cell infiltrate. Subsequently, an increase in collagen and other extracellular matrices are observed in the dermis and subcutaneous fat. In the atrophic phase, there is little cellular infiltrate, thinning of the epidermis, and increased collagen contraction. The etiology is unknown, but it is probably related to abnormalities of the vascular endothelium, and of both the immune and connective tissue systems.

Diagnosis: Diagnosis is clinical, based on criteria established by the American Rheumatism Association. Determination of choroidal vasculature abnormalities usually requires fluorescein and/or indocyanine green angiography.

Treatment: The two main modalities at present are organ-specific therapy (oriented to diminish symptoms caused by the disease) and disease-modifying agents to halt the fibrotic and inflammatory responses characteristic of scleroderma. Organ-specific treatment (emphasizing only ocular involvement management): Dry eye can be treated in the same way as in other entities using lubricating and anti-inflammatory agents in addition to temporary or permanent punctal occlusion. Topical and/or systemic corticosteroids may be helpful to manage orbital inflammation. The real hope for major advances in the care of patients with scleroderma probably lies in the area of immunomodulatory therapy. Promising results with cyclophosphamide bode well for significant improvement in the management of these patients.

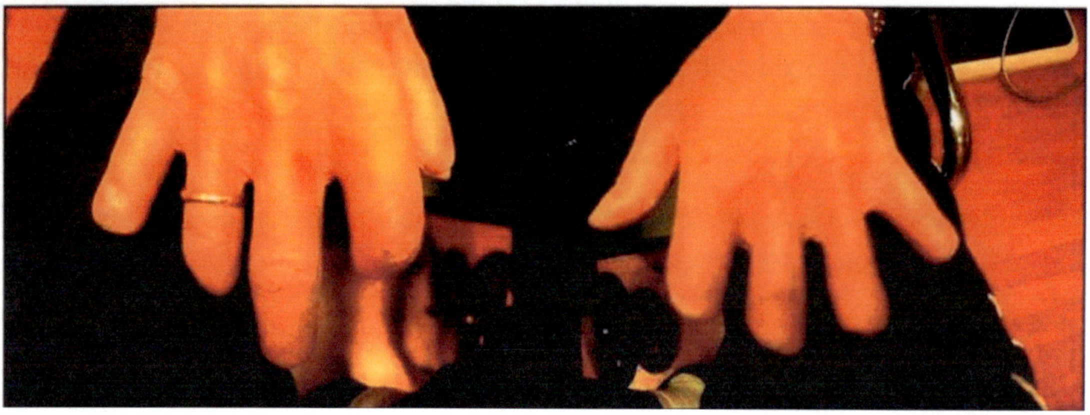

Figure 136: Digital deformity due to sclerodactyly in a patient affected by scleroderma.

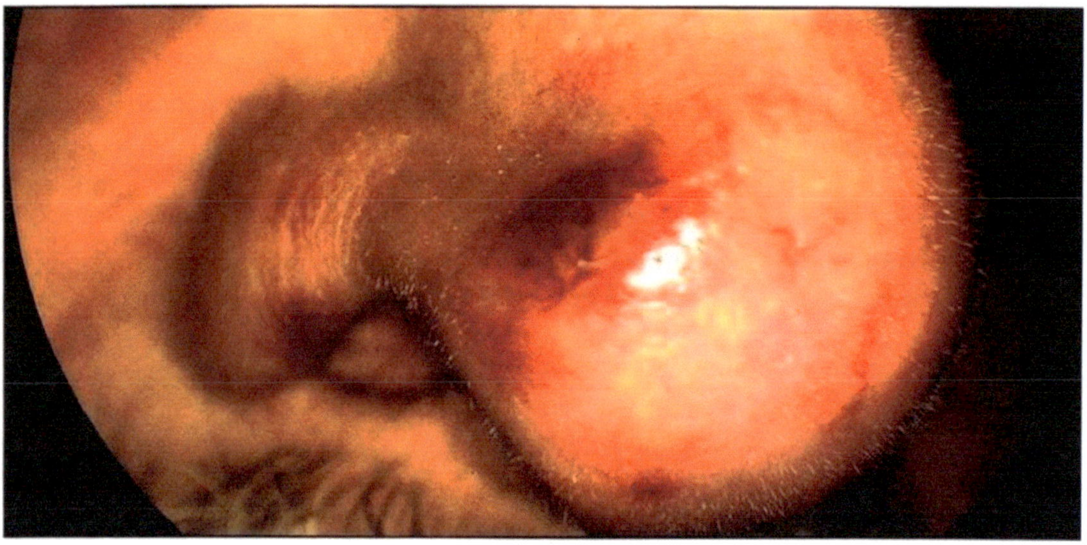

Figure 137: Red sink nodule secondary to scleroderma of the nose.

References:

1) Ekong A, Baltatzis S, Foster CS. Scleroderma; in: *Diagnosis and treatment of uveitis*. Saunders. Philadelphia 2002:610-8.
2) Chung L, Lin J, Furst DE, et al. Systemic and localized scleroderma. *Clin Dermatol.* 2006 Sep-Oct;24(5):374-92.
3) Charles C, Clements P, Furst DE. Systemic sclerosis: hypothesis-driven treatment strategies. *Lancet.* 2006; 367(9523):1683-91.

Ankylosing Spondylitis

Definition: Ankylosing spondylitis (AS) is a chronic and progressive systemic disease of unknown etiology that belongs to the group of seronegative spondyloarthropathies. It is characterized by inflammed sacroiliac joints, and ocular manifestations, most frequently anterior uveitis.

Epidemiology: Historically, AS was thought of as an entity which affected young men almost exclusively. More recent studies suggest a male-to-female ratio of 2 or 3 to 1, although there can be substantial geographic and ethnic variation. Disease onset is more frequent in the second or third decades of life. Prevalence is about 1% in the Caucasian population. Human leukocyte antigen (HLA) B27 is strongly linked to disease susceptibility, and there is a close correlation between the frequency of several subtypes of this allele in a population and the prevalence of AS.

Clinical features:

Articular manifestations: Low back pain and stiffness are the most typical presenting symptoms, along with gluteal pain (sacroiliac involvement) Peripheral arthritis may also be seen and involves hips, shoulders, and knees.

Extra-articular manifestations:

Ocular manifestations: Anterior uveitis (AU) is the most common extra-articular manifestation in AS. AU is typically unilateral, although the fellow eye is frequently affected in other attacks, and often shows prominent cellular reaction, fibrinous exudates, and posterior synechiae formation. (Figure 138). AU does not correlate with the severity of AS and AU often leads to diagnosis of the AS, especially in women. Hypopyon may be seen. Other common features are conjunctivitis and scleritis (which usually occurs after years of active disease).

Non-ocular manifestations: Aortic regurgitation, upper lobe pulmonary fibrosis, and chronic prostatitis may occur.

Pathogenesis: The etiology of AS remains unknown. Enthesitis (inflammation at the point of attachment of skeletal muscles to bone, which often causes fibrosis and calcification) is the hallmark of AS and may involve synovial or cartilaginous joints, syndesmoses, and extra-articular entheses. These lesions lead to a process of ossification in the apophyseal and sacroiliac joints as well as in the intervertebral discs.

Diagnosis: The diagnosis of AS is mainly based on history, clinical evaluation, and radiologic confirmation. Radiographs or magnetic resonance imaging (MRI) of the affected joints show joint space narrowing, erosions with new bone formation, and synovitis. HLA-B27 typing in AS is a useful adjunct to diagnosis. The classic 'bamboo spine' appearance is seen on X ray.

Treatment: Acute episodes usually respond to short courses of topical corticosteroids and cycloplegic/mydriatic agents. Recalcitrant cases may need regional and/or systemic use of corticosteroids. Systemic NSAID maintenance therapy, may prevent or reduce the frequency of recurrences. In refractory cases, immnosuppressive agents such as methotrexate or azathioprine may prove helpful.

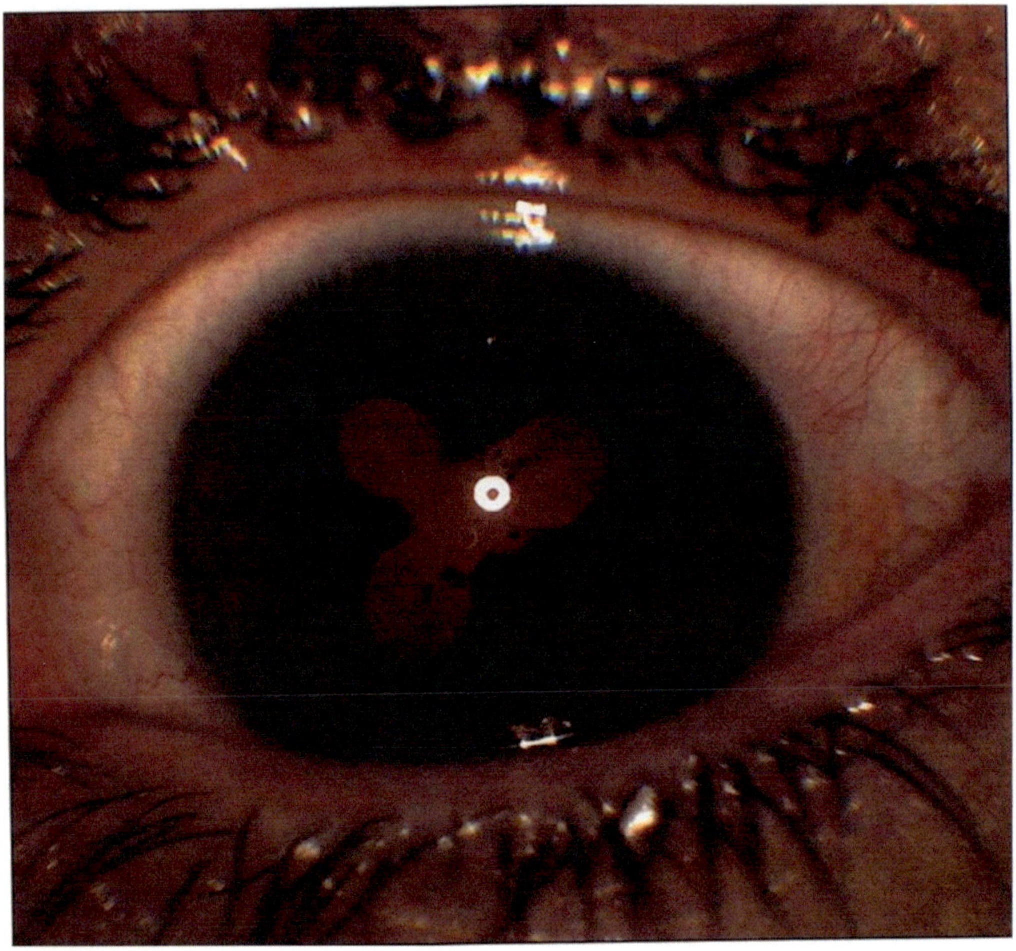

Figure 138: Posterior synechiae in an eye affected by reactive arthritis associated uveitis. Note the irregular pupil (with a clover-leaf appearance) which in a number of cases is the first sign of uveitis in these patients. Note also the diminished red reflex secondary to vitreous debris.

References:

1) Sainz de la Maza M. Seronegative Spondyloarthropathies; in: Foster CS, Vitale AT. *Diagnosis and Treatment of Uveitis*. Saunders. Philadelphia 2002.
2) Elyan M, Khan MA. Diagnosing ankylosing spondylitis. *J Rheumatol Suppl.* 2006; 78:12-23.
3) Zochling J, Braun J. Management and treatment of ankylosing spondylitis. *Curr Opin Rheumatol.* 2005; 17(4):418-25.

Inflammatory Bowel Disease

Definition: Inflammatory Bowel Disease (IBD) is divided into Ulcerative Colitis (UC) and Crohn's Disease (CD), which may affect any part of the gastrointestinal tract from the mouth to the anus.

History: The first description of ulcerative colitis was reported in 1793. Crohn described a series of patients with inflammation of the Terminal ileum in 1932.

Epidemiology: IBD may affect individuals at any age. The incidence of UC displays a bimodal distribution with peak onset at ages 15 to 30 and 50 to 70. Smoking increases the risk for CD but is protective against UC.

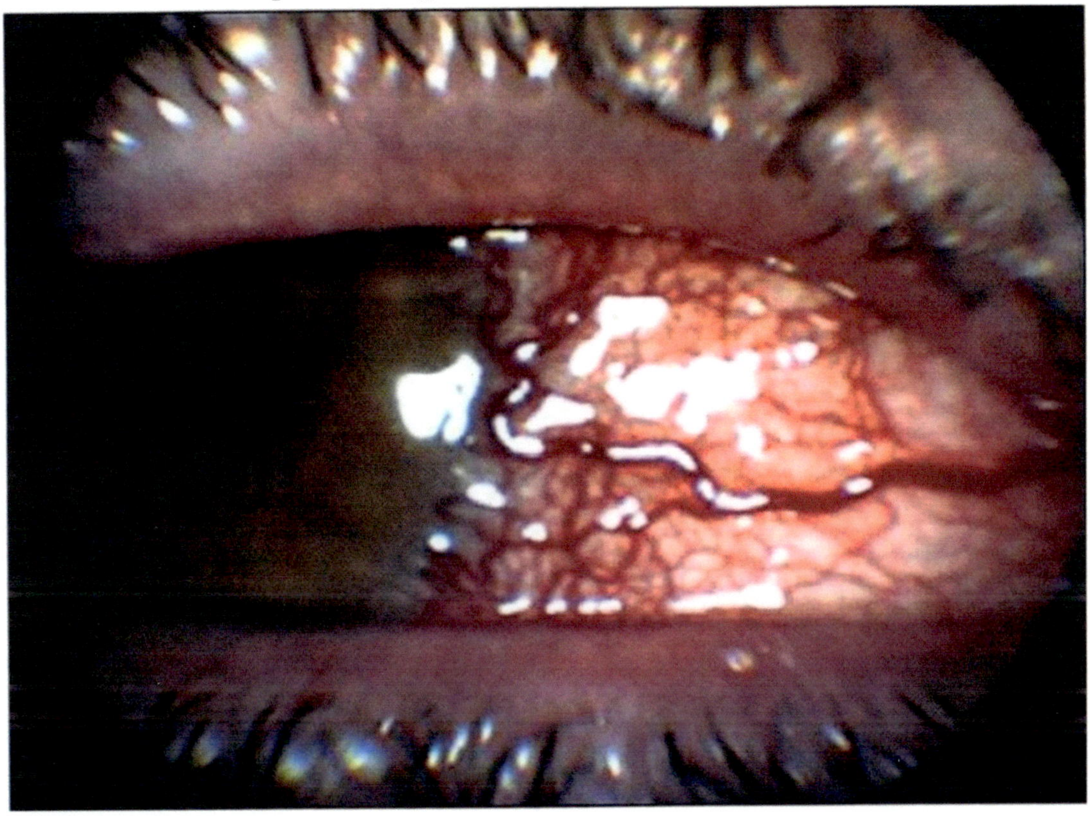

Figure 139: Inflammatory bowel disease-associated scleritis. Note the engorged, tortuous vessels.

Clinical Features:

Systemic manifestations: Abdominal pain, bloody diarrhea, constipation, nausea, emesis, anorexia, and weight loss are the most common symptoms. The prevalence of peripheral arthritis is 10% in UC and 20% in CD; sacroiliitis can occur. Erythema nodosum and pyoderma gangrenosum are associated with IBD.

Ocular manifestations: Ocular involvement occurs in 10% or less of IBD patients. Bilateral, chronic, non-granulomatous anterior uveitis is the most common manifestation. Episcleritis, scleritis, (Figure 139) and peripheral keratitis (Figure 140) are less common. Conjunctivitis and orbital involvement are rare.

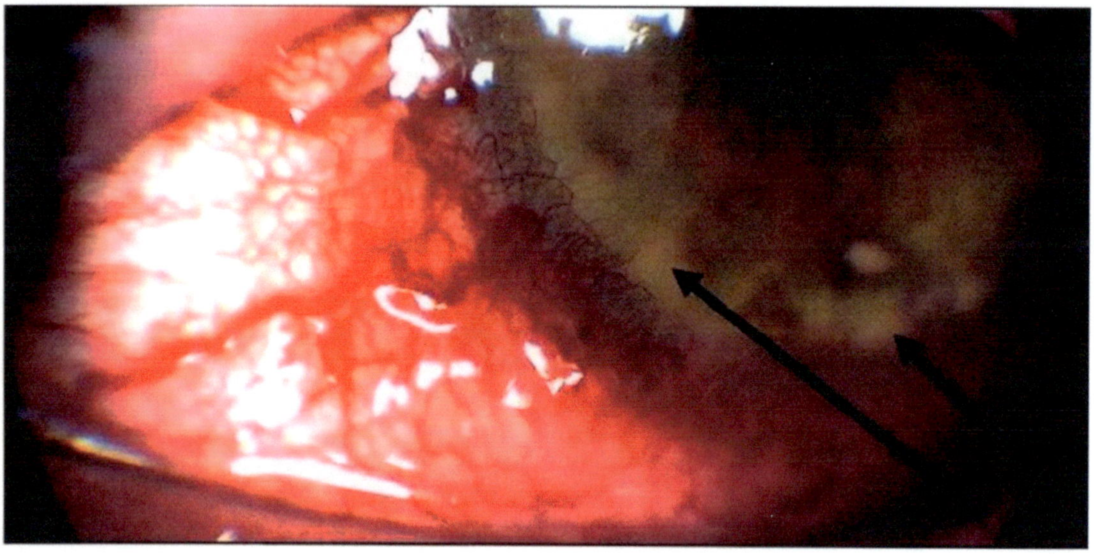

Figure 140: Peripheral areas of neovascularization, interstitial keratitis, and scleritis in a patient affected by inflammatory bowel disease.

Pathology/Pathogenesis:. The etiology is unknown. Increased gut mucosal permeability to antigens leading to abnormal immunoregulation is thought to play a role.

Diagnosis: IBD is associated with HLA-B27 in 50-70% of cases. An anti-neutrophil cytoplasmic antibody is present in 70% of UC patients. Characteristic findings on upper gastrointestinal series or barium enema support the diagnosis. Endoscopy with tissue biopsy demonstrating characteristic granulomatous inflammation in the absence of pathogenic organisms is diagnostic.

Treatment: Oral non-steroidal anti-inflammatory drugs, 5-acetyl salicylic acid products, oral corticosteroids, disease modifying anti-rheumatic drugs (DMARDs), and biologic response modifiers (BRMs) are efficacious therapies for systemic manifestations. DMARDs and BRMs are effective for steroid dependent scleritis, peripheral ulcerative keratitis (Figure 141) and chronic uveitis.

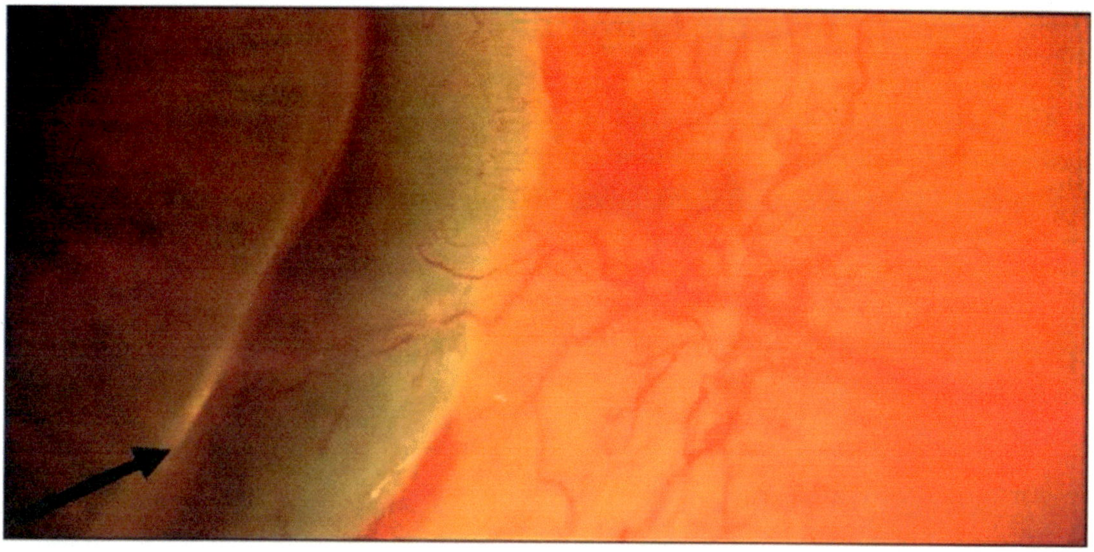

Figure 141: Peripheral ulcerative keratitis secondary to inflammatory bowel disease.

Reference:

Sainz de la Manza M. Inflammatory Bowel Disease, in: Foster CS, Vitale AT. *Diagnosis and treatment of uveitis*. Saunders. Philadelphia 2002:589-591

Juvenile idiopathic arthritis (JIA)

Definition: Juvenile idiopathic arthritis (JIA), previously called juvenile rheumatoid arthritis (JRA, is defined as persistent arthritis for more than 6 weeks with an onset at less than 16 years of age, after excluding all other causes. JIA consists of various subtypes, representing a heterogeneous group of autoimmune diseases of unknown etiology, and it is the most common rheumatic disease of childhood.

History: In 1897, G.F. Still was the first to provide the basis to establish the disease as JRA. A few years later, in 1910, Ohm gave the first report of ocular inflammation secondary to JIA.

Epidemiology: JIA has an estimated prevalence of more than 100 per 100,000 children in the United States. It affects girls predominantly (3:1). No race or geographical predisposition has been identified. The oligoarticular onset type is the most common (50%), followed by the polyarticular (40%) and the systemic (10%) onsets. Genetic factors play a role in the association between arthritis and uveitis. HLA-DR5 is associated with uveitis in children with oligoarticular JIA. Conversely, both HLA-DR1 and HLA-DR4 seem to protect from uveitis.

Clinical Features: There are 3 subtypes of JIA attending to the type of onset: Oligoarticular (previously called pauciarticular), polyarticular, and systemic.

Oligoarticular-onset JIA: It is characterized by arthritis of four or fewer joints during the first 6 months of the disease. It occurs more frequently in girls with a peak of onset at 2 years of age. Knees are the most frequently affected joints. About 75% of the patients have positive antinuclear antibodies (ANA).

Polyarticular-onset JIA: Involves 5 or more joints during the first 6 months of the disease. It occurs more frequently in girls with a peak of onset at 3 years of age. Small joints of the hand are the most commonly affected joints. 10% of the patients show positive rheumathoid factor (IgM) and 40% positive ANA.

Systemic-onset JIA: Equal frequency in boys and girls and can appear at any age. They characteristically have fever, macular rash, leukocytosis, lymphadenopathy, and hepatomegaly. Articular disease is symmetric. There is ANA positivity in 10% of the patients. Ocular manifestations: About 20% of children with oligoarticular JIA and 5% of the children with polyarticular JIA develop uveitis. Known risk factors for JIA-associated uveitis are: Female gender, young age, ANA positive, seronegativity of rheumatoid factor, and oligoarticular onset.

Ocular Manifestations:

Anterior segment: JIA-associated uveitis is usually chronic, nongranulomatous, bilateral, and often asymptomatic. Keratic precipitates (small to medium-sized, localized in the inferior half of the corneal endothelium), and posterior synechiae (with distorted pupil) are common findings. Anterior chamber reaction and associated flare is characteristic. Frequent complications are cataract, glaucoma, and band keratopathy.

Posterior segment: Vitreous inflammatory cells are commonly seen. Cyclitic membrane formation (with or without associated hypotony), cystoid macular edema, and optic disc atrophy may develop as a consequence of uncontrolled inflammation.

Diagnosis: This is mainly based on clinical examination. Some laboratory tests (especially serologic determination of ANA positivity) may also be helpful. Periodic ocular examination of children with JIA is mandatory, especially those who have known risk factors to develop uveitis.

Since JIA is a diagnosis of exclusion, it is important to be familiar with alternative diagnoses. Ocular sarcoidosis in children, seronegative spondyloarthropathy-associated anterior uveitides, herpetic uveitis, and Kawasaki disease-associated uveitis are the main diseases to consider in the differential diagnosis.

Treatment: Therapeutic options for children and adolescents with chronic arthritis are increasing dramatically. Intraarticular corticosteroid injections, together with oral non-steroidal anti-inflammatory drugs (or low-dose systemic methotrexate if not respondent to NSAIDs) are the mainstay of treatment for children with oligoarthritis. Tumor necrosis factor-alpha receptor blockers (such as infliximab and etanercept) are also promising therapies.

The mainstay of treatment for ocular inflammation consists of topical corticosteroids and cycloplegics, used in combination with previously mentioned systemic agents if the inflammation persists or recurs.

Collaboration between the ophthalmologist and rheumatologist is crucial for optimal management.

References:

1) Ravelli A, Martini A. Juvenile Idiopathic arthritis. *Lancet* 2007; 369:767-78.
2) Sainz de la Maza M. Seronegative spondyloarthropathies; in: Foster CS, Vitale AT. *Diagnosis and treatment of uveitis*. Saunders. Philadelphia 2002:581-600.

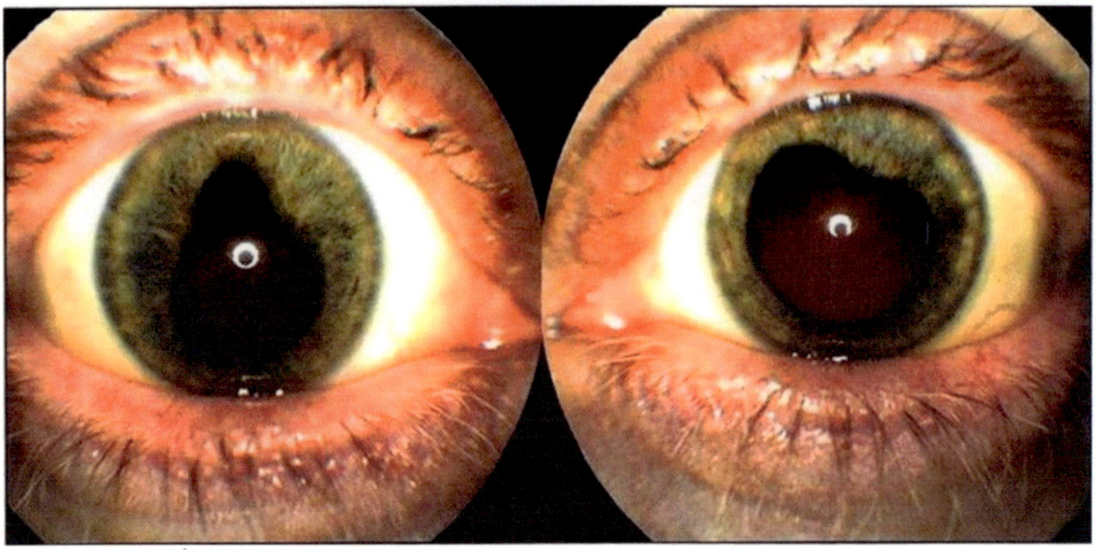

Figure 142: Bilateral posterior synechiae in JIA-associated anterior uveitis

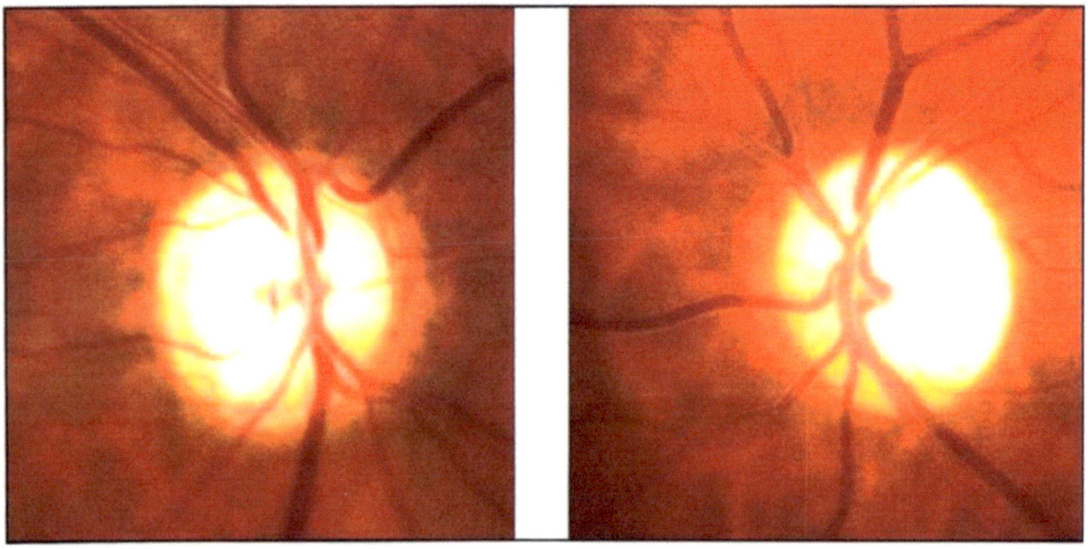

Figure 143: Bilateral, severe optic disc atrophy secondary to inflammation and glaucoma in a patient affected by JIA.

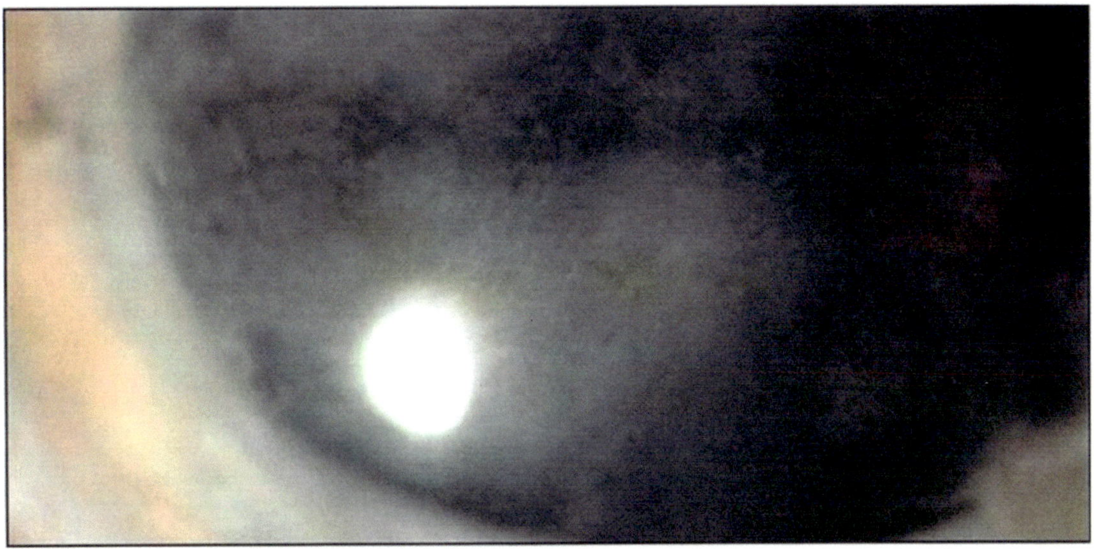

Figure 144: Band keratopathy in an aphakic eye of an eight-year-old male with JIA-associated uveitis.

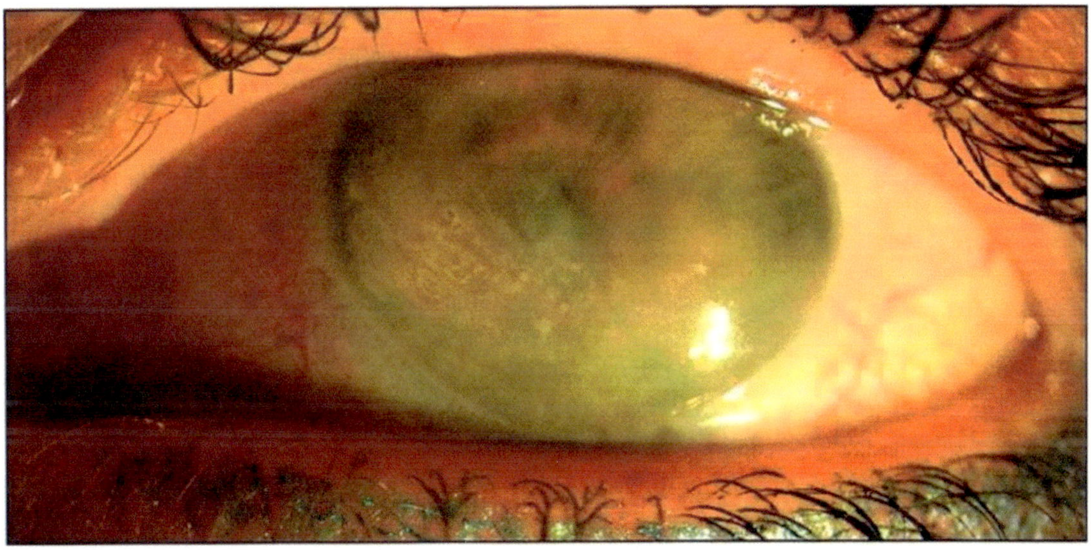

Figure 145: Pre-phthisical hypotonous eye resulting from inflammation by juvenile idiopathic arthritis-associated chronic uveitis treated solely with corticosteroids for twenty-one years.

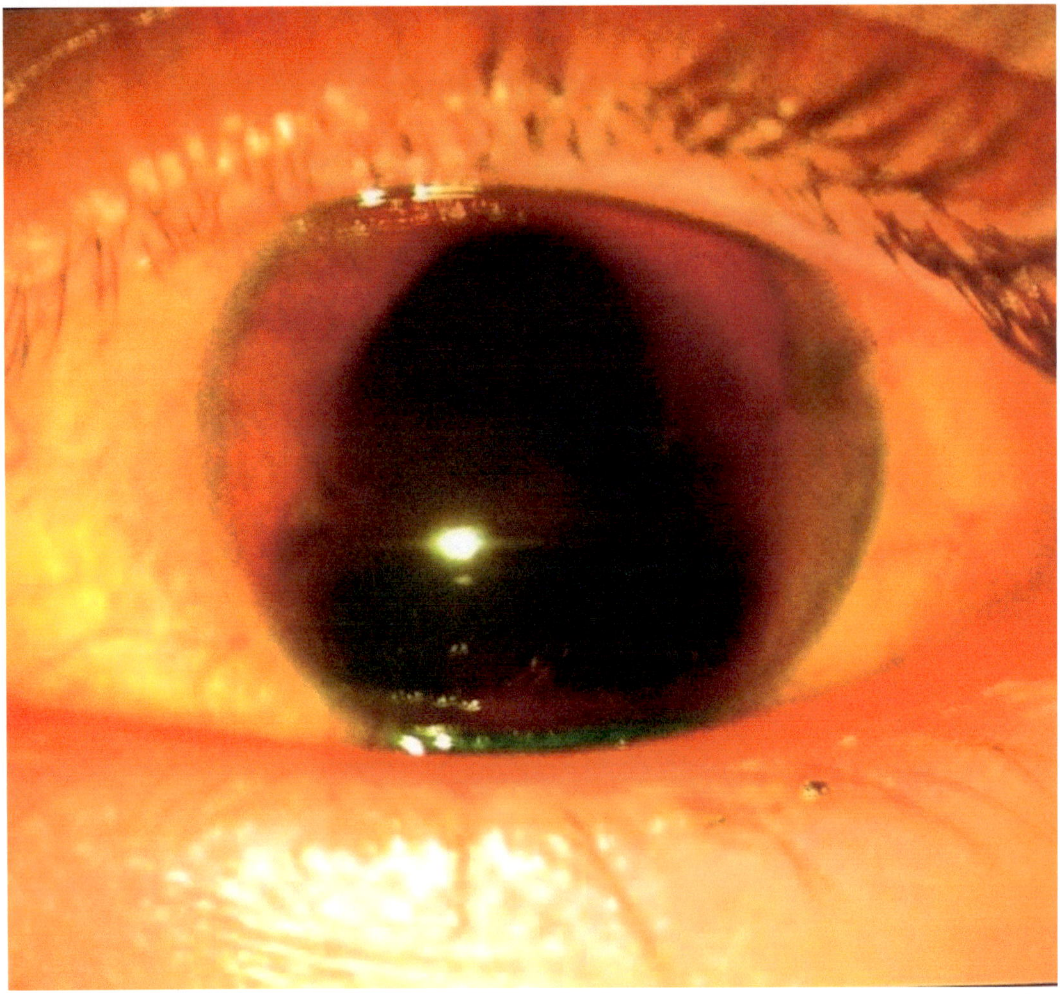

Figure 146: Rubeosis iridis secondary to recalcitrant inflammation caused by sub-optimally treated chronic juvenile idiopathic arthritis-associated uveitis

Psoriatic Arthritis

Definition: Psoriatic arthritis (PA) is a serongeative arthritis associated with psoriasis.

History: PA emerged as a clinical entity separate from rheumatoid arthritis (RA) following the discovery of the rheumatoid factor in 1948 and, years later, with the separate observations of Wright and Baker.

Epidemiology: Arthritis occurs in 2-3% of the general population, but among patients with psoriasis (which affects 1-2% of the white population), the prevalence of arthritis varies from 6% to 42%. The onset is most frequent between the 4th and 5th decades of life and there is a slight predilection for women. A positive family history is present in about one third of the cases. Both PA and psoriasis are associated with human leukocyte antigen (HLA) A2, B17, B38, B39, Cw6, and DR7a genes.

Clinical features: Although by definition all patients with PA must have psoriasis, the arthritis may precede the psoriasis by many years. The common scenario is that psoriasis has its onset about 10 years before PA. Nail lesions are very common (40% in patients with psoriasis, 85% in patients with PA) and help distinguish between patients with RA, and those with PA. They are characterized by onycholisis, pitting, ridging, and nail discoloration or fragmentation.

At least five patterns of joint involvement in PA have been described:
(1) Asymmetric monoarticular arthritis
(2) Chronic asymmetric oligoarticular arthritis
(3) Chronic symmetric polyarthritis
(4) Spondyloarthritis
(5) Arthritis mutilans

Ocular manifestations: Anterior uveitis is probably the most frequent ocular feature, occurring in 7% to 20% of patients with PA. It is usually acute, non-granulomatous, with fine endothelial keratic precipitates. This is more frequent in patients who are HLA-B27 positive or those who have the spondyloarthritis pattern of PA. Conjunctivitis associated with PA is also frequent. Other less common associated ocular manifestations are episcleritis and scleritis (usually associated with many years of active disease) and (rarely) retinal vasculitis.

Pathogenesis/Pathology: The disease mechanism remains unknown. However, a specific genetic background and some infective agents appear to play a role. The primary pathologic lesion in the arthritis of PA is a synovitis, similar to that of rheumatoid arthritis.

Diagnosis: The diagnosis is mainly based on the clinical picture: Presence of psoriasis and/or psoriatic nail changes, in addition to a seronegative arthritis, with or without spondyloarthritis. Radiologic studies demonstrate the erosive and osteolytic tendency of PA. HLA-B27 positivity, although it increases the probability of severity, it does not establish the diagnosis. Differentiating between reactive arthritis and PA may be challenging given that both diseases are associated with HLA-B27 positivity, both involve sacroiliac joint and spine, and because pustular psoriasis and keratoderma blennorrhagicum is indistinguishable both clinically and histopathologically.

Treatment: Anterior uveitis can generally be easily managed with topical corticosteroids and mydriatics/cycloplegics in a substantial proportion of cases. Refractory cases or those who show posterior segment involvement may also be treated with regional and/or systemic corticosteroid therapy; but most such cases are better served with earlier rather than later introduction of an immunomodulatory agent with or without a TNF-alpha inhibitor.

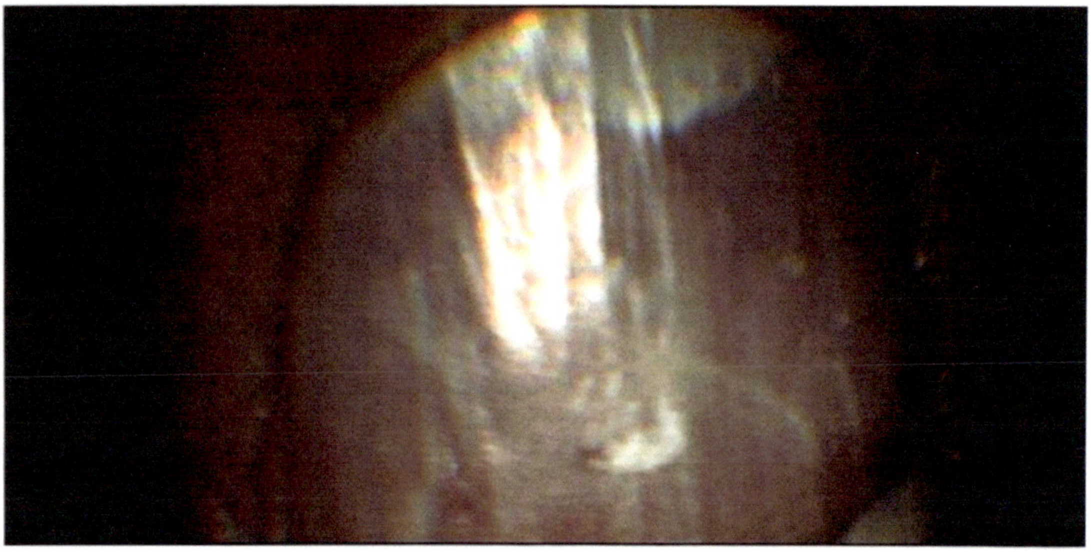

Figure 147: Nail pitting and ridging in a patient with psoriatic arthritis.

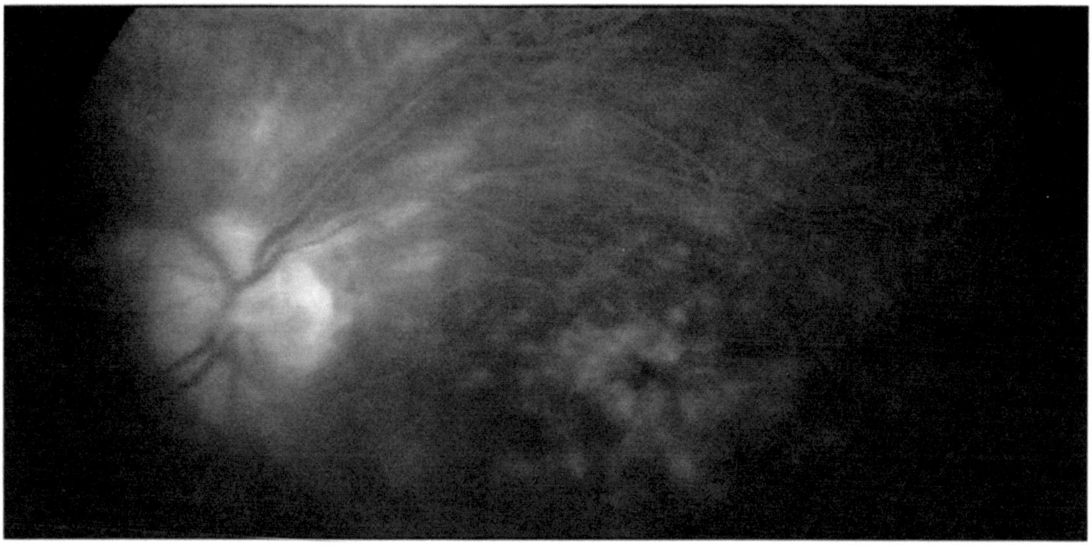

Figure 148: Late venous phase of a fluorescein angiogram in an eye affected by retinal vasculitis. Observe the petaloid pattern of hyperfluorescence due to cystoid macular edema. Diffuse capillary leakage at the optic disc is secondary to associated papillitis.

References:

1) Sainz de la Maza M. Seronegative Spondyloarthropathies; in: Foster CS, Vitale AT. *Diagnosis and Treatment of Uveitis*. Saunders. Philadelphia 2002.
2) Mease P. Psoriatic arthritis update. *Bull NYU Hosp Jt Dis*. 2006; 64(1-2):25-31.

Reactive Arthritis

Definition: Reactive Arthritis (RA) is classically defined as a clinical triad consisting of arthritis, urethritis, and conjunctivitis.

History: Stoll was most likely the first to describe the classic triad of arthritis, nongonococcal urethritis, and conjunctivitis following a dysenteric episode.

Epidemiology: RA develops in 1% to 3% of men following non-gonococcal urethritis (caused by *Chlamydia trachomatis* and others), up to 4% of individuals following enteric infections caused by *Shigella, Salmonella*, and *Campylobacter*, and in a higher proportion of patients with *Yersinia* enteric infections. RA usually affects middle-aged individuals showing a clear male predilection. However, postdysenteric RA affects both men and women equally. This syndrome is highly associated with the human leukocyte antigen B27 (HLA-B27) and is present in about 75% to 90% of the patients.

Clinical Features:

Systemic manifestations: These normally appear within one month of the inciting episode of urethritis or diarrhea. The systemic manifestations of RA may produce four syndromes:

(1) Peripheral arthritis syndrome: knees, ankles, and toes are primarily affected
(2) Enthesopathic syndrome: involves localized painful ligaments, tendons, and fascias. This includes dactylitis (sausage digits) and plantar fasciitis.
(3) Pelvic and axial syndrome: frequent in the most severely affected patients and associated with HLA-B27 positivity. This includes sacroileitis and spondylitis.
(4) Extra-articular involvement: which includes mucocutaneous, genitourinary, and ocular involvement (less common).

Ocular manifestations: Mucopurulent conjunctivitis is the most common ocular problem, occurring in approximately 58% of patients. It is usually mild and bilateral, and cultures are typically negative. Anterior uveitis is also common (although less frequent than conjunctivitis). It is usually mild, nongranulomatous, and occurs with fine to medium-sized white keratic precipitates. It is more frequent in patients who are HLA-B27+ and in those who have sacroiliitis. Scleritis (especially the diffuse and anterior type), episcleritis, and keratitis may occasionally occur. Involvement of the posterior segment is not common.

Pathogenesis: The disease mechanism is unknown. However, several hypotheses (as the molecular mimicry or the peptide presenting theories) have been formulated to explain the connection between RA and enteric or urogenital infections caused by certain agents. The reason for the association between HLA-B27 and RA remains unknown.

Diagnosis: This is principally based on established clinical criteria:

A) ***Major criteria:*** Polyarthritis, conjunctivitis /anterioruveitis, urethritis /cervicitis, balanitis circinata / keratoderma blennorrhagicum.

B) ***Minor criteria:*** Plantar fasciitis, Achilles tendonitis, lower back pain, sacroiliitis, spondylitis, keratitis, cystitis, prostatitis, psoriasiform eruptions, oral ulcers, nail changes, diarrhea, leukocytosis, increased serum globulins, inflammation in the synovial fluid.

Definitive diagnosis of RA requires presence of arthritis and two or more other criteria. The diagnosis of RA thus depends on history, clinical evaluation, and radiologic studies. Presence of HLA-B27 increases the probability of RA, but does not directly establish the diagnosis.

Treatment: Oral NSAIDs are often helpful in eliminating the systemic signs and symptoms. Those patients with sexually acquired disease may benefit from a systemic course of antibiotics (those used to treat non-gonococcal urethritis like doxycycline or azithromycin are recommended). Anterior uveitis often requires topical treatment with corticosteroids and mydriatics. Occasionally, regional and/or systemic administration of steroids is also needed. In those severe corticosteroid-intolerant or recalcitrant cases, other immunosuppressive agents as methotrexate or azathioprine may be necessary.

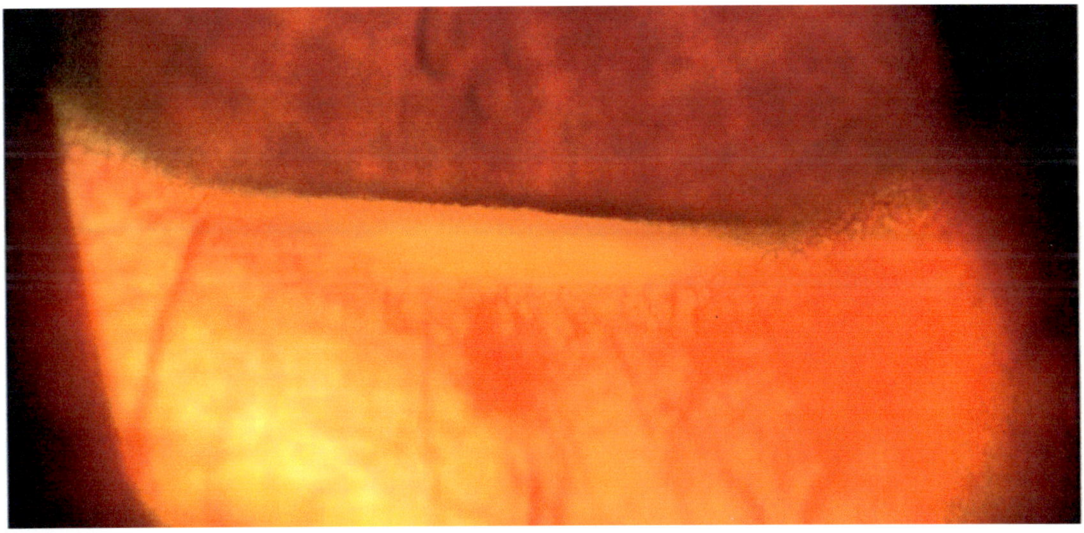

Figure 149: Hypopyon as seen in a patient with reactive arthritis.

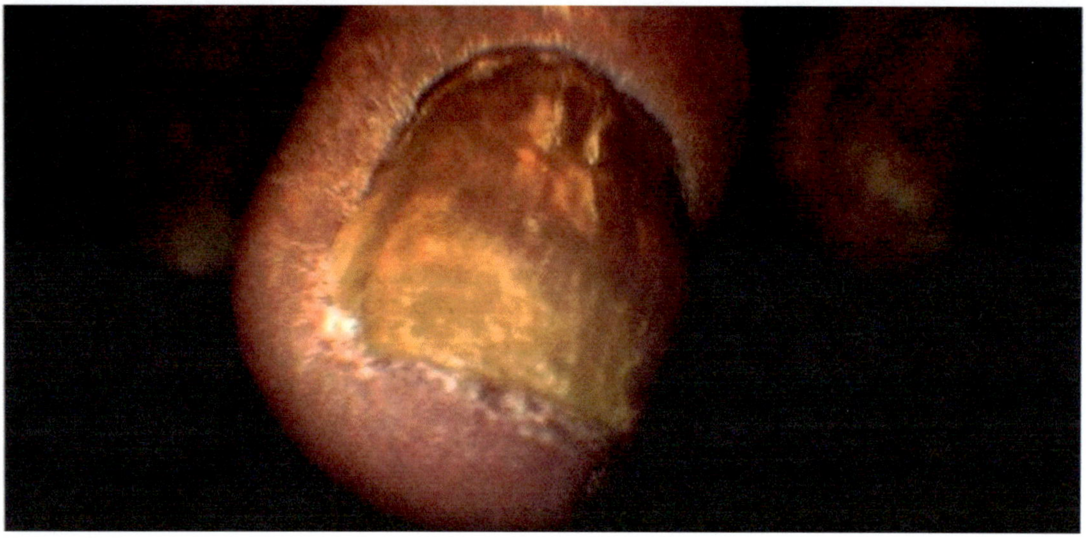

Figure 150: Onycholysis as seen in a patient with reactive arthritis.

References:

1) Sainz de la Maza M. Seronegative Spondyloarthropathies; in: Foster CS, Vitale AT. *Diagnosis and Treatment of Uveitis*. Saunders. Philadelphia 2002. 581-600.
2) Leirisalo-Repo M. Reactive arthritis. *Scand J Rheumatol.* 2005 Jul-Aug;34(4):251-9.

Subretinal Fibrosis and Uveitis syndrome

Definition: Subretinal fibrosis and uveitis syndrome (SFU) is a rare disease presenting with uni- or bilateral posterior uveitis that can progress to subretinal fibrosis. It belongs to a group of posterior uveitides characterized by the presence of multifocal lesions in the RPE and choroid, including such entities as punctate inner choroidopaty (PIC) and multifocal choroiditis and panuveitis (MCP).

History: In 1949, Ernest Fuchs described a clinical picture characterized by large areas of connective tissue formed on the inner side of the choroid, which he named choroiditis proliferans, which probably corresponds to the first reported case of this entity. However, in 1984, Palestine and colleagues described it clinically, histopathologically and immunohistopathologically.

Epidemiology: This is an extremely uncommon entity which predominantly affects young, otherwise healthy myopic women. There appears to be no racial predilection.

Clinical Features: Patients usually complain of acute progressive unilateral visual loss.

Anterior segment: Usually, mild to moderate anterior chamber inflammation is present in the early stages.

Posterior segment: In the early stage of the syndrome, mild to moderate vitritis usually coexists with multiple small (50-500μm), round, discrete, whitish, lesions with indistinct borders at the level of the retinal pigment epithelium (RPE) or inner choroid in the posterior pole and mid-periphery. RPE disturbances at the posterior pole may also be seen.

Many of the acute lesions enlarge and coalesce, forming stellate, irregular areas of subretinal fibrosis scattered throughout the posterior pole and mid- periphery.

Pathology/Pathogenesis: The cause of SFU is unknown. Histopathologic and immunohistopathologic findings in eyes with SFU seem to indicate that the disease is a result of inflammation leading to RPE destruction and transformation, with consequent fibrotic tissue formation, and existence of Muller cells.

Diagnosis: The diagnosis is based on the clinical picture. Patient characteristics (female, young, healthy and myopic) and early ocular manifestations (acute-progressive unilateral visual disturbances), help to establish the diagnosis. other tests may be helpful:
Fluorescein angiogram (FA): Acute lesions show hyperfluorescence in the early phases with later staining of the lesions (with or without leakage) and of the areas with subretinal fibrosis.

Visual Field: Sometimes shows marked scotomas that encompass a zone slightly larger than that of subretinal lesions.

Electroretinogram (ERG) and electrooculogram (EOG): During the early stages of the disease, several entities may be confused with SFU (Acute posterior multifocal placoid pigment epitheliopathy, Birdshot retinochoroidopathy, MCP, PIC, presumed ocular histoplasmosis syndrome and multifocal evanescent white dot syndrome are the major members of this group of syndromes). However, the distinctive subretinal fibrosis, which appears over time, helps to differentiate SFU from other conditions.

Treatment: Systemic corticosteroids may be of benefit during the acute phase, but once the subretinal fibrosis occurs, there is no evidence concerning effective treatment. Some immunomodulatory agents (cyclophosphamide, cyclosporine A, and azathioprine) have also been found to lack evidential efficacy.

Prognosis: The visual prognosis of patients with SFU is poor, and recurrences are common, typically involving previous affected sites. In most series reported, visual acuities range from 20/200 to no light perception.

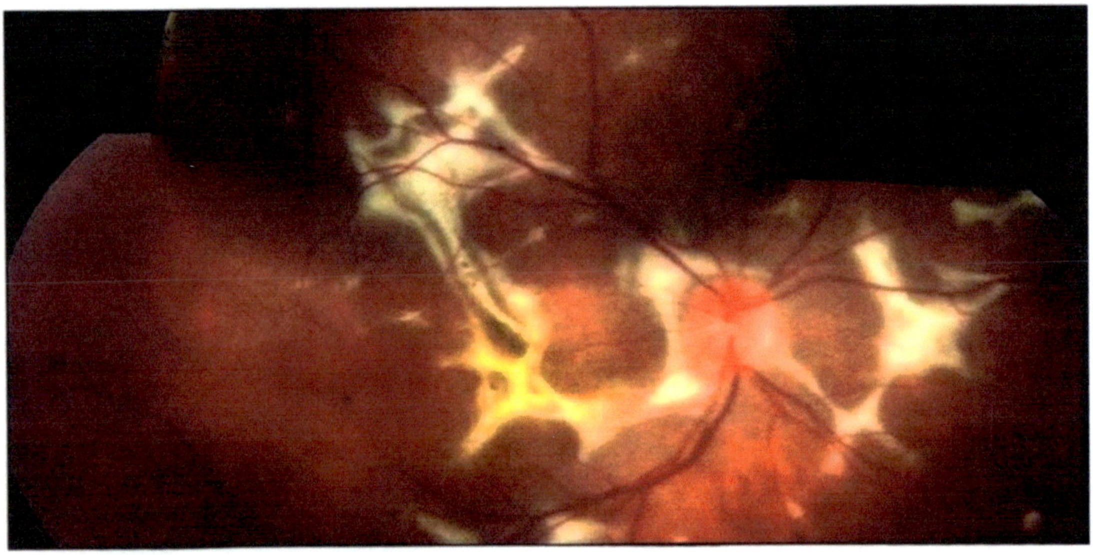

Figure 151: 26 year-old white female affected by SFU. Note the large areas of subretinal fibrosis affecting the posterior pole.

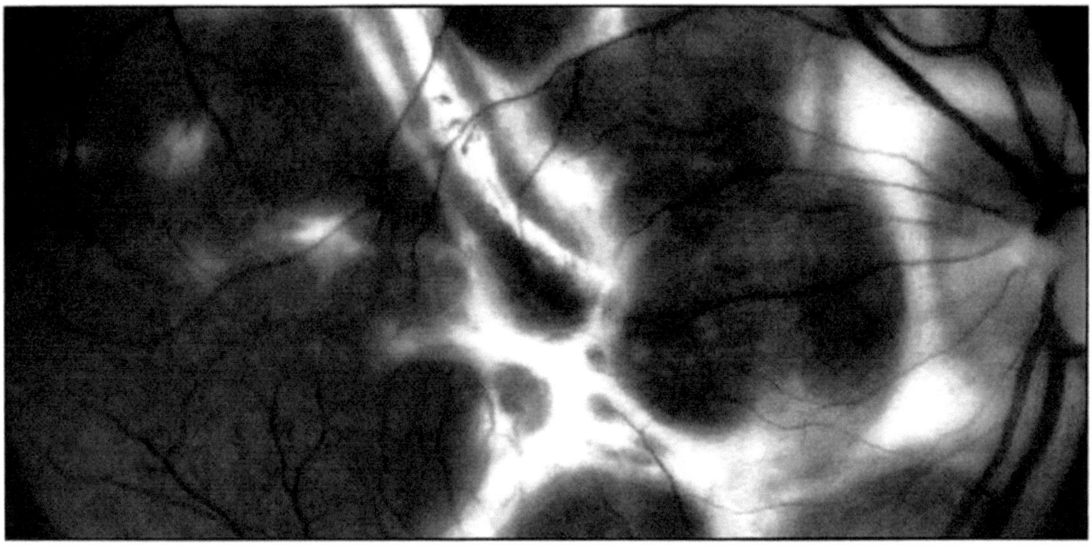

Figure 152: Same patient. Red-free image shows the extensive nature of the fibrotic lesions. Her visual acuity was 20/400.

References:

1) Rojas B. Subretinal fibrosis and uveitis syndrome; in: Foster CS, Vitale AT. *Diagnosis and treatment of uveitis*. Saunders. Philadelphia 2002:797-805.
2) Kaiser PK, Gragoudas ES. The subretinal fibrosis and uveitis syndrome. *Int Ophthalmol Clin.* 1996; 36(1):145-52.

Sympathetic Ophthalmia

Introduction: Sympathetic ophthalmia (SO) is a bilateral granulomatous uveitis occurring days to decades after either surgery or penetrating trauma to one eye. The time from ocular trauma to onset of SO ranges from 10 days to 66 years, but most cases manifest within a year after the trauma.

The first detailed characterization of the disease was provided by McKenzie in the 19th century. In 1905, Ernest Fuchs gave the first detailed histopathologic description of the disease and established it as a separate disease entity.

The incidence of SO is less than 0.5% after penetrating trauma and even lower after surgery.

Pathophysiology: SO is an autoimmune inflammatory reaction that occurs in the eye following uveal antigen exposure to conjunctival lymphatics. A diffuse granulomatous infiltration is seen throughout the uveal tract with marked thickening in the posterior choroid.

Clinical Manifestations:

Systemic manifestations: All of the systemic findings related to Vogt-Koyanagi Harada (VKH) syndrome (i.e., poliosis, vitiligo, dysacusia, cerebrospinal fluid pleocytosis) may be present.

Anterior segment: "Mutton fat" keratic precipitates with a varying degree of inflammation are the most prevalent findings in the anterior chamber. Iris nodules may also be present. Other common findings are posterior synechiae and conjunctival injection.

Posterior segment: This is more characteristically involved and may include vitreous cells, retinal vasculitis, papillitis, choroiditis and serous retinal detachment. Dalen-Fuchs nodules (whitish-yellowish infiltrates usually arising from the peripheral choroid) are classically associated with but not pathognomonic of SO.

As in other chronic uveitides, persistent inflammation can result in a wide spectrum of complications including cataract, secondary glaucoma, retinal and optic nerve atrophy (see figure), choroidal neovascularization, and phthisis bulbi.

Diagnosis: Clinical diagnosis is based on the history of ocular trauma and the clinical findings. Other tests helpful in diagnosing and monitoring this entity:

Fluorescein angiography (acute phase): Shows small hyperfluorescent spots during the venous phase with extensive late diffuse leakage. Less commonly seen are hypofluorescent areas that later become hyperfluorescent.

Indocyanine Green Angiography: May be helpful, especially in cases of choroidal neovascularization.

B-scan Ultrasonography: Can show choroidal thickening (characteristic of SO).

Chorioretinal biopsy: Is not commonly needed, but if done shows a predominant T-cell inflammatory infiltrate in the uvea, early phagocytosis of pigment granules, and the presence of Dalen-Fuchs nodules.

Other tests: Lumbar puncture is useful to distinguish between SO and Vogt Koyanagi Harada Syndrome early in the course of the disease.

Treatment: Enucleation or evisceration of the injured eye before the inflammatory response begins can possibly prevent SO. It is generally agreed that once infection is excluded, immunosuppressive therapy is necessary to achieve good final visual acuity in eyes affected by SO. Systemic corticosteroids are used for the initial control of active inflammation and immunomodulatory therapy is usually necessary for long term control of the chronic inflammation and prevention of vision loss . Cyclosporine (alone or in combination with other IMT) has been reported to be an alternative regimen in corticosteroid-resistant cases of SO with varying success. Chlorambucil has been especially effective in SO that is recalcitrant to more conventional therapy. Other IMT agents used, alone or in combination, are methotrexate, mycophenolate mofetil, azathioprine and tacrolimus.

References:

1) Power WJ. Sympathetic ophthalmia. In: Foster CS, Vitale AT. *Diagnosis and Treatment of Uveitis.* Philadephia: WB Saunders, 2001;pp 742-747.
2) Cordero Coma M, Sobrin L, Foster CS. Sympathetic Ophthalmia. *Contemporary Ophthalmol* 2006; 5 (5):1-6.
3) D'Amico FM, Kiss S, Young LH. Sympathetic Ophthalmia. *Semin Ophthalmol* 2005; 20(3): 191-7.

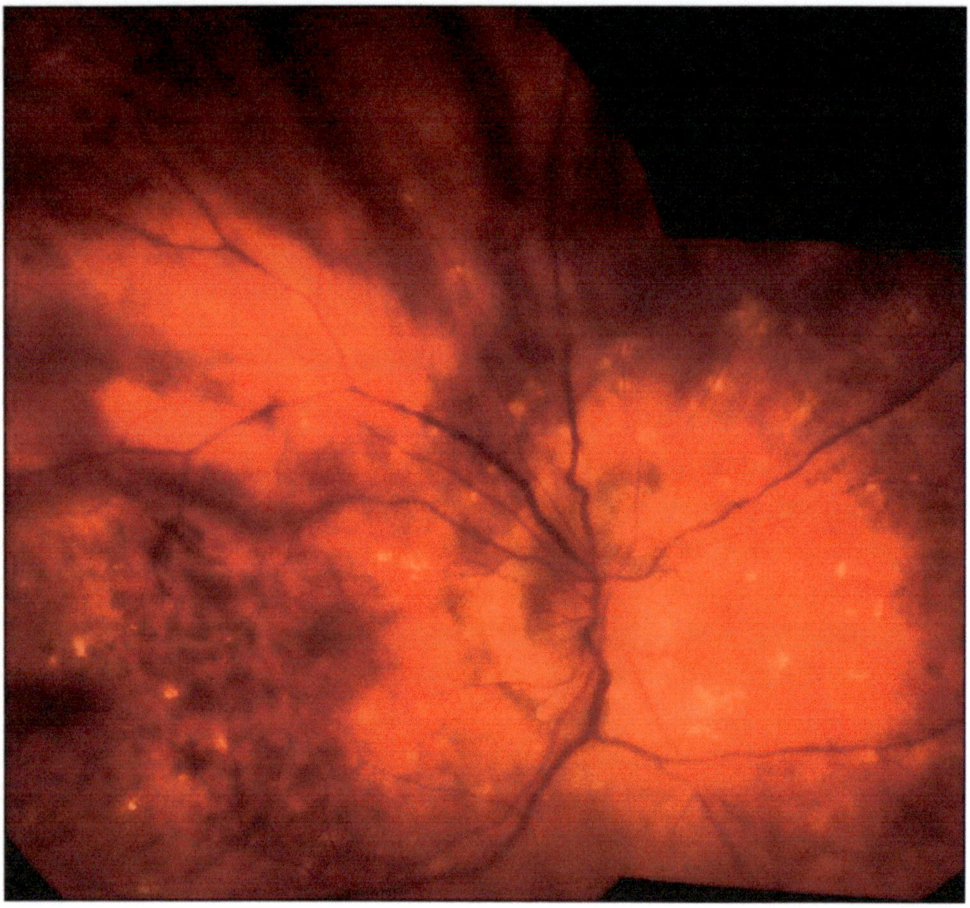

Figure 153: Widespread Dalen-Fuchs nodules, vessel attenuation, and RPE changes in a patient with sympathetic ophthalmia. Note the optic nerve hyperemia.

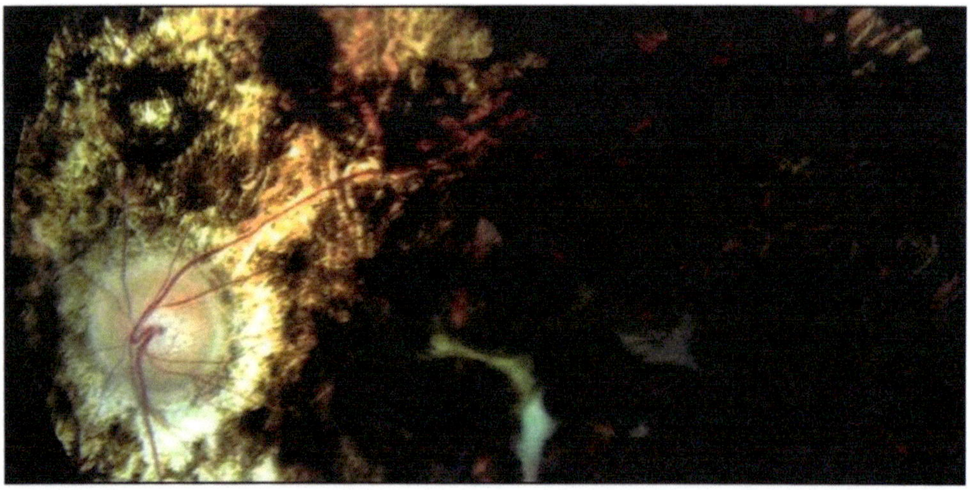

Figure 154: Extensive chorioretinal atrophy located in areas of previous choroidal infiltration in a 61 year-old Hispanic female. Note the optic nerve pallor and the atrophy of the retinal vasculature as a consequence of persistent inflammation.

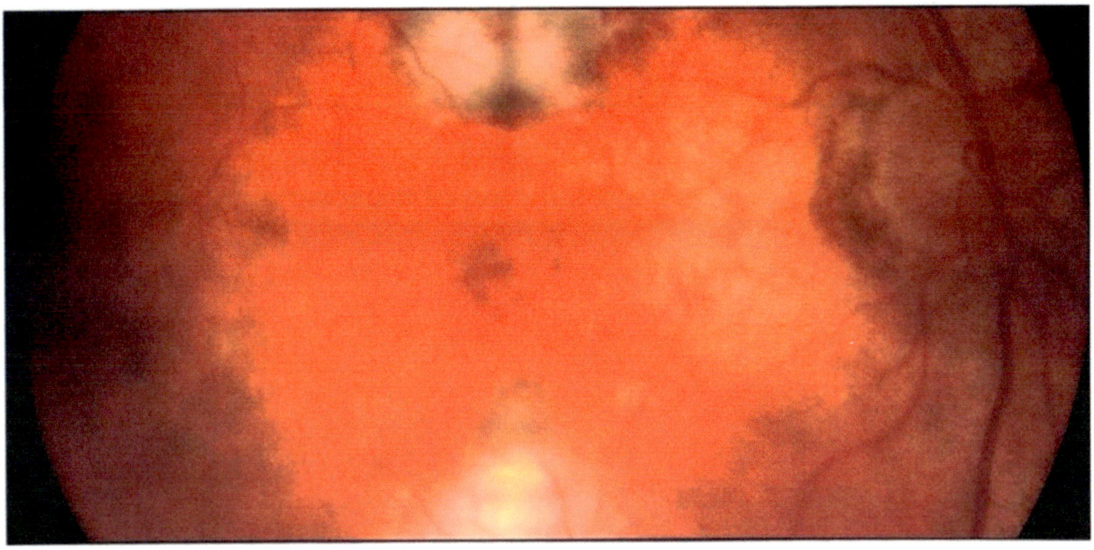

Figure 155: Two focal areas of old choroidal neovascular membranes secondary to SO.

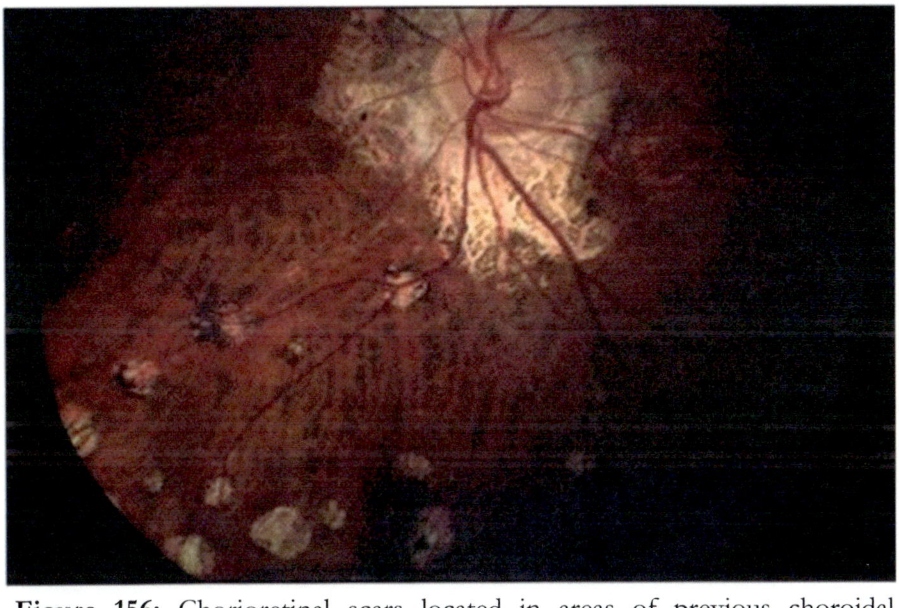

Figure 156: Chorioretinal scars located in areas of previous choroidal infiltration in an eye affected by sympathetic ophthalmia. Note the extensive peripapillary atrophy.

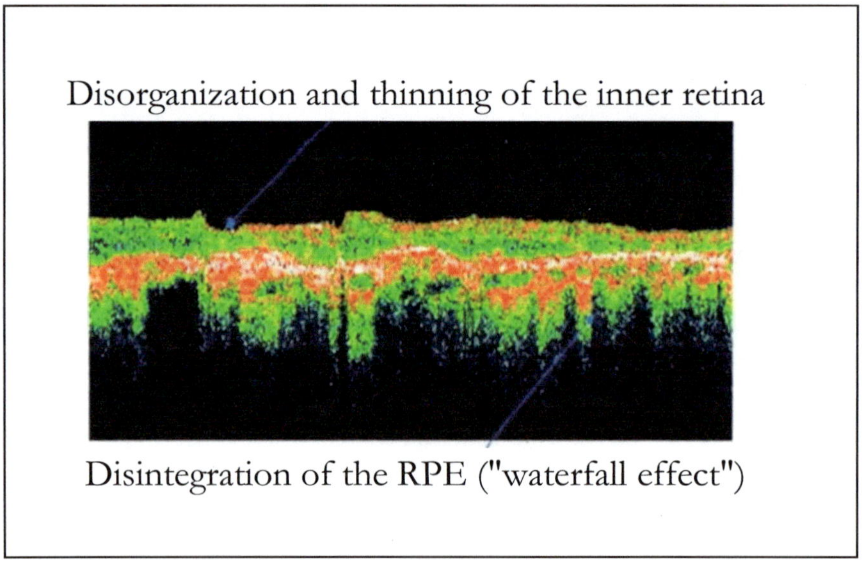

<u>Figure 157:</u> Optical coherence tomography image displaying a thinned retina in a patient with SO.

Systemic Lupus Erythematosus

Introduction: Systemic lupus erythematosus (SLE) is an autoimmune disease characterized by the production of numerous autoantibodies targeting joints, skin, kidneys, brain and the eye.

Lupus dermatitis was first described in 1845 by Hebra, who regarded it as a benign, local skin condition. Years later, Kaposi reported that this condition was in fact a systemic disease with potential life-threatening consequences. The first description of ocular lesions (classic retinal findings) in a patient with SLE was in 1929 by Bergmeister. In 1971, the American Rheumatic Association published a report which provided the first published criteria for the diagnosis of SLE. These criteria were revised (incorporating serologic abnormalities) in 1982 and are now widely accepted, thus currently providing the basis for the standardized diagnosis of SLE.

The prevalence of SLE varies worldwide with an incidence of 40 in 100,000 people in North America and Northern Europe. A clear gender preference is observed, with women representing up to 90% of the cases. Black Americans and Hispanics appear to have higher incidence rates. Over 80% of the cases involve women in their childbearing years.

Clinical Manifestations:

Systemic manifestations: The systemic manifestations of SLE are diverse. The 1982 revised criteria for the classification of SLE included skin findings (malar rash, discoid rash, photosensitivity), oral ulcers, non-erosive arthritis, serositis (pleuritis, pericarditis), renal disorder (proteinuria, nephritis), neurological disorder (seizures, psychosis), hematologic disorder (hemolytic anemia, leukopenia, lymphopenia, thrombocytopenia), and an immunologic disorder (anti-Sm and/or anti-native DNA antibodies, false positive test for syphilis, antinuclear antibody (ANA)).

Ocular manifestations:

External involvement: The periocular skin can be especially involved in discoid lupus erythematosus (DLE). These lesions may be confused for chronic blepharitis or eczema and, therefore, remain undiagnosed for years. Involved areas have a tendency to heal with scarring. Atrophy with loss of lashes and periorbital edema (sometimes violaceous) are other oculocutaneous presentations. Other rare ophthalmic involvement includes orbital myositis, orbital pseudotumor, orbital apex syndrome, Brown's syndrome or ocular ischemic syndrome.

Anterior segment: The most common ocular manifestation of SLE is keratoconjunctivitis sicca (KCS), presenting in approximately 25-35% of the patients. Corneal involvement in KCS may manifest as punctate epithelial erosions, filamentary keratitis, and in severe cases, KCS predisposes the patient to bacterial keratitis and sterile ulceration. Secondary Sjogren's syndrome may be the underlying cause of KCS in patients with systemic autoimmune diseases, such as SLE. In addition, the inflammatory process in SLE can also affect the perilimbal capillary arcades producing a clinical picture called peripheral ulcerative keratitis (PUK), which is frequently accompanied by a necrotizing sderitis, and usually reflects the presence of severe systemic vaso-occlusive disease. Recurrent episodes of episcleritis are common. Scleritis is less common, but it can cause severe ocular morbidity. Conjunctival involvement in the form of chronic conjunctivitis (developing scarring and pathological adhesions in severe cases) is infrequent in SLE.

Posterior segment: Retinal involvement is considered the second, after the KCS, most common manifestation of lupus. The classic finding in SLE-retinopathy is a cotton-wool spot, which is an ischemic infarct in the retinal nerve fiber layer. It may be isolated or seen in association with areas of retinal edema, ischemia, hard exudates, hemorrhages, vascular sheathing, capillary and venous dilatation, tortuosity and microaneurysms. These findings, similar to the clinical picture of hypertensive retinopathy, can occur as an independent manifestation of the underlying disease in the absence of hypertension. Severe occlusive retinopathy or vasculitis is a rare form of retinopahy in SLE affecting smaller retinal arteries and arterioles (often associated with similar changes in the central nervous system), and can be associated with proliferative retinopathy (and retinal neovascularization), occlusions of larger diameter retinal vessels, and/or exudative macular edema. Lupus choroidopathy is associated with multifocal serous detachments of the RPE and neural retina, with the transudation of the accumulated fluid through Bruch's membrane and RPE affected by choroidal ischemia and inflammation. The dysfunction of the choroidal vasculature can also lead to choroidal neovascularization or central serous chorioretinopathy.

The incidence of neuro-ophthalmological manifestations ranges from 3% to 30% in various studies. The most common manifestation is that of optic nerve damage (papillitis, ischemic optic neuropathy, retrobulbar optic neuritis, etc.). Lesions of the posterior visual pathways are relatively uncommon, but can lead to severe disability.

Diagnosis: This is based on a combination of clinical and laboratory findings. Detection of antinuclear antibodies (present in 95% of the patients) is a good screening test. More specific antibodies for the diagnosis of SLE include antibodies to double-stranded DNA and to the Smith (Sm) antigen. Antiphospholipid antibodies are present in approximately 17% of SLE patients; these are associated with thrombotic events.
Fluorescein angiogram (FA): Angiographic findings in lupus retinopathy are nonspecific, but may be used to evaluate retinal perfusion or detect retinal neovascularization or macular edema that may be amenable to treatment. Angiography is also useful in confirming lupus choroidopathy.

Skin or conjunctival biopsy: In unusual cases of DLE, isolated eyelid involvement needs to be seen in order to make the correct diagnosis. Biopsy is also extremely helpful in cases of chronic conjunctivitis with conjunctival scarring.

Image tests (MRI): Performed in cases of neuro-ophthalmological manifestations.

Treatment: Since the ocular complications of SLE are generally associated with active disease elsewhere in the body, control of the systemic disease may lead to resolution of ocular manifestations.

Nonsteroidal anti-inflammatory agents or antimalarial therapy (especially hydroxychloroquine sulfate) may be sufficient in relatively mild ocular disease (episcleritis, eyelid involvement).

The presence of severe manifestations of SLE, such as scleral, retinal, choroidal, neuro-ophthalmological, or orbital involvement requires immunomodulatory therapy (IMT). Initial empiric treatment with steroids is typically oral, with or without initial pulse with intravenous corticosteroids. These may be supplemented with topical and/or regional corticosteroids, especially in cases of asymmetrical involvement. When corticosteroid therapy fails to control the disease or when therapy is expected to be required for longer than three months, other agents (alone or in combination) such as cyclophosphamide, azathioprine, methotrexate, cyclosporine, chlorambucil, mycophenolate mofetil, and tacrolimus, may be necessary.

Anti-platelet treatment and anticoagulation may have a role in the secondary prevention of thromboembolic events in the presence of antiphospholipid antibodies.

Laser photocoagulation and vitreoretinal surgical procedures may be necessary to treat complications associated with retinal vasculitis, such as persistent neovascularization and localized fluid accumulation in the retina.

Adjunctive therapy for KCS, such as tear supplements, punctal occlusion, and eyelid hygiene, is crucial. In severe cases, topical or even systemic immunomodulatory agents may be necessary.

References:

1. Mills JA: Systemic Lupus Erythromatosis. *N Engl J Med* 1994;330:1871.
2. Steinberg AD: Management of systemic lupus erythromatosis. In: Kelly WN, Harris ED, Ruddy S, et al, eds: *Textbook of Rheumatology*, 2nd ed. Philadelphia, W.B. Saunders, 1985, p 1130.
3. Gold DH, Morris DA, Henkind P: Ocular findings in systemic lupus erythromatosis. *Br J Ophthalmol* 1972;56:8m.

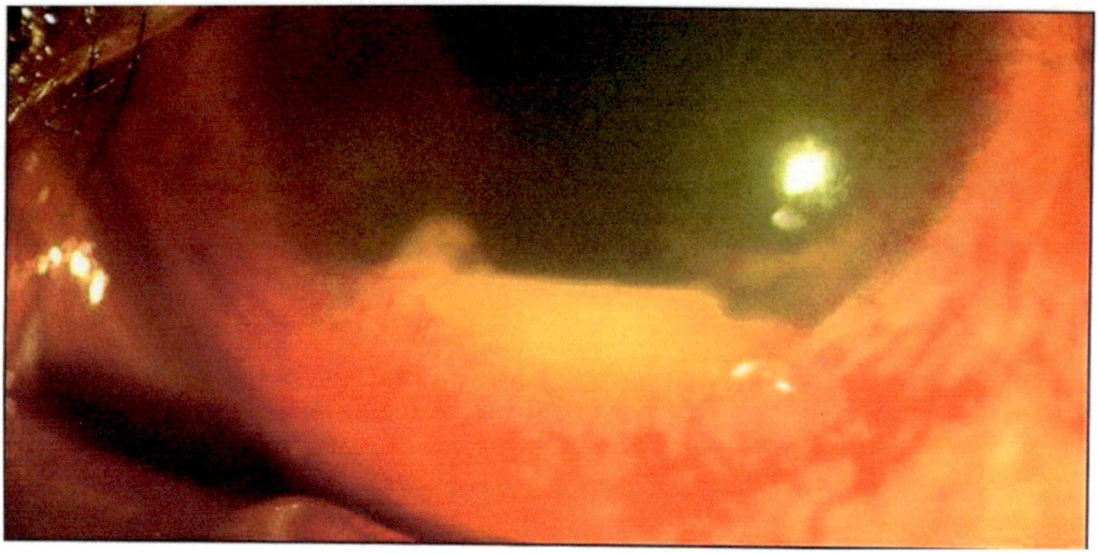

Figure 158: Hypopyon in an African-American patient with SLE.

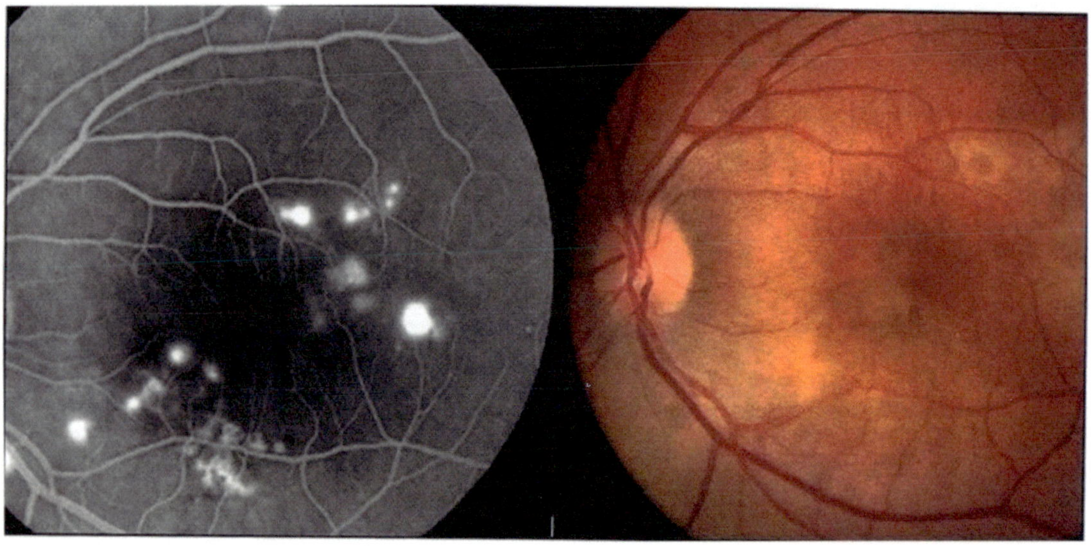

Figure 159: 36 year-old white female with lupus choroidopathy. Fluorescein angiography demonstrates multiple sites of leakage from the choroid into the sub-RPE and subretinal spaces. This pathological fluid deposition may also be observed in the color photograph.

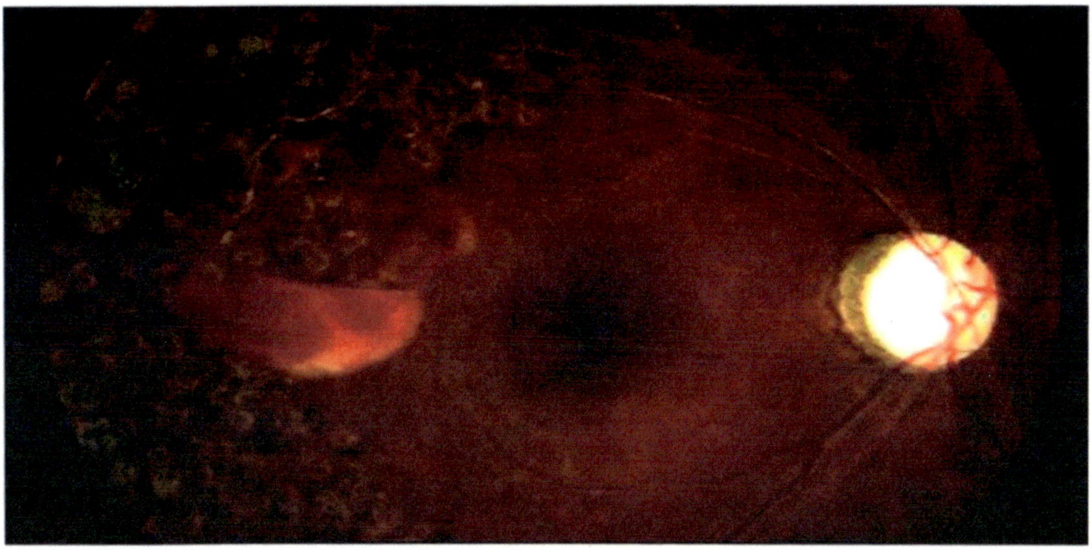

Figure 160: Regression of neovascularization elsewhere in the context of systemic lupus erythematosus. Note the sheathing of the superior retinal vein and optic nerve pallor.

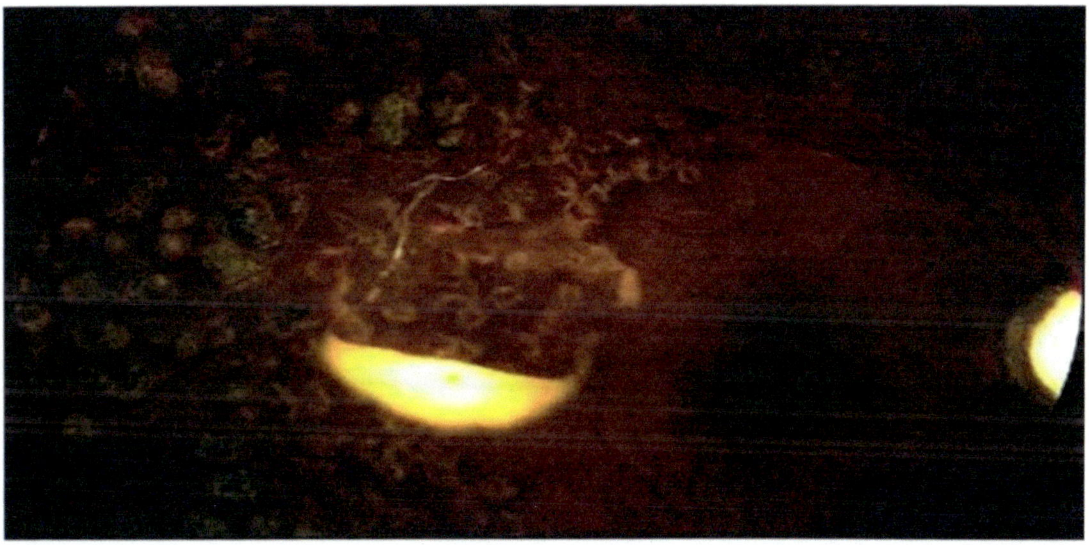

Figure 161: Fibrosed area of neovascularization secondary to SLE-associated vasculitis after an intravitreal bevacizumab injection.

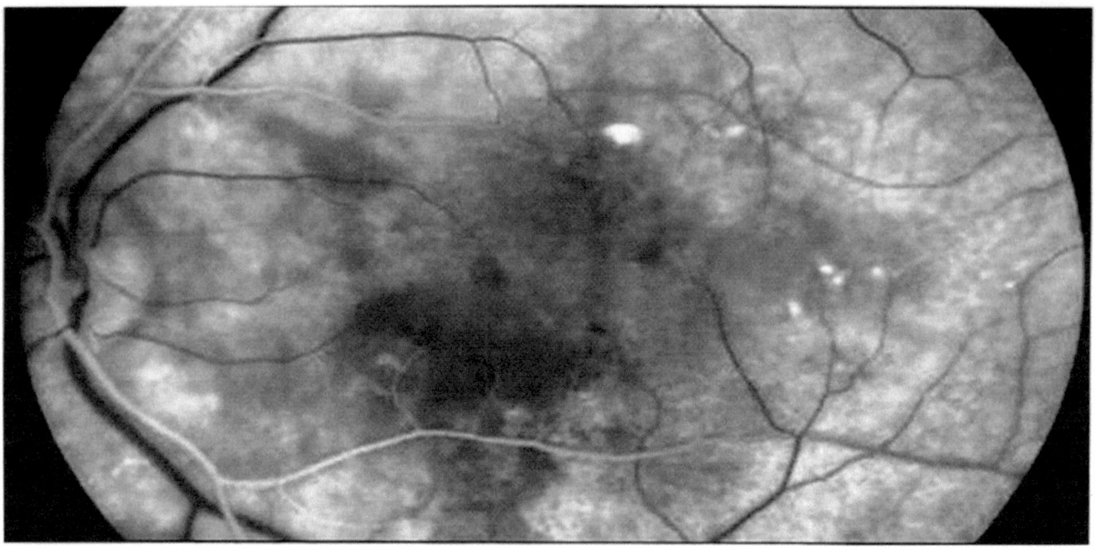

Figure 162: Patchy choroidal filling during the early phase of the fluorescein angiogram. This is indicative of underlying choroidopathy in a patient with SLE.

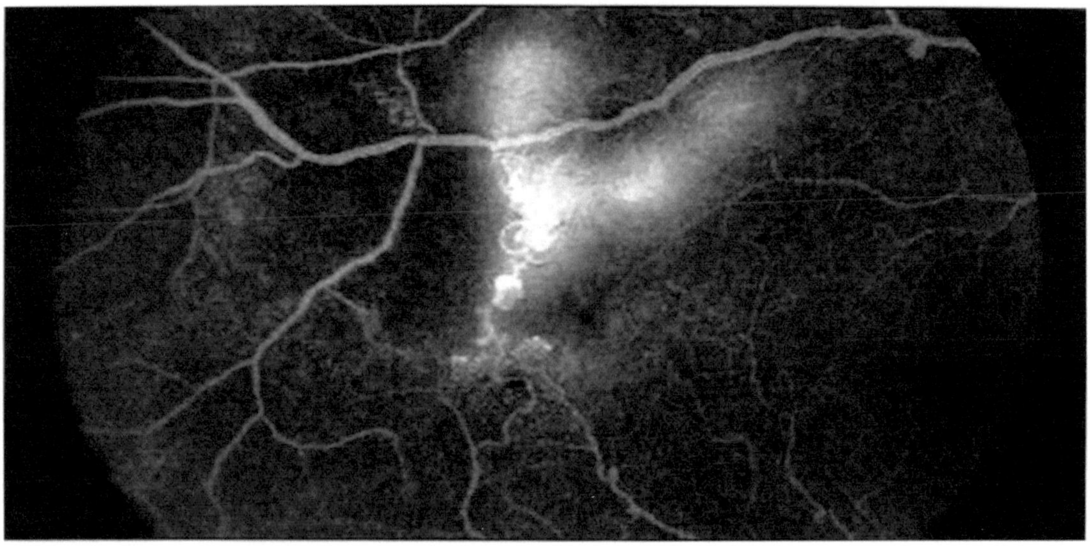

Figure 163: Temporal neovascularization elsewhere (NVE) in the right eye of a patient with SLE-associated vasculitis.

Tubulointerstitial Nephritis and Uveitis

Introduction: Tubulointerstitial nephritis and uveitis (TINU) is a rare condition characterized by acute tubulointerstitial nephritis preceding or concurrent with uveitis.

TINU was described in 1975 by Dobrin, Vernier, and Fish. Fewer than 200 reported cases exist in the world medical literature.

Because nephritis may remain subclinical, the true incidence is unknown. The average age of onset is 15 years with a range of 9 to 74 years. Females are affected 3 times more often than males.

Pathophysiology: Although the cause of nephritis is unknown, an immunoglobulin from the G class directed against a kidney protein was identified in the serum of one affected patient. Renal biopsy specimens reveals a cellular infiltrate of T lymphocytes, monocytes, and macrophages. Plasma cells, B lymphocytes, neutrophils, and eosinophils are rarely observed. Renal tubule edema, epithelial degeneration, and focal necrosis are frequent.

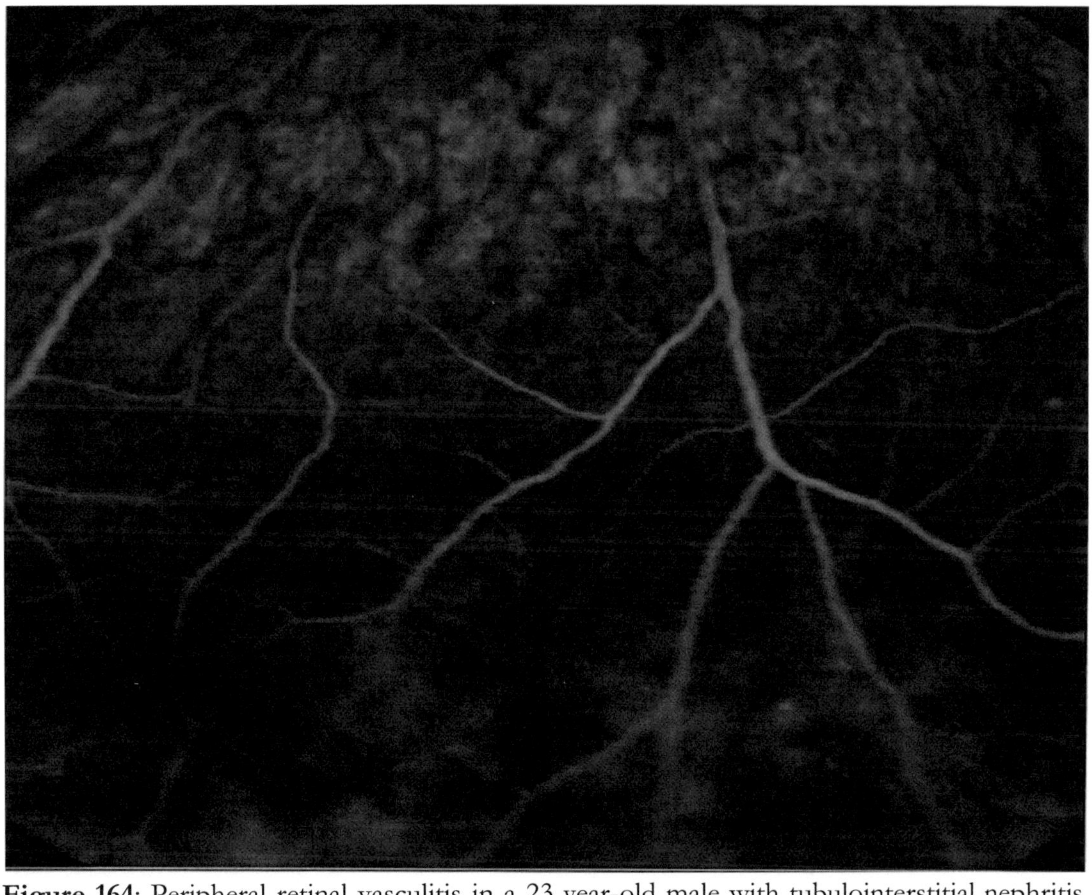

Figure 164: Peripheral retinal vasculitis in a 23 year-old male with tubulointerstitial nephritis and uveitis syndrome. The patient subsequently was started on oral mycophenolate mofetil therapy.

Clinical Manifestations: Fatigue, malaise, anorexia, headache, and abdominal pain are the most common symptoms. Fever, weight loss, nausea, and vomiting may be presenting signs. The classic triad consists of inflammatory syndrome (anemia, elevated erythrocyte sedimentation rate, and hypergammaglobulinemia), nephritis, and uveitis. Nephritis typically develops within a month. Uveitis may occur before, after, or concurrent with renal disease.

Diagnosis: Non-granulomatous anterior uveitis is the most common ophthalmic manifestation; however posterior segment involvement may include papillitis, cystoid macular edema, retinal vascular sheathing, vitritis, and multifocal choroiditis. Nodular episcleritis may be the initial manifestation.

Urinalysis including microscopic examination may reveal the presence of glycosuria, proteinuria, aminoaciduria, or microscopic hematuria and necessitates evaluation by a nephrologist. Twenty four hour urine collection for protein, beta-2 microglobulin, and N-acetyl-beta-D-glucosaminadase aid in the diagnosis.

Renal Gallium scanning is abnormal during the acute nephritic phase. Renal biopsy demonstrates necrosis of renal tubule epithelium. Interstitial edema, and CD4 positive lymphocytic infiltrates are the hallmark features.

Serum azotemia and normochromic, normocytic anemia are additional findings. Complement levels may be reduced during the acute phase; systemic corticosteroid therapy led to normalization in one case. HLA- DQA1*1/DQB1*05/DRB1*01 was present in 72% TINU patients from 3 U.S. uveitis centers.

Endocrine abnormalities of the thyroid and parathyroid glands have been described in association with TINU syndrome; thyroid stimulating hormone testing is recommended for all newly diagnosed patients.

Treatment: Interstitial nephritis typically resolves spontaneously. Corticosteroids are indicated to prevent structural damage resulting from acute renal failure. Nephropathy is chronic in 1.1% of cases and renal dialysis is necessary in less than 5% of patients.

Uveitis is seldom chronic in nature and responds to topical corticosteroids in most cases. Topical cycloplegics may prevent formation of posterior synechiae. Regional and rarely systemic corticosteroid therapy is indicated for moderate to severe acute uveitis. Mycophenolate mofetil is an efficacious steroid sparing agent in cases of chronic uveitis.

References:

Pinar V, Gion N, Foster CS. Tubulointerstitial Nephritis and Uveitis Syndrome; in: Foster CS, Vitale AT. *Diagnosis and treatment of uveitis*. Saunders. Philadelphia 2002:726-730.

Vogt-Koyanagi-Harada

Introduction: Vogt-Koyanagi-Harada syndrome (VKH), formerly known as uveomeningo-encephalitic syndrome, is a systemic disorder involving multiple organ systems, including the ocular, auditory, nervous, and integumentary systems. Severe bilateral panuveitis associate with exudative retinal detachment is the hallmark of ocular disease.

This syndrome was first described in the 10th century by a Persian doctor, Ali-Ibn-Isa. However, it was in the early 20th century when three independent physicians (Vogt, Koyanagi, and Harada) gave an accurate description of this entity and the term uveomeningitic syndrome was replaced by VKH.

VKH has a worlwide prevalence, but variable incidence among different geographical regions with predilection for darkly pigmented races. Women are more frequently affected than men and most patients are in the second to fifth decades of life at the onset of the disease.

Pathophysiology: The etiology is unknown. It is postulated to be a primarily inflammatory condition directed against a common antigen expressed by the skin, ear, eye, and meninges. Other hypothesis involving infectious agents as the primary cause have also been alternatively invoked. The main histopathologic findings of VKH are granulomatous inflammation of the uveal tract with lymphocytes and epithelioid cells as the predominant cellular lines. Dalen-Fuchs nodules (also seen in sympathetic ophthalmia) are often present in the chronic stage. The histopathological findings in these two entities (sympathetic ophthalmia and VKH) are similar, and standard histologic study cannot differentiate one from the other.

Clinical Manifestations: The natural history of VKH disease can be divided into four different stages:

The *prodromal* phase (few days), mimics a systemic viral infection. Symptoms include fever, headache, nausea, tinnitus (which is characteristic) and other less common neurological symptoms.

The *acute uveitic* phase (may last for several weeks), in which a severe bilateral (although sometimes there is a delay between first and second eye affection) uveitis develops. A thickening of the posterior choroid (with elevation of the peripapillary retinochoroidal layer), optic disc hyperemia, and multiple serous retinal detachments (due to retinal pigment epithelium breakdown) are usually seen. Eventually the inflammation may extend to the anterior segment showing granulomatous characteristics.

Bilateral uveitis (with the mentioned characteristics) and cerebrospinal fluid (CSF) pleocytosis with no other systemic manifestations are usually termed Harada' s form of the disease. Bilateral iridocyclitis accompanied by vitiligo, poliosis, and auditory problems are known as the Vogt-Koyanagi form of the disease.

The *convalescent* phase (may last for several months), is characterized by skin (perilimbal vitiligo is the earliest) and uveal depigmentation (in the choroid causes the classic sunset-glow fundus appearance).

The *chronic recurrent phase* (which may interrupt the previous stage), manifests as a recurrent and predominantly anterior uveitis, with characteristic development of iris nodules. Ocular complications of VKH usually develop during this phase (such as cataract, glaucoma, subretinal fibrosis and/or neovascularization, macular atrophy, pigmentary degeneration etc.).

Diagnosis: The following criteria are general guidelines for the diagnosis of VKH:

1) No history of ocular trauma or surgery.
2) At least three of four of the following signs:
   a) Bilateral chronic iridocyclitis.
   b) Posterior uveitis, including exudative retinal detachment, disc hyperemia, and sunset glow fundus.
   c) Neurologic signs of tinnitus, neck stiffness, headache, CSF pleocytosis, and/or central nervous system problems.
   d) Dermatologic manifestations of alopecia, poliosis, or vitiligo.

Some other tests may also be helpful for diagnosis and monitoring:

Fluorescein angiography(FA) and indocyanine green angiography (ICG): FA characteristically shows multiple punctate hyperfluorescent dots at the level of the retinal pigment epithelium (RPE) in the acute stage, which gradually enlarge and coalesce. This has been termed starry night appearance. Disc leakage is also very frequent. In the chronic phase RPE window defects or blockage (due to atrophy) give alternating hyper- and hypofluorescence giving a moth-eaten appearance. ICG classicaly shows extensive hypofluorescence in the early phase.

Ultrasonography (US) and ultrasound biomicroscopy (USBμ): US usually reveals choroidal thickening reflecting the serous retinal detachments. USBμ may reflect ciliochoroidal detachment.

Lumbar puncture: Usually reveals CSF pleocytosis between the first and eighth week.

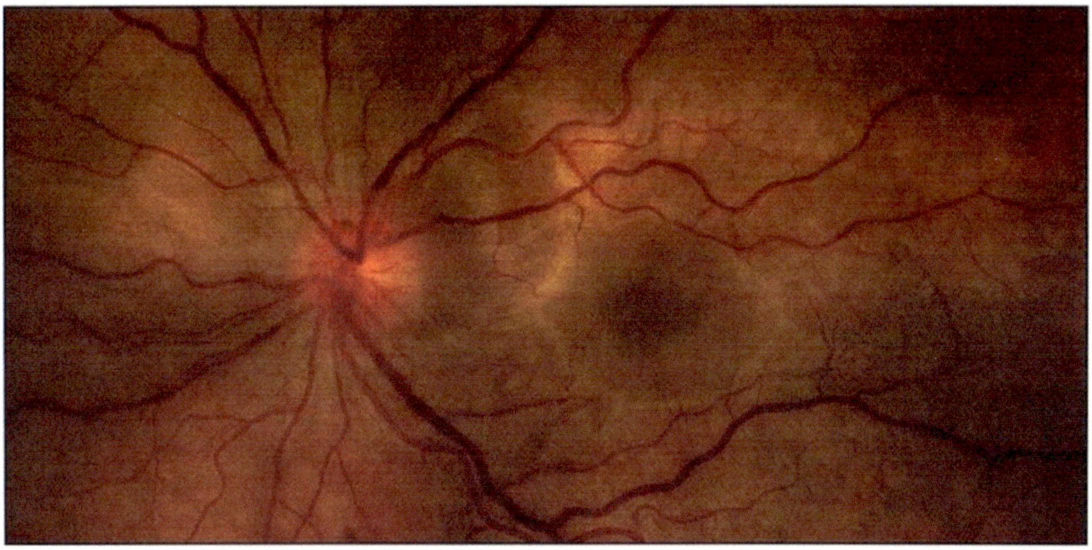

Figurc 165: Serous macular detachment in the left eye. Note the disc hyperemia and widespread choroidal infiltrates.

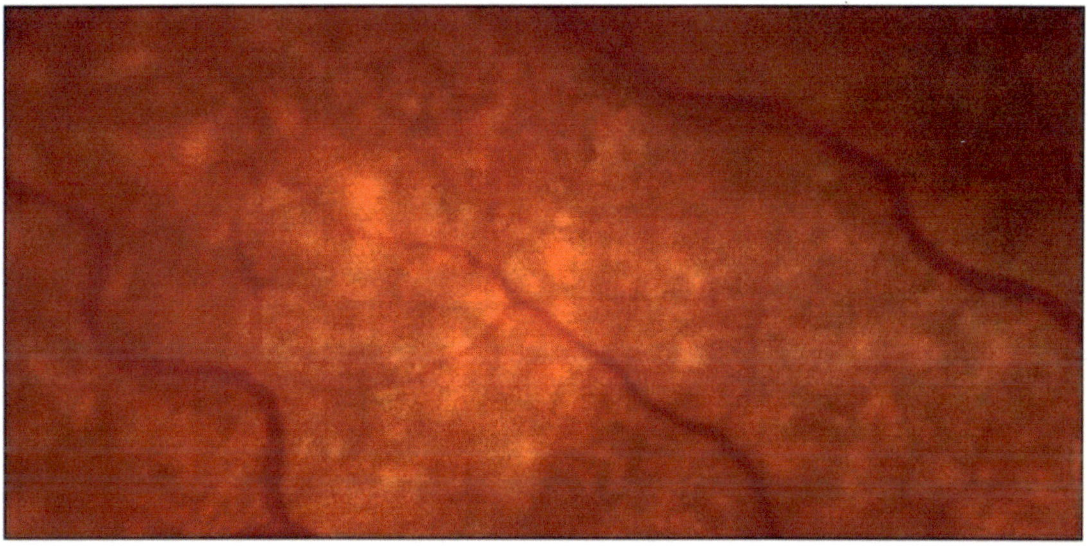

Figure 166: Same patient as in Figure 165. Characteristic finding of VKH: Multiple choroidal infiltrates spread diffusely in the retina.

Treatment: The typical treatment for VKH is high-dose corticosteroid therapy followed by a slow tapering of the drug over 3 to 6 months. In severe cases high-dose pulsed intravenous steroid therapy may be necessary. Patients who are intolerant or resistant to corticosteroid therapy may be treated with other immunomodulatory agents to minimize complications and to improve visual prognosis. Several agents such as Cyclophosphamide, Cyclosporine, and Tacrolimus have been used. Recent studies suggest that first line immunomodulatory therapy (IMT) with those aforementioned agents would achieve superior visual outcomes when compared to corticosteroid as monotherapy or with delayed addition of IMT for treatment of VKH-associated uveitis. Cataract and glaucoma are frequent complications, subretinal neovascularization is less frequent.

References:

1) Tesavibul N. Vogt-Koyanagi-Harada syndrome. In: Foster CS, Vitale AT. Diagnosis and Treatment of Uveitis. Philadelphia: WB Saunders, 2001;pp 748-56.
2) Andreoli CM, Foster CS. Vogt-Koyanagi-Harada disease. Int Ophthalmol Clin. 2006; 46(2):111-22.
3) Paredes I, Ahmed M, Foster CS. Immunomodulatory therapy for Vogt-Koyanagi-Harada patients as first-line therapy. Ocul Immunol Inflamm. 2006;14(2):87-90.

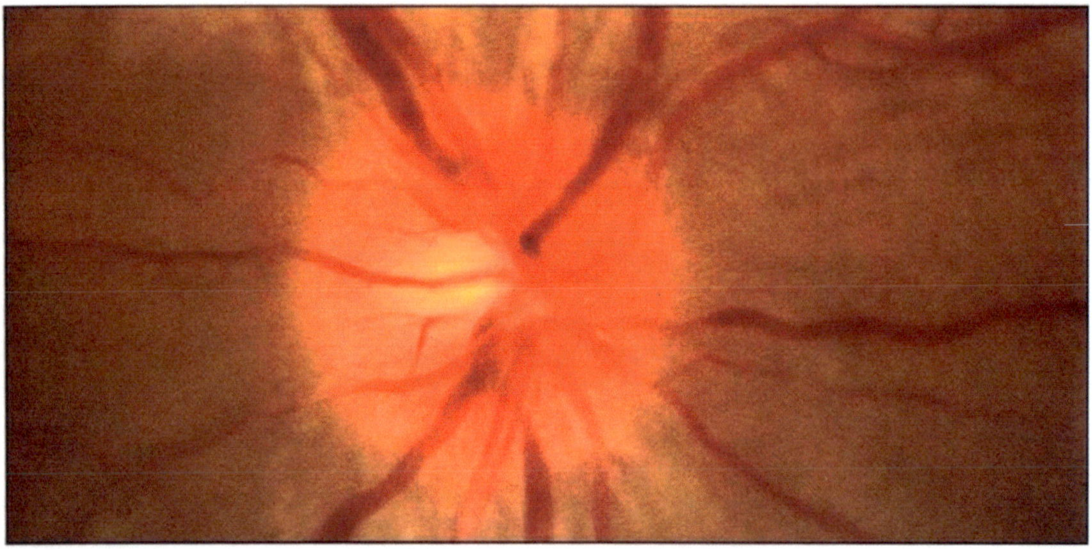

Figure 167: Same patient as in Figure 165. Optic nerve hyperemia in the acute phase of VKH with encircling serous retinal detachments.

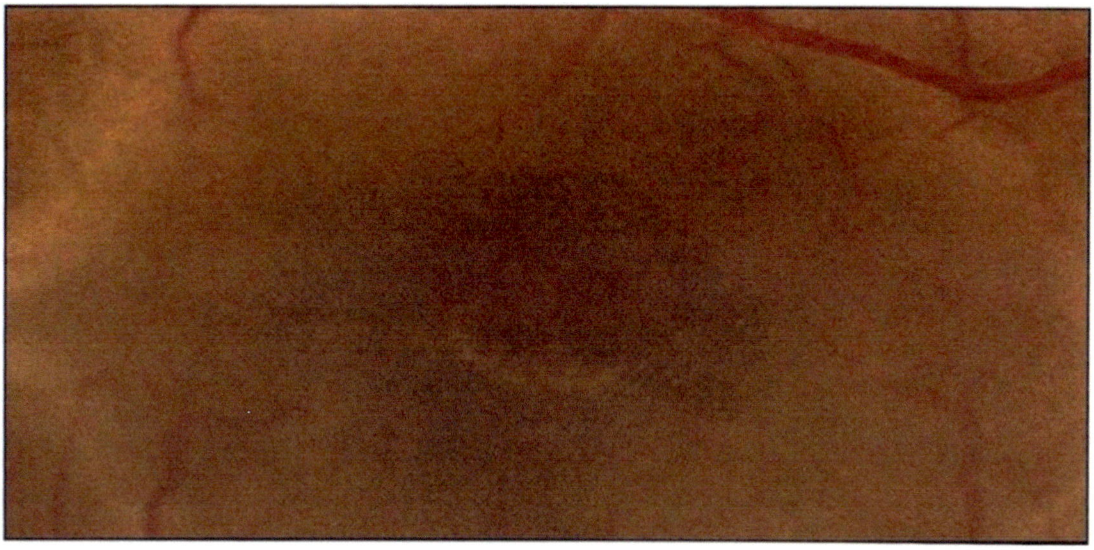

Figurc 168: Samc patient as in Figure 165. Serous macular detachment in the left eye. Note the elevation of the retinal vessels in the macular region

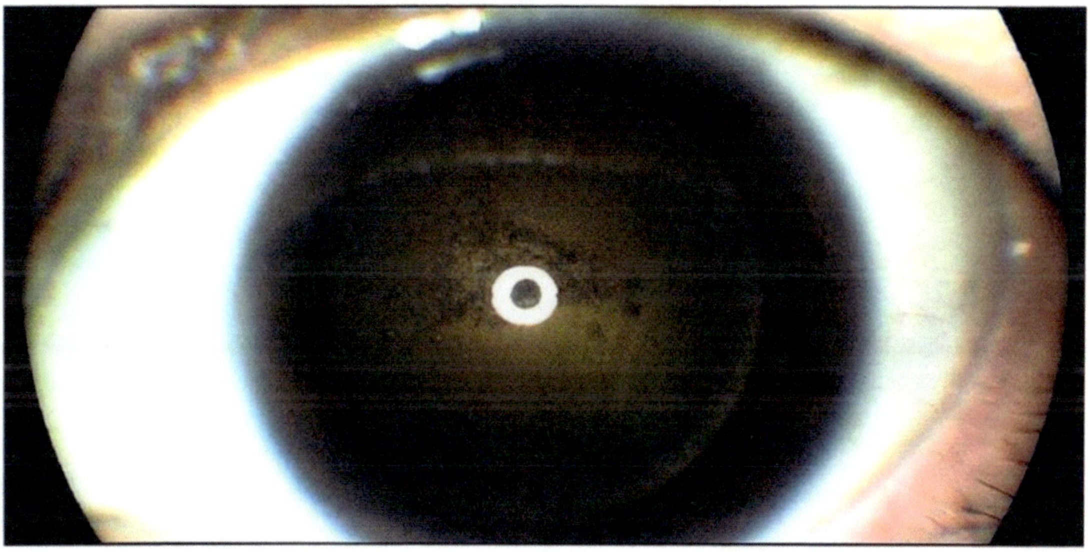

Figure 169: 2+ posterior subcapsular cataract in a patient with Vogt-Koyanagi-Harada Syndrome.

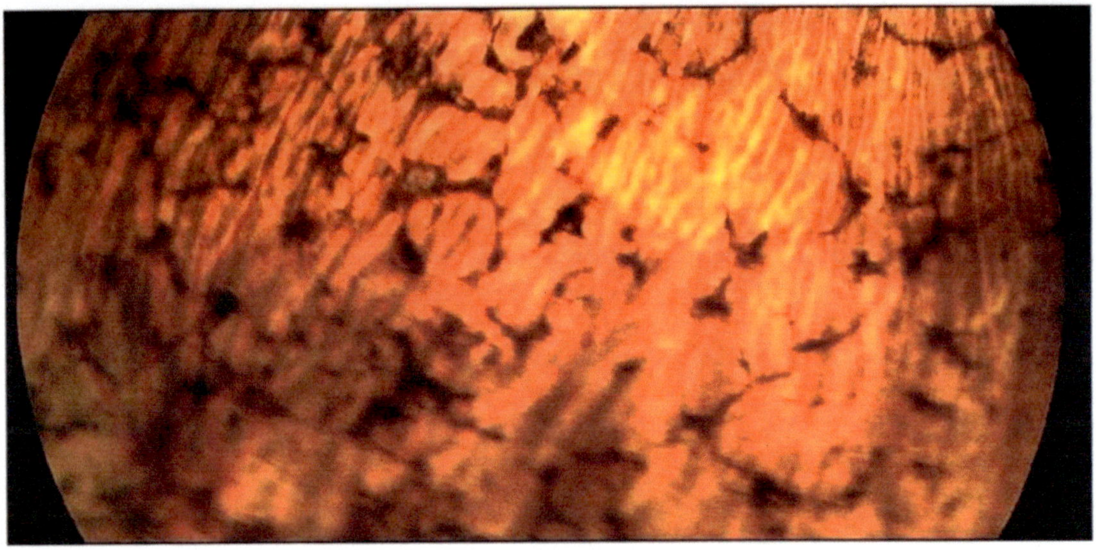

Figure 170: Diffuse chorioretinal scarring in the inferior periphery of a patient afflicted by Vogt-Koyanagi-Harada Syndrome.

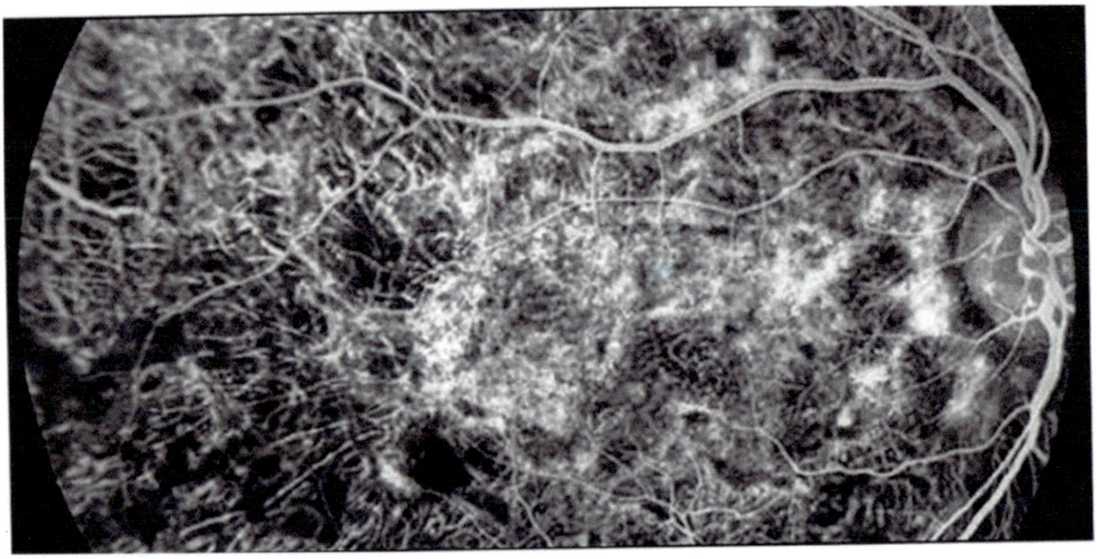

Figure 171: Diffuse RPE scarring secondary to recalcitrant inflammation as seen on a fluorescein angiogram. Note the visible choroidal vasculature.

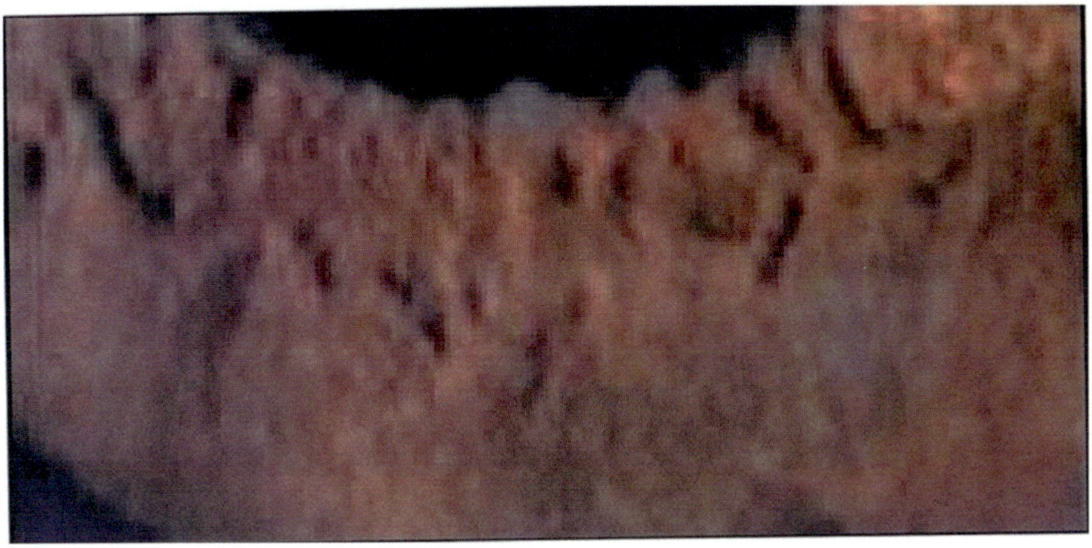

Figure 172: Iris nodules in a patient with VKH.

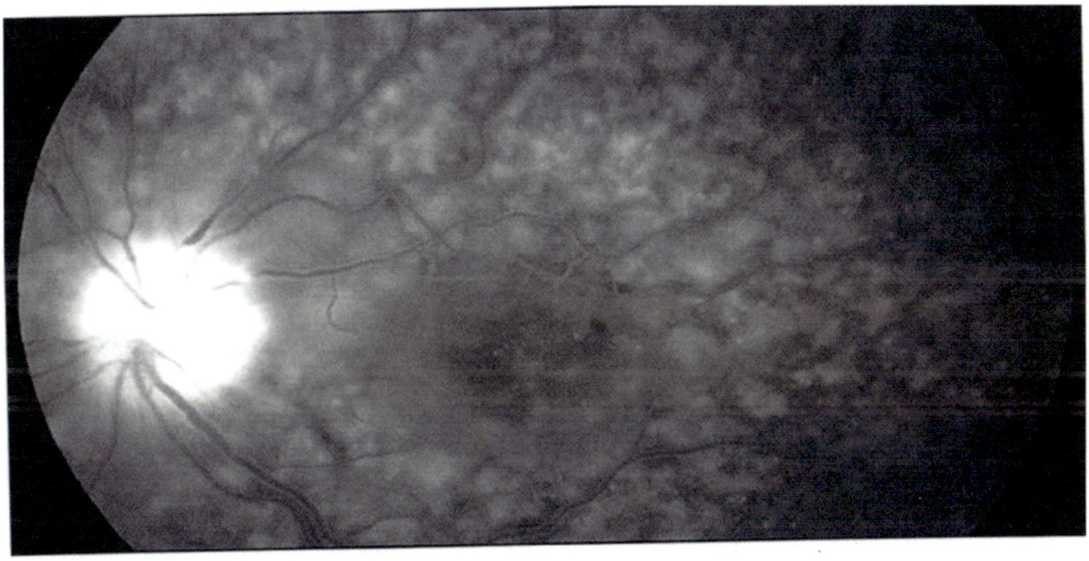

Figure 173: Same patient as in Figure 158. Characteristic "starry-night appearance" with late-stage optic disc hyperfluorescence as revealed by fluorescein angiography.

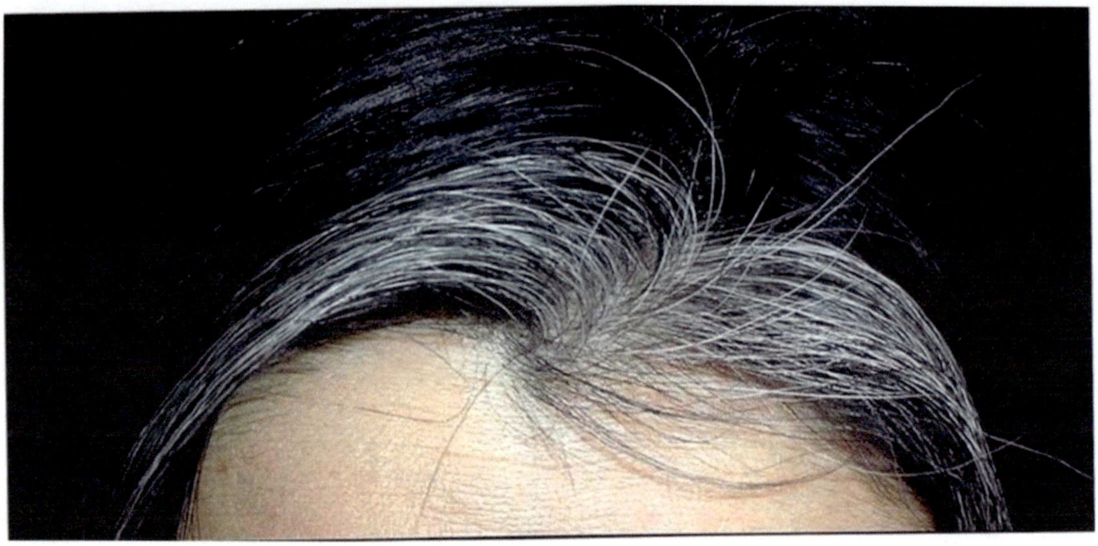

Figure 174: Characteristic white forelock of hair as seen in a patient with VKH.

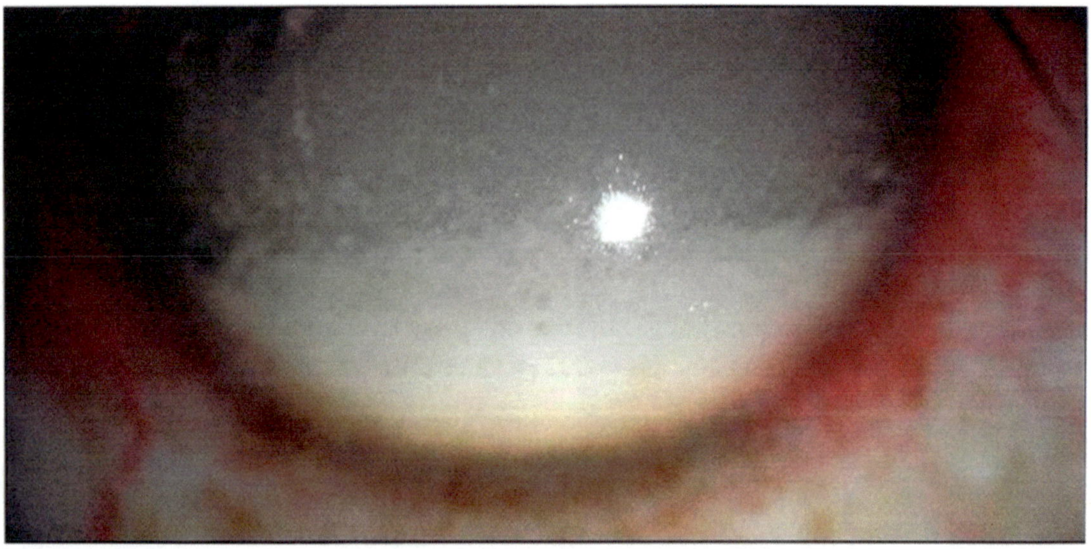

Figure 175: Anterior chamber deposition of triamcinolone acetonide secondary to Vogt-Koyanagi-Harada syndrome-related hypopyon.

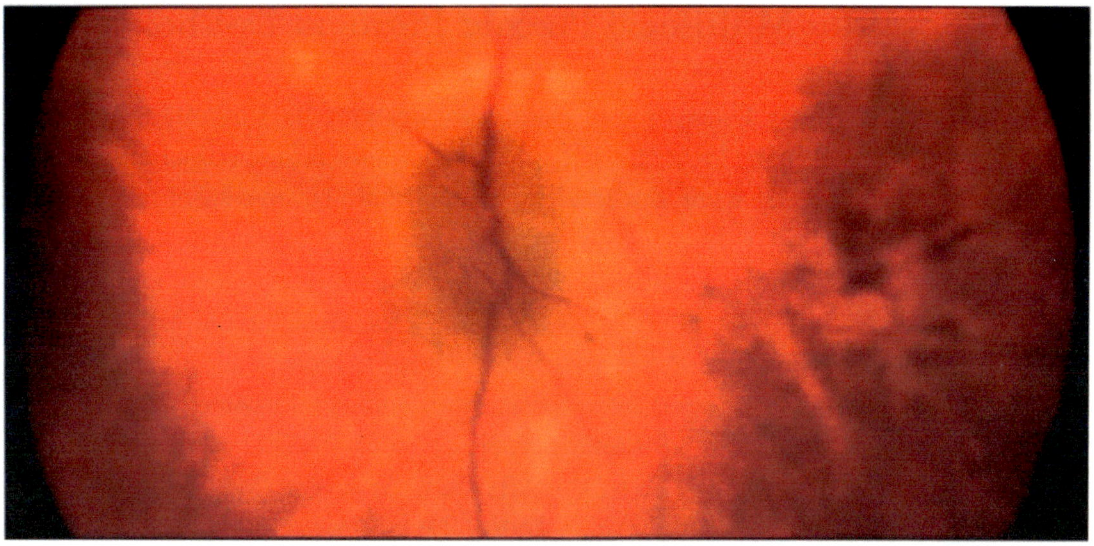

Figure 176: Depigmentation of the choroid causing the characteristic "sunset-glow" appearance of the fundus in an eye affected by Vogt-Koyanagi-Harada syndrome.

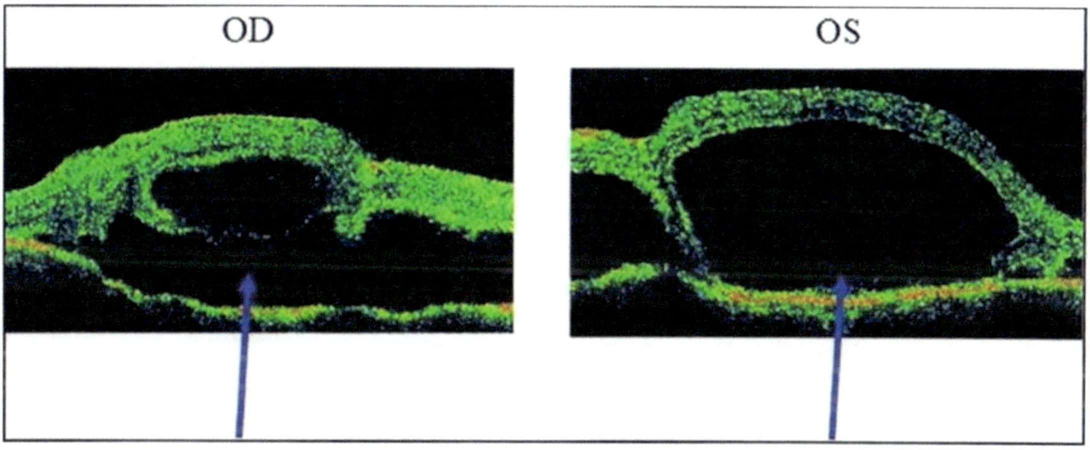

Figure 177: Massive amounts of serous fluid which has disrupted the retinal architecture.

Acute Posterior Multifocal Placoid Pigment Epitheliopathy

White Dot Syndromes: These unique entities are characterized by multiple whitish-yellow inflammatory lesions located at the level of the outer retina, retinal pigment epithelium, and choroid. The white dot syndromes may share some clinical features. The majority of individuals are less than 50 years of age with exception of BSRC and serpiginous choroiditis. MEWDS, BSRC, and MFC occur most frequently among women. They can be unilateral (DUSN, MEWDS) or bilateral (APMPPE, BSRC, MCP, serpiginous choroiditis). Positive ocular complaints include blurry vision, visual field loss (blind spot enlargement), photopsias, nyctalopia, and floaters. Mild presence of posterior vitreous cells can be found, except in cases of BSRC and MCP. The degree of ocular inflammation can be subtle (MEWDS) or severe (MCP). The white dot lesions may be discrete (MEWDS, MCP, BSRC, DUSN) or more placoid in appearance (APMPPE and serpiginous choroiditis).

Introduction: APMPPE is an inflammatory chorioretinal disease characterized by a sudden loss of vision caused by acute inflammatory lesions that are typically yellowish-white at the level of the retinal pigment epithelium and the choriocapillaris.

Gass was the first to describe this clinical entity in 1968. He reported three cases. Maumenee in 1970 reported six females, who presented with sudden central visual loss associated with similar clinical findings as those described by Gass. In a large epidemiologic study, APMPPE patients only accounted for 2% of those with posterior uveitis. It commonly presents in patients between the ages of 20 and 50 years with no sex predilection.

Pathophysiology: The prodromal illness characterized by flu-like symptoms may indicate a viral-triggered autoimmune response. Some patients have developed APMPPE after swine flu vaccination, hepatitis B vaccination, mumps, or bacterial infection. Associations with HLA-B7 and HLA-DR2 also have been reported.

Clinical features: APMPPE produces a rapid onset of blurred vision associated with central and paracentral scotomas that can be asymmetrical. The fellow eye usually becomes involved within a few days. Approximately one-third of individuals report a pre-existing viral illness. Patients may complain of headache, fever, malaise, myalgia or upper respiratory symptoms weeks before the onset of eye symptoms. Mild vitreous cells are usually present. Bilateral, multifocal yellowish-white placoid lesions, usually less than 1 disc diameter in size, are located primarily in the posterior pole at the level of the retinal pigment epithelium. The lesions fade gradually over the course of 1 to 2 weeks. Atypical findings include papillitis, periphlebitis, central retinal vein occlusion, disc neovascularization, exudative neurosensory retinal detachment, and subhyaloid hemorrhage.

Most individuals have a good visual prognosis, with spontaneous recovery of visual acuity to 20/40 or better within 3 to 6 weeks. Although extremely rare, there are reports of death associated with central nervous system vasculitis that developed within several weeks after the onset of APMPPE.

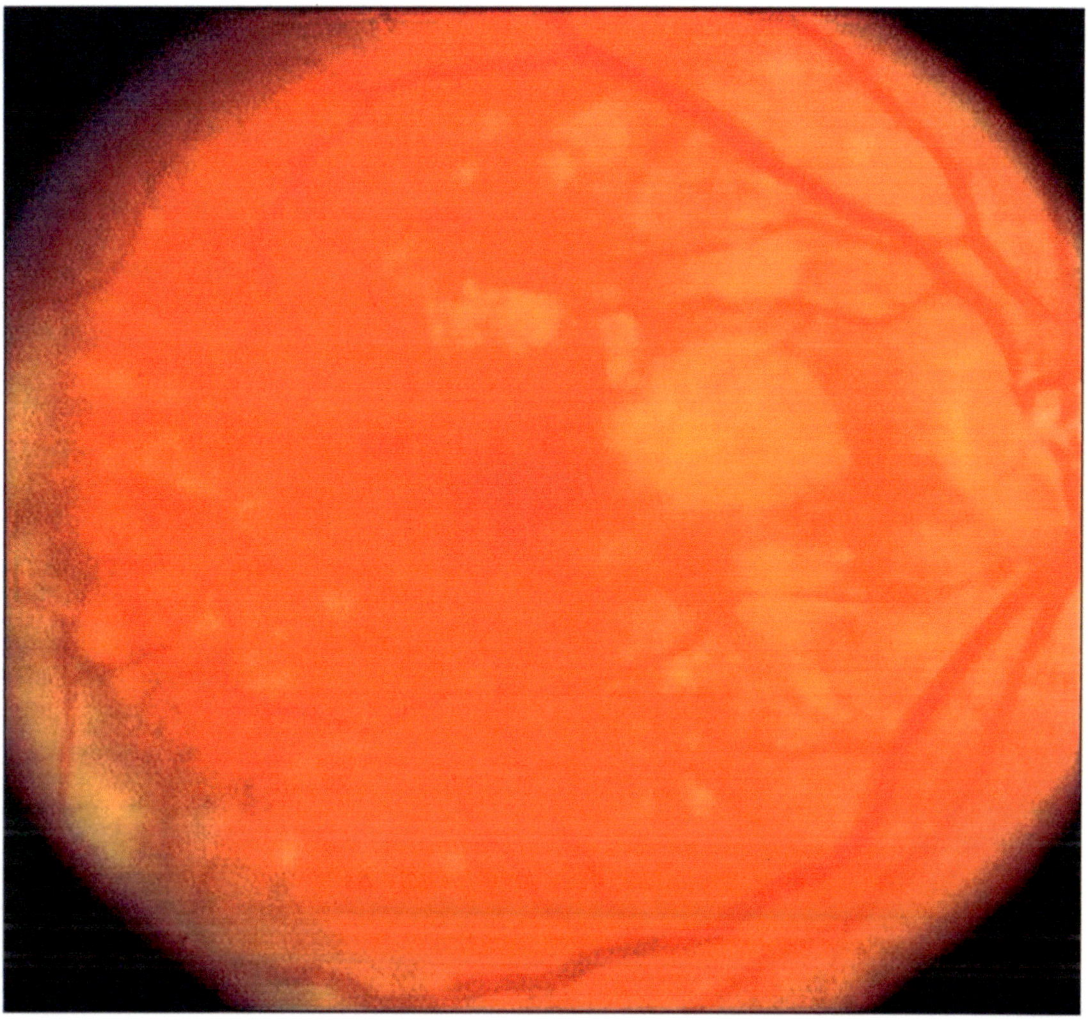

Figure 178: Numerous discrete yellow lesions involving the macula and peripheral retina in a patient with APMPPE.

Diagnosis: The diagnosis is clinically supported by a thorough diagnostic evaluation including medical history, review of systems, and meticulous ocular examination. Fluorescein angiography (FA) reveals typical early hypofluorescence and late staining. If a patient relates the presence of neurologic symptoms, magnetic resonance or computed tomography along with cerebrospinal fluid analysis is advised to rule out CNS involvement.

Treatment: APMPPE has a self-limiting clinical course. Without treatment, 80% of the patients obtain 20/40 visual acuity. Steroid systemic therapy may reasonably be considered for the treatment of APMPPE, especially for those with macular involvement.

References:

1) Gass JDM. Acute posterior multifocal posterior placoid pigment epitheliopathy. *Arch Ophthalmol* 1968;80:177-185
2) Maumenee AE. Clinical entities in "uveitis": An approach to the study of intraocular inflammation. *Am J Ophthalmol* 1970;69:1-27
3) Rodriguez A. Calongne M, Pedroza-Seres M, et al. Referral Patterns of uveitis in a tertiary eye care center. *Arch Ophthalmol* 1996;114:593-599
4) Hector RE. Acute posterior multifocal placoid pigment epitheliopathy, *Am J Ophthalmol* 1978; 86:424-425
5) Brezin AP, Massin-Korobelnik P, Boudin M, et al. Acute posterior multifocal placoid pigment epitheliopathy after hepatitis B vaccine. *Arch Ophthalmol* 1995:113:297-300

Acute Zonal Occult Outer Retinopathy (AZOOR)

Introduction: Acute zonal occult outer retinopathy (AZOOR) is the acute loss of outer retinal function in one or more zones associated with photopsia, mild vitritis, blind spot enlargement, electroretinographic abnormalities, and minimal initial fundoscopic changes in one or both eyes.

The term acute zonal occult outer retinopathy was coined by Gass in 1993 when he reported 13 cases, predominantly women, with an acute loss of the outer retinal function in one or more zones. AZOOR occurs in young to middle aged patients with higher frequency in young myopic women. It is bilateral on long-term follow-up in 76% of the cases.

Pathophysiology: AZOOR is an inflammatory autoimmune disease of unknown etiology. Gass speculated about a viral infection causing acute retinal dysfunction.

Clinical Manifestations: Patients with AZOOR experience an acute visual field loss and photopsias in one or both eyes. Classical photopsias in AZOOR can be described as moving colors or lights within the area of visual field loss. Symptoms may be exacerbated by bright light, exercise, stress, and fatigue. Mild vitritis is present in 50% of the cases. Optic disc edema can be present, but is rare. Retinal pigment epithelial atrophy and intraretinal pigment migration (retinitis pigmentosa-like fundus) in the areas of visual field loss can occur in advanced stages. AZOOR can be associated with cerebrospinal pleocytosis and brain magnetic resonance imaging abnormalities.

Diagnosis: The diagnosis can be challenging as most of the patients do not have retinal findings in early stages. Suggestive findings on ancillary testing include:

Visual fields: Show progressive loss involving mainly the blind spot and temporal field. In late stages, the defect can include most of the central field and move towards the periphery.

Fluorescein angiography: shows no abnormalities in patients with AZOOR.

ERG: May show both rod or cone photoreceptor dysfunction with delayed 30-Hz-flicker latency. This is helpful in making the diagnosis in the presence of classic symptomatology.

Treatment: No effective treatment for AZOOR is available to date and the disease can have a variable course and outcome. Gass reported best corrected visual acuity of 20/40 or better in 88% of patients in at least one eye on final follow-up. He also reported the stabilization of visual field loss in 78% and improvement of the visual field in 20% of patients with AZOOR within the first 6 months.

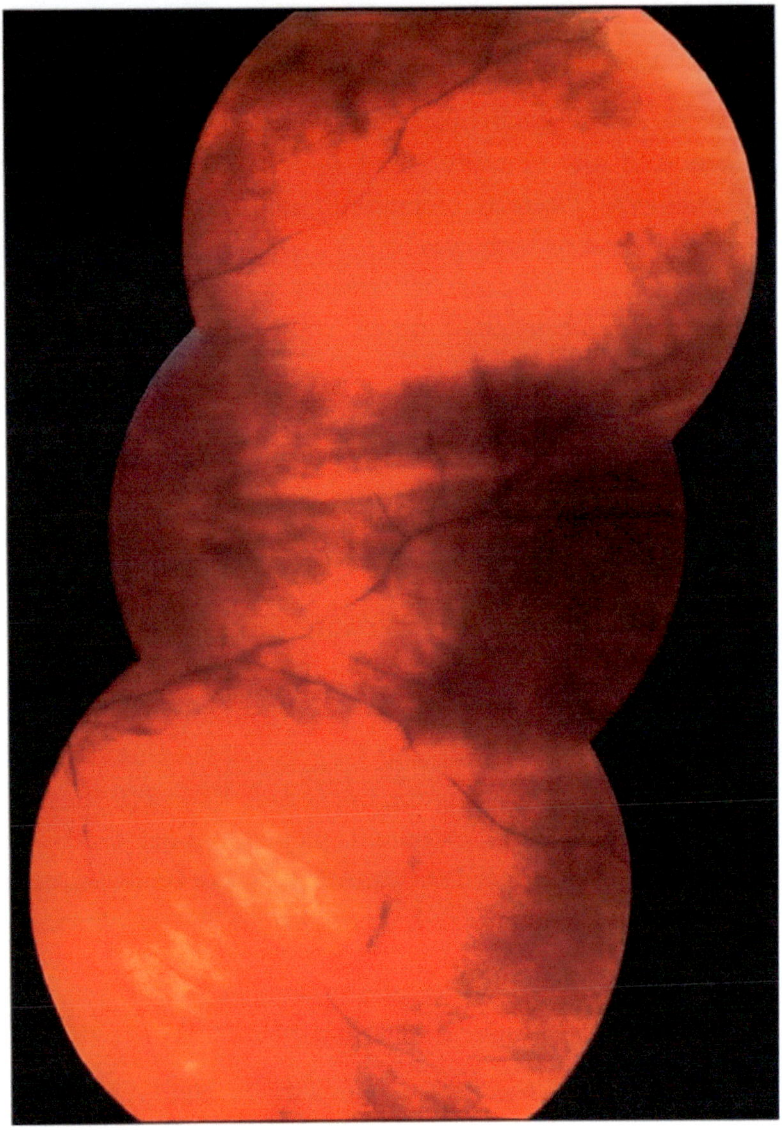

Figure 179: Area of demarcation in the temporal periphery of the left eye in a 38 year-old male with AZOOR. The patient also complained of a scotoma of varying size.

References:

1) Gass JD. Acute zonal occult outer retinopathy. Donders Lecture: The Netherlands Ophthalmological Society, Maastricht, Holland, June 19, 1992. *J Clin Neuroophthalmol.* 1993 Jun;13 : 79-97.
3) Jacobson DM. Acute zonal occult outer retinopathy and central nervous system inflammation. *J Neuroophthalmol.* 1996 Sep;16 (3):172-7.
4) Gass JDM. *Stereoscopic Atlas of Macular Diseases: Diagnosis and Treatment*, vol 2, 4th ed. St. Louis, CV Mosby, 1997, pp 682-687.
7) Gass JDM, Agarwal A, Scott IU. Acute zonal occult outer retinopathy: a long-term follow-up study. *Am J Ophthalmol* 2002;134:329-339.
8) Fekrat S, Wilkinson CP, Chang B, et al. Acute annular outer retinopathy (AAOR). *Am J Ophthalmol* 2000;130: 636-44

Birdshot Retinochoroidopathy

Introduction: BSRC is a chronic intraocular inflammatory disease manifesting as vitritis and multiple bilateral hypopigmented and postequatorial fundus lesions. Ryan and Maumenee described this disease entity in 1980 as a distinctive, posterior uveitis that included the presence of multiple depigmented spots at the level of the choroid and retinal pigment epithelium in 13 patients. It represents an uncommon disease that accounts for only about 8% of all cases of posterior uveitis. BSRC typically occurs during middle age, and is almost exclusively present in the Caucasian population, with a high incidence in those of northern European descent. Women are affected in 70% of the cases.

Pathophysiology: HLA-A29 is found in up to 98% of the cases. The relative risk for diseasc development of an individual who has HLA-A29 ranges from 50 to 224 times greater than with other phenotypes.

Clinical Features: Patients often complain of poor vision despite good visual acuity assessment. Nyctalopia and paracentral scotomas are common. Patients can also experience floaters, photopsias, and problems with color vision. Anterior segment inflammation is generally minimal or absent Vitritis is moderate and present in all cases. The yellowish-orange lesions with indistinct borders that appear to radiate from the optic nerve head are the most reliable diagnostic features. The spots are seen mainly in the nasal retina and are symmetrically distributed in both eyes. Retinal vasculitis is an important component of the disorder. Retinal hemorrhaging or exudation is rare and most of the retinal vascular change is limited to arteriolar and venular narrowing. Macular edema is the most common complication of BSRC and occurs in 50% of the cases. Progressive optic nerve pallor often indistinguishable from glaucoma is characteristic of chronic disease. Choroidal neovascularization can occur as a consequence of disruption of Bruch's membrane.

Diagnosis: The presence of a moderate vitritis and cystoid macular edema without pars plana exudation is suggestive of the diagnosis of BSRC. Fluorescein (FA) and indocyanine green angiography (ICGA) are two exceptional tools to document BSRC pathology and progression. FA may detect active leakage along the retinal vessels and cystoid or diffuse macular edema. Prolonged fluorescein arterio-venous transit times seem to be a characteristic feature of BSRC that does not however reflect the actual intravascular hemodynamics. ICGA reveals areas of blockage in the early to mid-phases of the angiogram, which may persist into the late stages. Electroretinography (ERG) is usually abnormal with reduced rod and cone amplitudes and increased latencies. The ERG is useful to monitor disease activity.

<u>Treatment:</u> Require long-term immunomodulatory therapy. Dramatic response to high-dose oral or periocular steroids is observed, but corticosteroids do not induce durable remission.

References:

1) Ryan SJ, Maumenee AE. Birdshot retinochoroidopathy. *Am J Ophthalmol.* 198o Jan;89(1):31-45.
2) Rodriguez A. Calongne M, Pedroza-Seres M, et al. Referral Patterns of uveitis in a tertiary eye care center. *Arch Ophthalmol* 1996;114:593-599
3) Priem H. [Vascular manifestations in birdshot chorioretinopathy] *Bull Soc Belge Ophtalmol.* 1989;230:41-8.
4) Nussenblatt RB, Whicup SM, Palestine AG. Birdshot retinochoroidopathy. In: Nussenblatt RB, Whicup SM, Pelastine AG, eds: *Uveitis: Fundamentals and Clinical Practice*, 2nd ed. St Louis, Mosby Year Book, 1996, p 325
5) Cassoux N, Lehoang P. [Birdshot retinochoroidopathy]. *Ann Med Interne* (Paris) 2000;151(1 Suppl):S45-S47.
6) Fardeau C, Herbort CP, Kullmann N, et al. Indocyanine green angiography in birdshot chorioretinopathy. *Ophthalmology* 1999;106: 1928-1934.
7) Zacks DN, Samson CM, Loewenstein J, Foster CS. Electroretinograms as an indicator of disease activity in birdshot retinochoroidopathy. Graefes *Arch Clin Exp Ophthalmol* 2002;240:601-607.

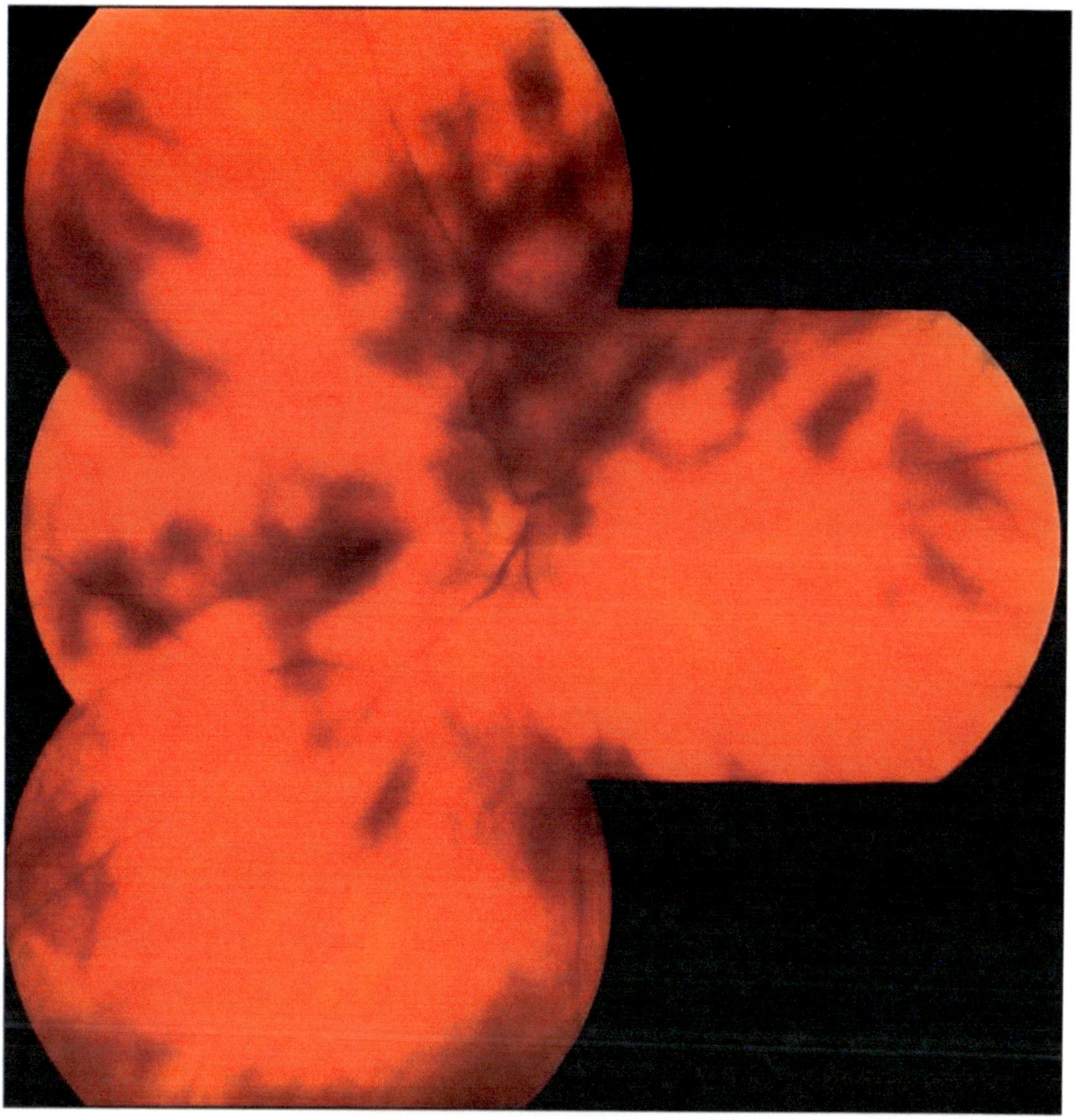

Figure 180: Characteristic cream-colored, scattered lesions in birdshot retinochoroidopathy.

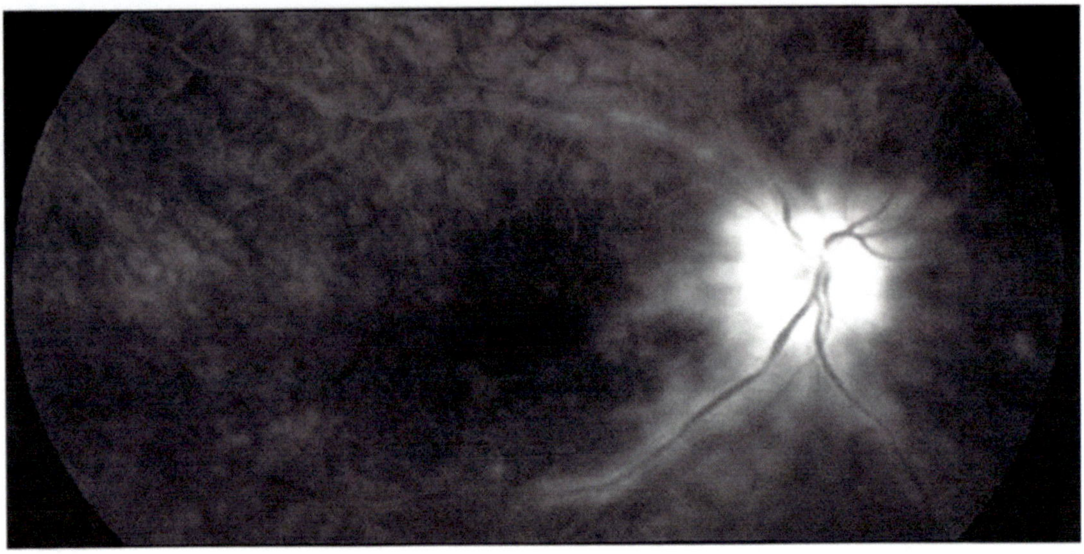

Figure 181: Papillitis and vasculitis predominantly along the inferior arcade in a forty-seven year old white female with birdshot BSRC.

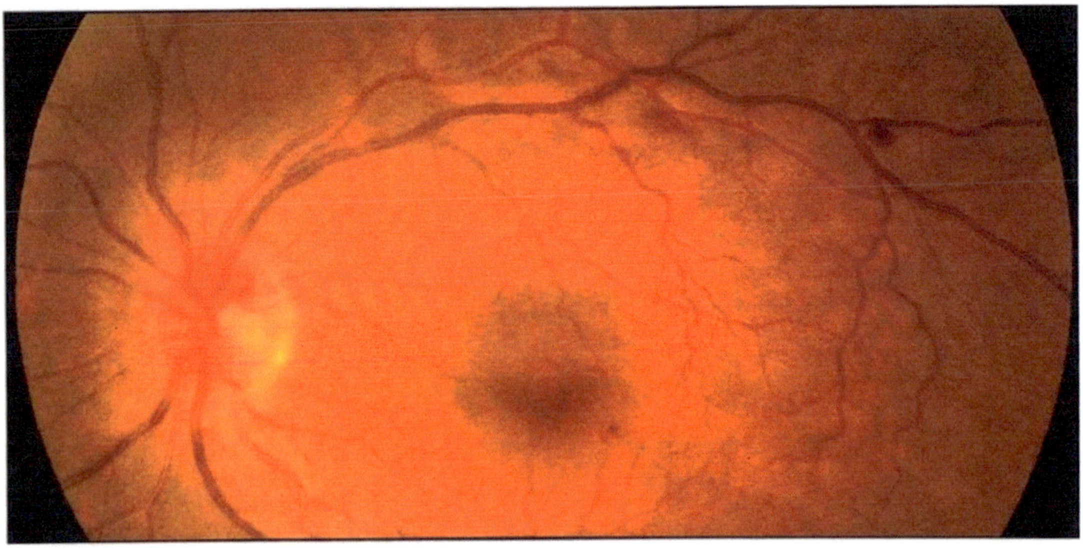

Figure 182: Intraretinal hemorrhages alongside the superior arcade in a patient with BSRC.

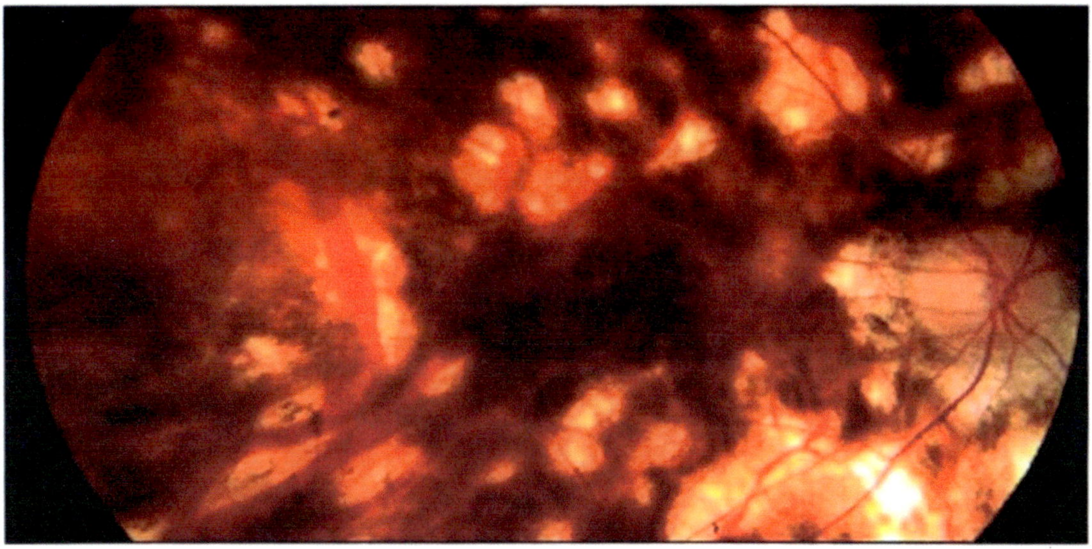

Figure 183: Vessel attenuation, peripapillary atrophy, and diffuse, extreme retinal pigment epithelium atrophy in a patient with birdshot retinochoroidopathy.

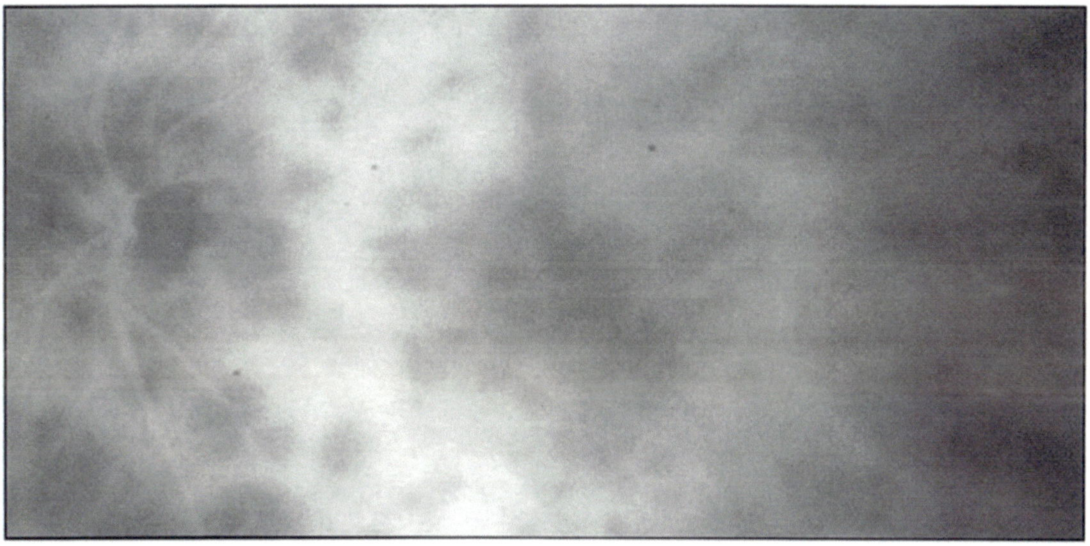

Figure 184: Typical appearance of BSRC during the mid-phase of the ICG study.

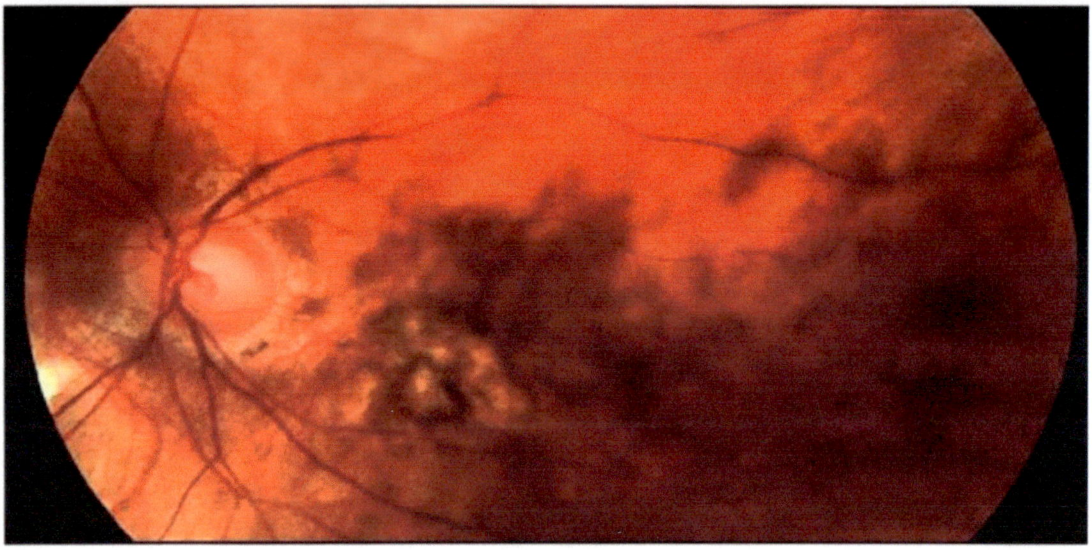

Figure 185: Old choroidal neovascular membrane in a patient with birdshot retinochoroidopathy. Note the myopic disc tilt, peripapillary atrophy, and inferior atrophic birdshot lesions.

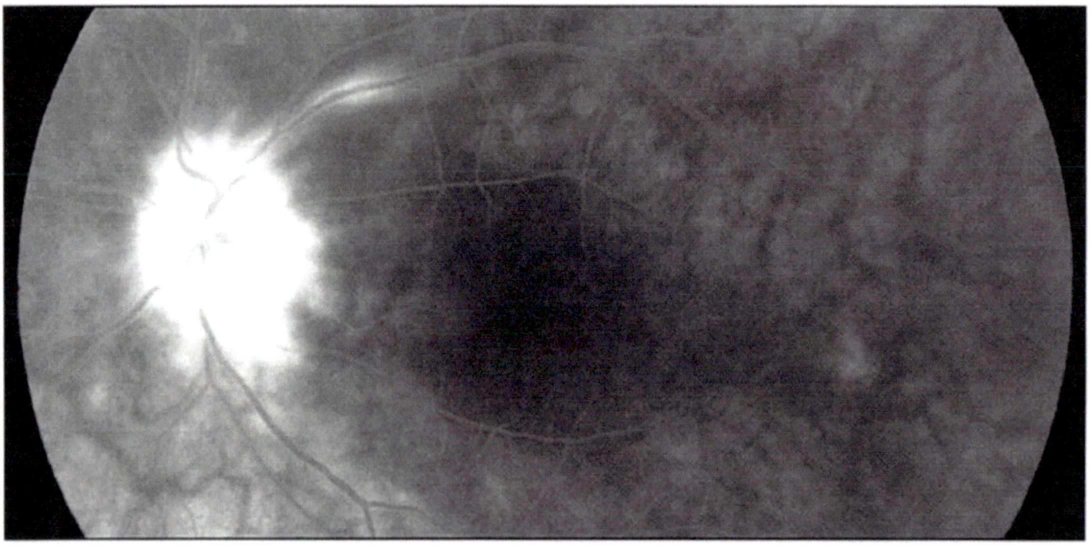

Figure 186: Late-phase fluorescein angiogram demonstrating optic disc staining and vasculitis along the superior vein in BSRC.

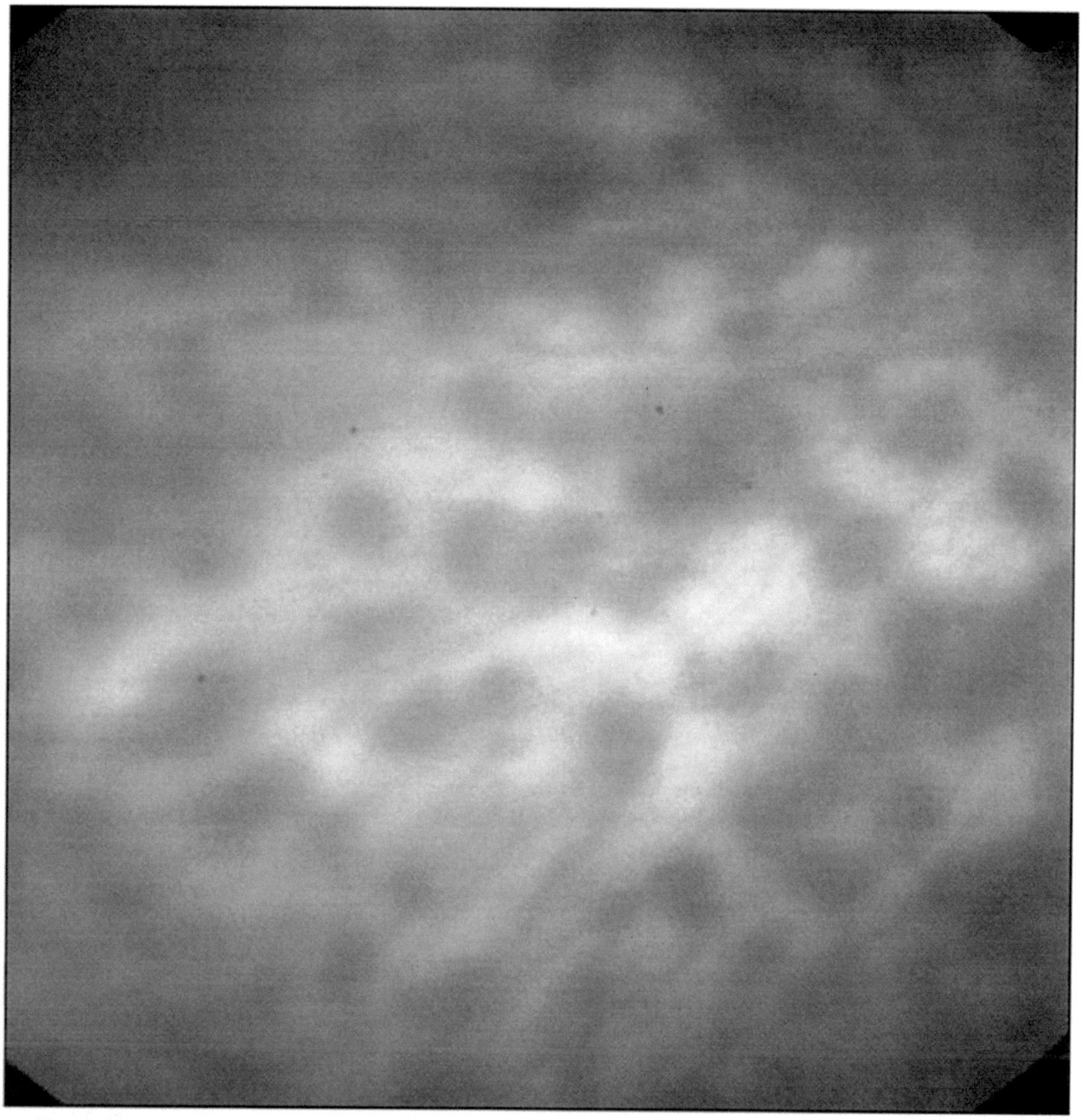

Figure 187 Scattered birdshot lesions in the peripheral fundus during an ICG angiogram, which are not as numerous clinically or on FA.

Multifocal Choroiditis and Panuveitis

Introduction: Multifocal choroiditis and panuveitis (MCP) is a chorioretinal inflammatory disease of unknown etiology associated with significant vitritis and anterior segment inflammation.

It was first described by Nozik and Dorsch in 1973 in two cases with bilateral inflammatory chorioretinopathy and anterior uveitis that resembled (the chorioretinal lesions) presumed ocular histoplasmosis syndrome.

MCP is commonly seen in young adults in their third decade of life. The ratio of females to males is 3:1. There is no racial or geographical predilection.

Pathophysiology: The pathogenesis of this disease is unknown. One hypothesis is that the presence of an inciting external agent (viral, bacterial, etc.) triggers the inflammatory process.

Clinical Manifestations: The common features are bilateral vitreous inflammation, anterior uveitis, and active choroidal lesions. Some cases are asymmetric. Some eyes with MCP can also develop diffuse subretinal fibrosis (DSF) in the late stage of the disease. DSF is characterized by a coalescence of lesions and broad zones of subretinal fibrosis. Patients chiefly complain of decreased vision and floaters (as a consequence of vitritis). The main cause of decreased vision includes choroidal lesions beneath the macula, macular edema, and choroidal neovascularization in the macular area. DSF and retinal pigment epithelium hyperplasia and metaplasia also are important components that lead to decreased visual acuity. Punched-out chorioretinal scars with pigmented borders within the posterior pole and periphery are typically found in patients with MCP. These lesions are usually 50 μm to 100 μm in diameter.

Diagnosis: The diagnosis is clinical. Fluorescein angiography: Shows lesions within the macula, which are not visible clinically. Acute lesions show early hypofluorescence with late hyperfluorescent staining as in other white dot syndrome lesions. Macular edema, leakage from acute lesions within the macula, and choroidal neovascularization arising from juxtapapillary or macular scars might also be present.

Visual Field testing: Shows an enlarged blind spot.

Indocyanine green angiography: Can be useful in detecting lesions that are undetectable by other means. Lesions may be more numerous and extensive on indocyanine green angiography compared to fluorescein angiography.

Treatment: Corticosteroids by oral and periocular route are effective in the acute control of intraocular inflammation and prevention of permanent visual loss in some patients with MCP. Immunomodulatory therapy including methotrexate, azathioprine, cyclosporine, cyclophosphamide, chlorambucil, tacrolimus, and mycophenolate mofetil have been effective in treating patients with MCP.

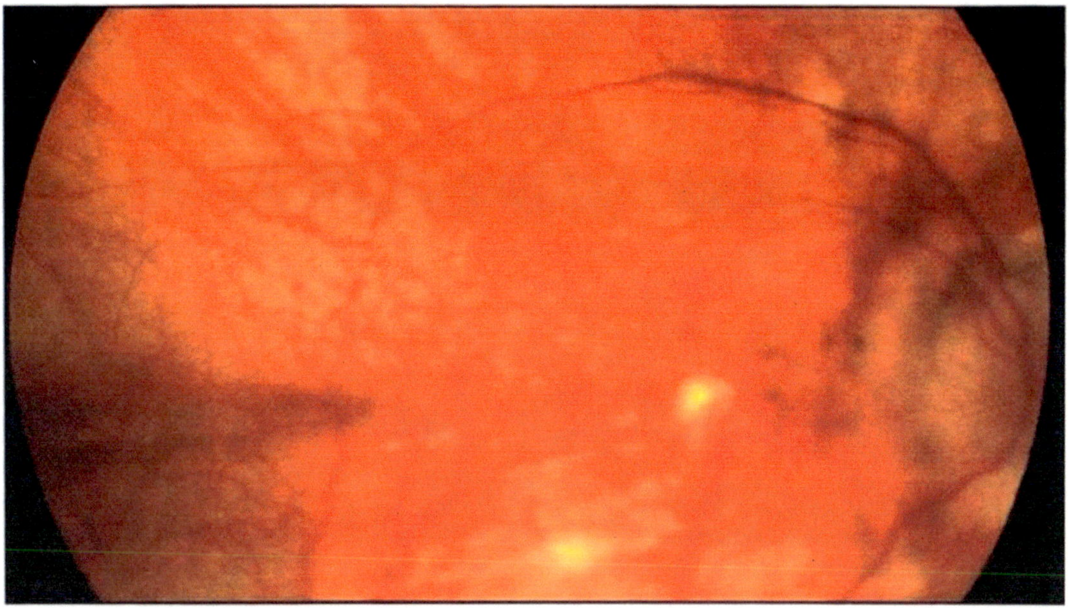

<u>Figure 188:</u> Multifocal lesions of choroidal inflammation with associated retinal striae, prominent choroidal vasculature, and extensive peripapillary atrophy.

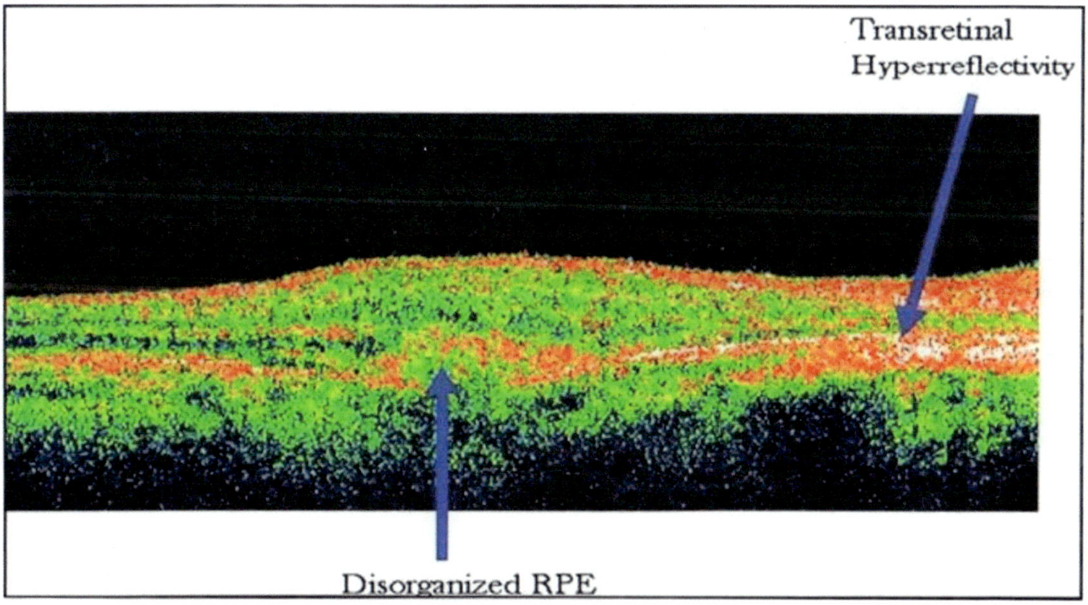

<u>Figure 189:</u> Active Multifocal Choroiditis and Panuveitis on OCT.

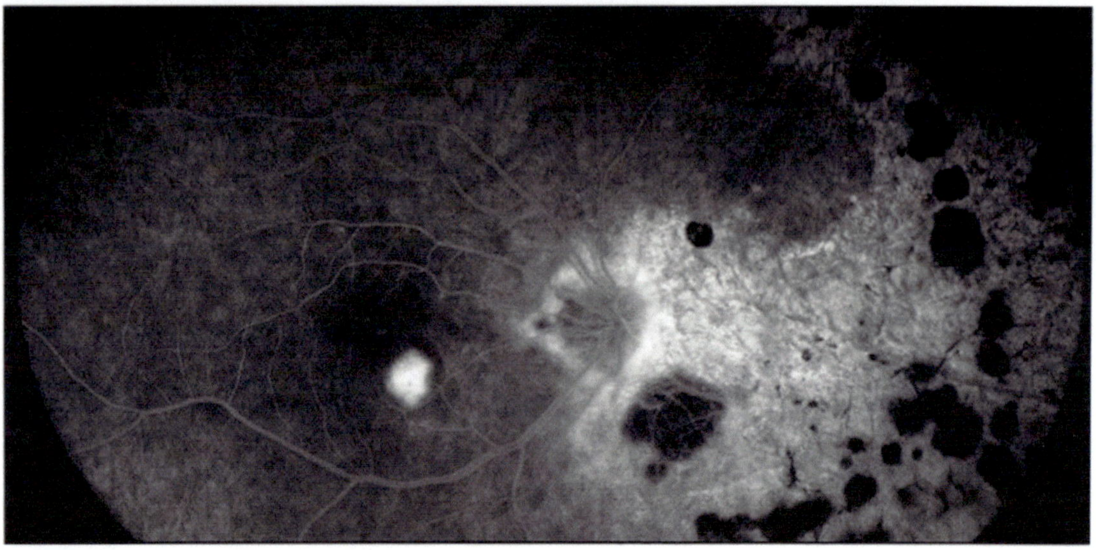

Figure 190: Old, diffuse chorioretinal scarring nasal to the optic disc and active choroidal neovascular membrane in a patient with multifocal choroiditis and panuveitis.

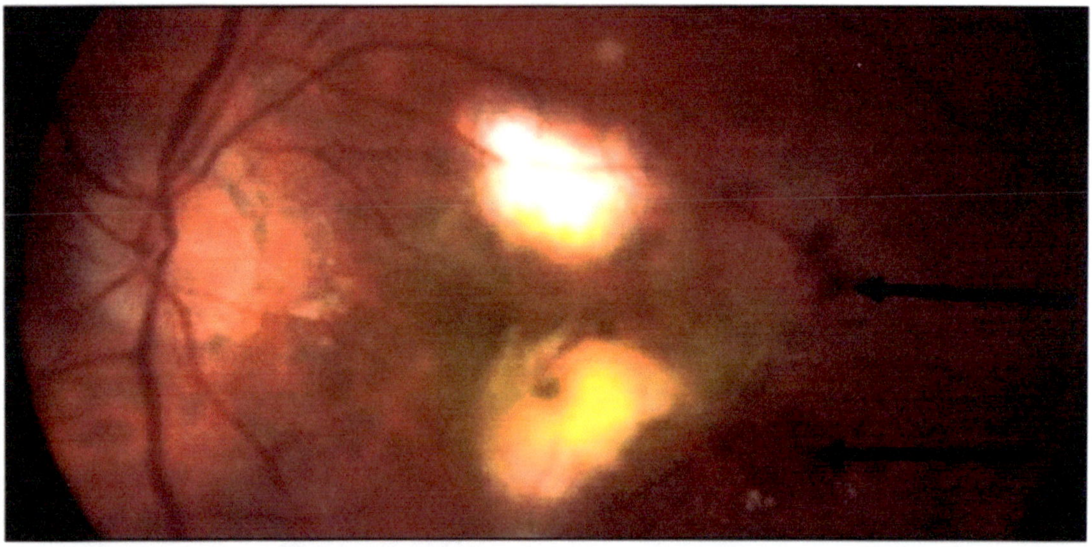

Figure 191: Two large areas of subretinal fibrosis in a patient affected by multifocal choroiditis and panuveitis. Note the areas of hemorrhages.

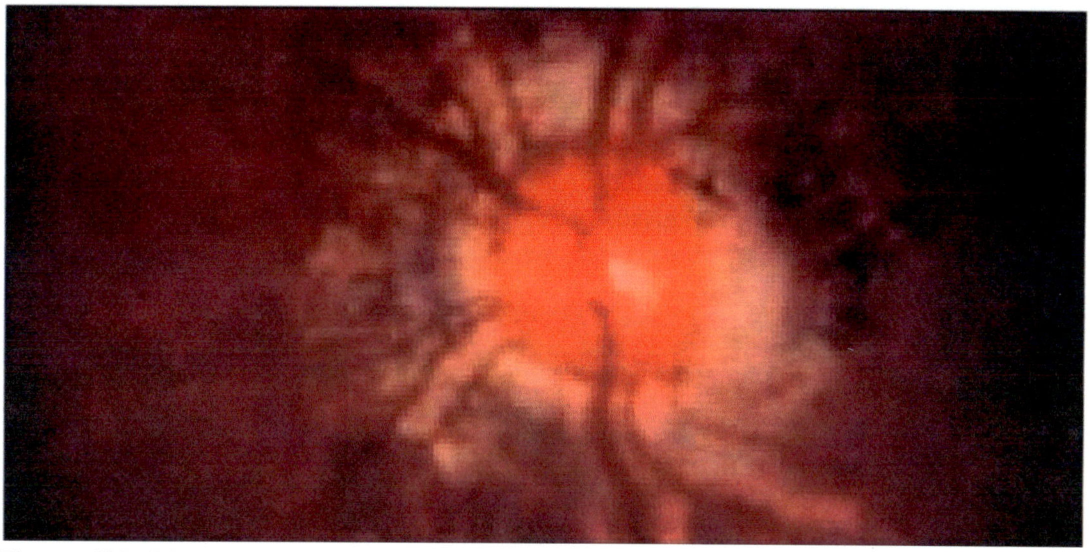

Figure 192: Most patients with MCP develop peripapillary scarring similar to that seen in POHS.

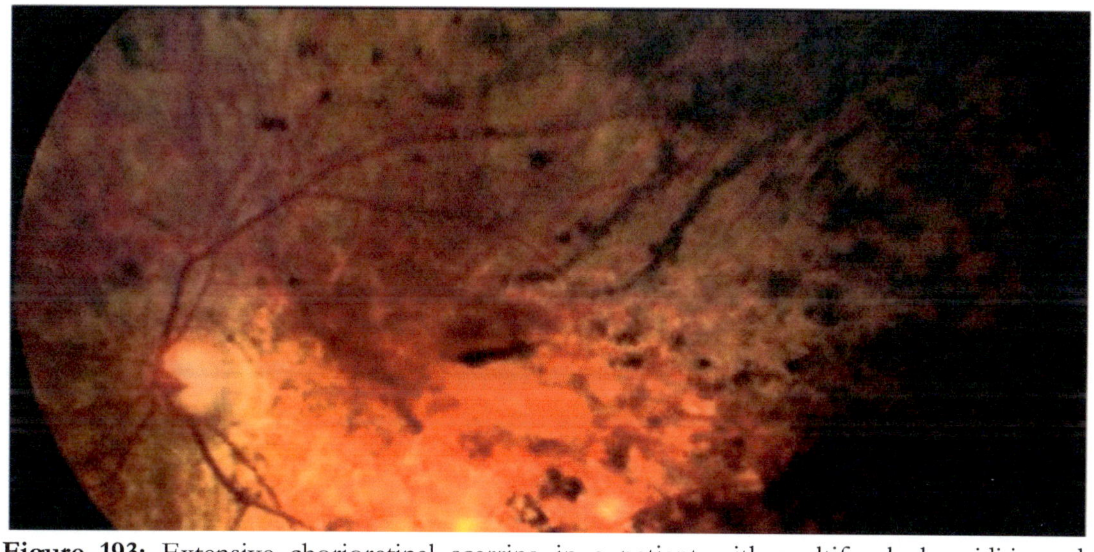

Figure 193: Extensive chorioretinal scarring in a patient with multifocal choroiditis and panuveitis.

References:

1) Nozik RA, Dorsch W. A new chorioretinopathy associated with anterior uveitis. *Am J Ophthalmol.* 1973 Nov;76(5):758-62.
2) Dreyer RF, Gass JDM. Multifocal choroiditis and panuveitis: a syndrome that mimics ocular histoplasmosis. *Arch Ophthalmol* 1984;102: 1776-1784.
3) Morgan CM, Schatz H. Recurrent multifocal choroiditis. *Ophthalmology* 1986;93:1138-1147.
4) Cantrill HL, Folk JC. Multifocal choroiditis associated with progressive subretinal fibrosis. *Am J Ophthalmol* 1986;15:101:170-180.
5) Brown J Jr., Folk JC, Reddy CV, Kimura AE. Visual prognosis of multifocal choroiditis, punctate inner choroidopathy, and the diffuse subretinal fibrosis syndrome. *Ophthalmology* 1996;103:1100-1105.
6) Reddy CV, Brown J Jr., Folk JC, Kimura AE, Gupta S, Walker J. Enlarged blind spots in chorioretinal inflammatory disorders. *Ophthalmology* 1996;103:606-617
7) Slakter JS, Giovannini A, Yannuzzi LA, Scassellati-Sforzolini B, Guyer DR, Sorenson JA, Spaide RF, Orlock D. Indocyanine green angiography of multifocal choroiditis. *Ophthalmology.* 1997 Nov;104(11):1813-9.
8) Oh KT, Folk JC, Maturi RK, Moore P, Kardon RH.Multifocal electroretinography in multifocal choroiditis and the multiple evanescent white dot syndrome. *Retina* 2001;21:581-589.
9) Michel SS, Ekong A, Baltatzis S, Foster CS. Multifocal choroiditis and panuveitis: immunomodulatory therapy. *Ophthalmology.* 2002 Feb;109(2):378-83

Multiple Evanescent White Dot Syndrome

Introduction: Multiple evanescent white dot syndrome (MEDWS) is an inflammatory disorder characterized by the presence of white lesions deep in the outer retina or at the retinal pigment epithelium.

Jampol and colleagues described this syndrome in 1984 in 11 young adults with transient visual loss associated with white dots in the fundus.

The mean age of presentation is 28 with a range of 17 to 47 years. Females are more affected than males with an approximate rate of 3:1 and with no race predilection.

Pathophysiology: The etiology of this disease is unknown. An infectious etiology has been postulated by the presence of flu-like symptoms that some patients experience before the onset of this disease that might trigger an autoimmune mechanism of inflammation. An elevation of serum IgM and IgG can also be present.

Clinical Manifestations: The main clinical feature is the presence of multiple small lesions ranging from 100 to 200 μm with a whitish-yellow color located over the posterior fundus, especially at the perifoveal and peripapillary regions. This disease is typically unilateral, but bilateral cases of MEWDS have been reported. The disease onset is sudden with blurred vision, temporal or paracentral scotomas, photopsias, and dyschromatopsia. A history of viral illness is present in one-third of the cases,. Initial visual acuity can range from 20/20 to 20/400. There is a slight tendency of myopia among affected patients. A relative afferent pupillary defect may be present. In most of the cases, a quiet anterior segment is evident. The grade of vitritis is commonly mild. Optic nerve inflammation can be present. The lesions are multiple small, well-defined white dots located at the level of the outer retina or retinal pigment epithelium. The fovea may have a yellowish-orange granularity; this granularity may persist after resolution of the white dot lesions. Patients may develop choroidal neovascularization. Visual field testing reveals enlargement of the blind spot and temporal or paracentral scotomas as well.

Diagnosis: Fluorescein angiography is a useful diagnostic tool that demonstrates the classic early and late hyperfluorescence of the white dots. Late-phase hyperfluorescence of the optic head disc can be also present during the acute stage of the disease. On indocyanine green angiography, the number of spots may be more numerous than those seen clinically or with fluorescein angiography. Electrophysiology testing may demonstrate a reduced a-wave on the ERG. The EOG may be subnormal. The ERG and EOG changes can improve after the total remission of the disease.

Treatment: The disease is self-limiting and requires no specific treatment. Most of the patients retain good visual acuity.

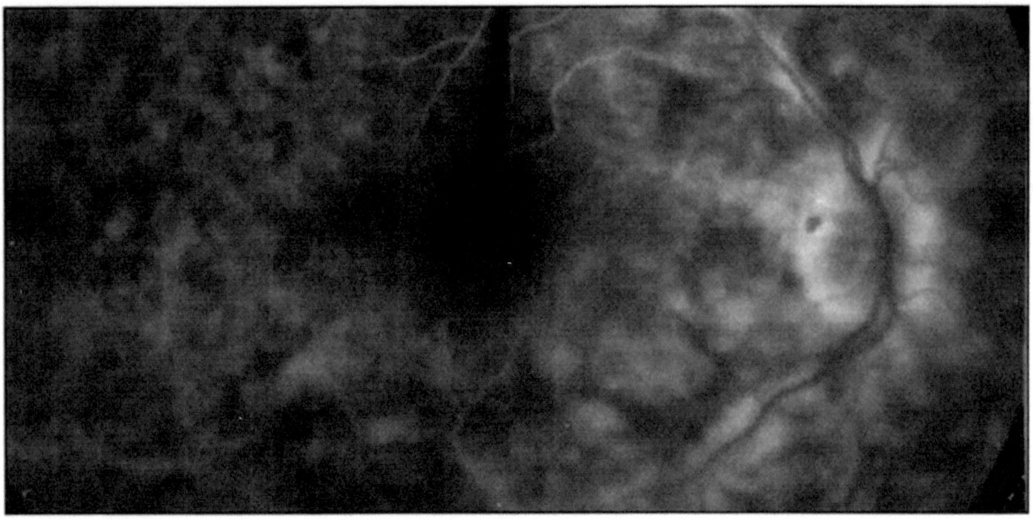

Figure 194: Mid-phase fluorescein angiogram of a patient with MEWDS. Note the optic disc hyperfluorescence and vasculitis.

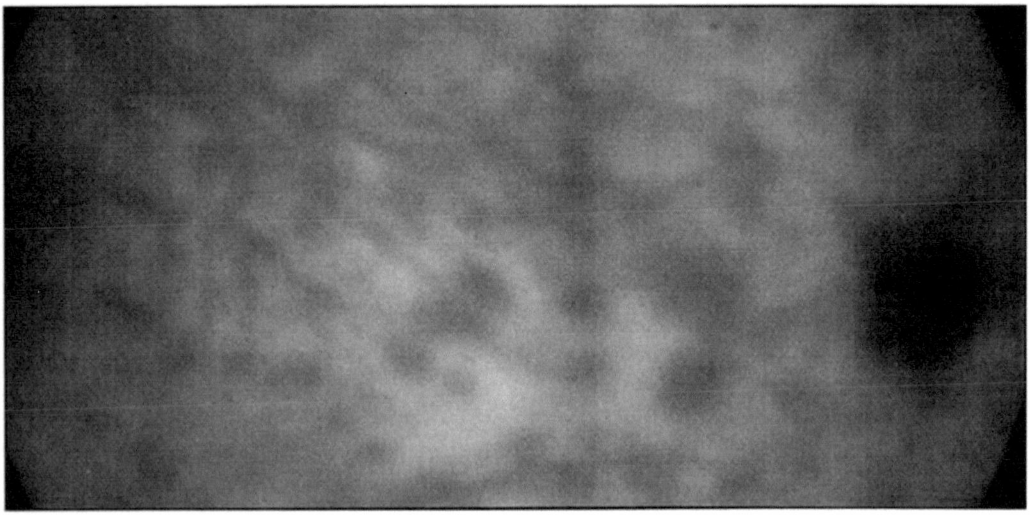

Figure 195: Late-phase indocyanine green angiography demonstrating multiple hypofluorescent spots in the paramacular region seen in multiple evanescent white dot syndrome. These same spots appear hyperfluorescent on clinical examination and FA.

References:

1) Jampol LM, Sieving PA, Pugh D, Fishman GA, Gilbert H. Multiple evanescent white dot syndrome. I. Clinical findings. *Arch Ophthalmol.* 1984 May;102(5):671-4.
2) Aaberg TM, Campo RV, Joffe L. Recurrences and bilaterality in the multiple evanescent white-dot syndrome. *Am J Ophthalmol* 1985; 100:29-37.
3) Oh KT, Christmas NJ, Russell SR. Late recurrence and choroidal neovascularization in multiple evanescent white dot syndrome. *Retina* 2001;21:182-184.
4) Chung YM, Yeh TS, Liu JH. Increased serum IgM and IgG in the multiple evanescent white-dot syndrome. *Am J Ophthalmol.* 1987 Aug 15; 104(2):187-8
5) Sieving PA, Fishman GA, Jampol LM, Pugh D. Multiple evanescent white dot syndrome. II. Electrophysiology of the photoreceptors during retinal pigment epithelial disease. *Arch Ophthalmol* 1984;102:675-679.

Punctate Inner Choroidopathy

Introduction: Punctate inner choroidopathy (PIC) is an autoimmune multifocal chorioretinopathy of unknown etiology.

In 1984, Watzke and co-workers described 10 patients, predominantly women, with moderate myopia, who presented with photopsias, paracentral scotomas, and blurry vision. Fundus examination revealed small, yellowish-white lesions at the level of the inner choroid with associated subretinal detachments. Most of the patients had bilateral disease.

The incidence of this disease is estimated to be about 100 to 200 cases per year. Many cases may be subclinical and these numbers may be underestimated. PIC tends to affect otherwise healthy white women with an average age of 27 to 30 years.

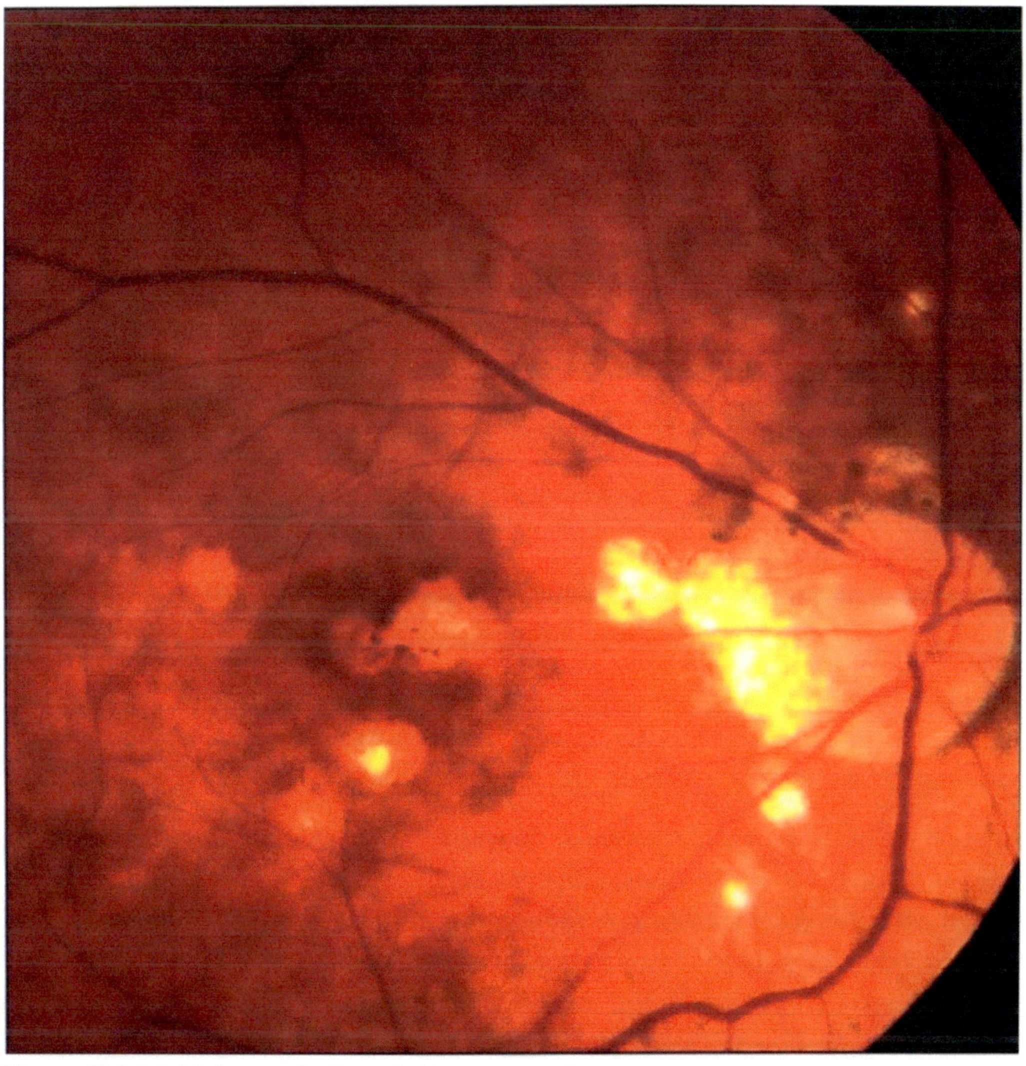

Figure 196: Multiple punched-out lesions as seen in punctate inner choroidopathy

Pathophysiology: The etiology is unknown. Histopathologic examination shows lymphocyte infiltration around the neovascular membranes.

Clinical Manifestations: At presentation, the main symptoms are blurry central vision and/or scotomas. These patients can also experience photopsias and floaters. Seventy-five percent of the patients have a visual acuity of 20/40 or better. Anterior segment examination reveals a quiet chamber. The absence of vitreous cells is a hallmark of PIC. The lesions are small and confined to the posterior pole at the level of the inner choroid and retinal pigment epithelium. Choroidal neovascularization develops in 69% of patients with PIC.

Diagnosis: A key feature to diagnose PIC is the absence of anterior or posterior segment inflammation. The absence of peripapillary atrophy also rules out presumed ocular histoplasmosis syndrome. The presence of serous detachments is also distinctive from similar entities, such as multiple evanescent white dot syndrome. During the acute phase, fluorescein angiography shows early hyperfluorescence and leakage in the late arterio-venous phase. Some lesions may also present early hypofluorescence and stain in the later phases. On indocyanine green angiography, PIC lesions may present as hypofluorescence in the posterior pole.

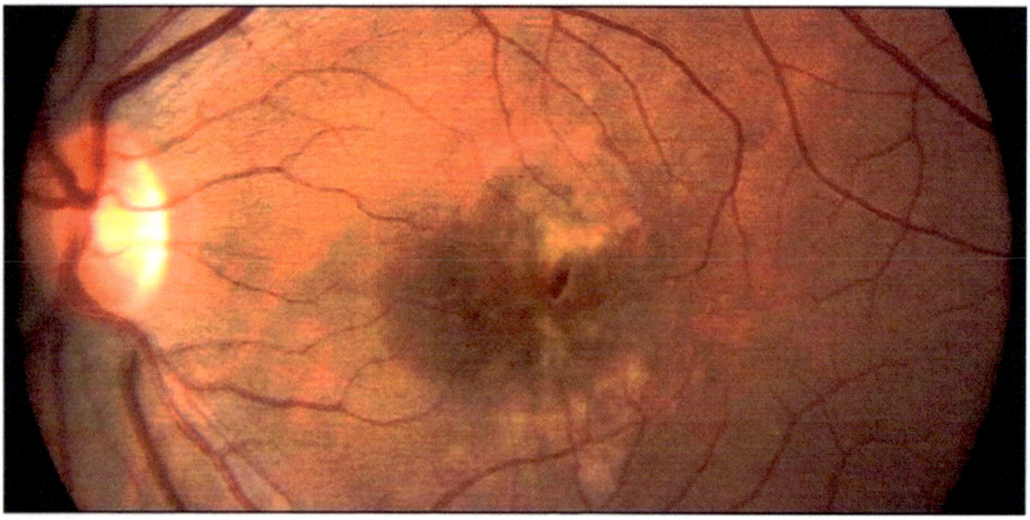

Figure 197: Twenty-three year-old myopic female with a fibrovascular choroidal neovascular membrane in the fovea as seen in punctate inner choroidopathy.

Treatment: In the absence of choroidal neovascularization, no treatment is advised since the prognosis is good. In cases with poor visual acuity (20/200 or less) at presentation, oral corticosteroids may be considered to prevent permanent visual loss and to prevent disruption of Bruch's membrane that may lead to choroidal neovascularization. Some experts also consider the use of immunomodulatory therapy for the prevention of disease relapse. Treatment options for choroidal neovascularization are thermal laser, photodynamic therapy, submacular surgery and intravitreal bevacizumab.

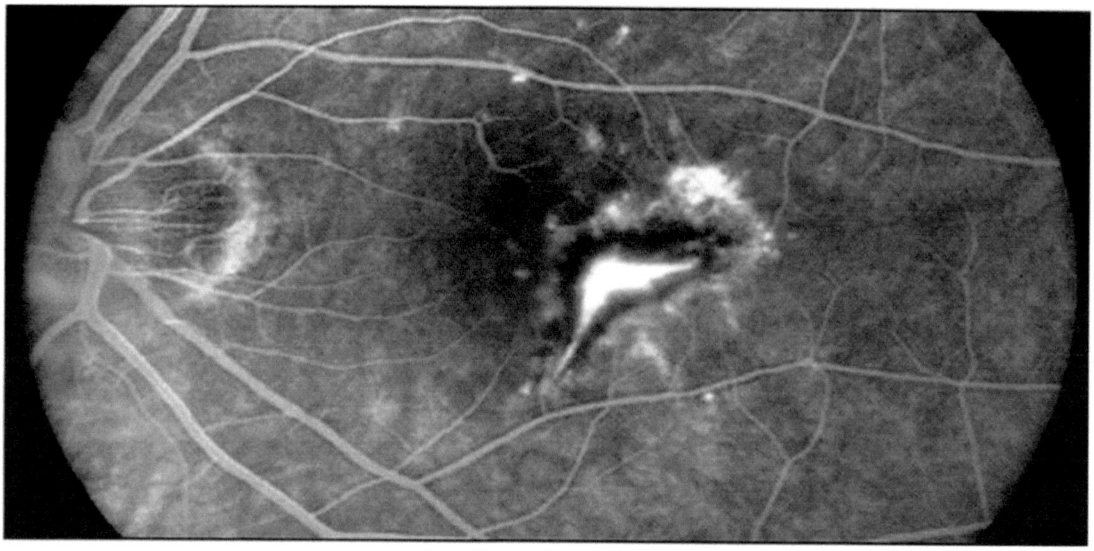

Figure 198: Choroidal neovascular membrane with faint atrophic spots in punctate inner choroidopathy.

References:

1) Watzke RC, Packer AJ, Folk JC, Benson WE, Burgess D, Ober RR. Punctate inner choroidopathy. *Am J Ophthalmol.* 1984 Nov;98 (5):572-84.
2) Brown J Jr, Folk JC, Reddy CV, Kimura AE. Visual prognosis of multifocal choroiditis, punctate inner choroidopathy, and the diffuse subretinal fibrosis syndrome. *Ophthalmology.* 1996 Jul;103(7):1100-5.
3) Reddy CV, Brown J Jr, Folk JC, Kimura AE, Gupta S, Walker J. Enlarged blind spots in chorioretinal inflammatory disorders. *Ophthalmology.* 1996 Apr; 103(4): 606-17
4) Gerstenblith AT, Thorne JE, Sobrin L, Do DV, Shah SM, Foster CS, Jabs DA, Nguyen QD. Punctate Inner Choroidopathy A Survey Analysis of 77 Persons. *Ophthalmology.* 2007 Apr 13; [Epub ahead of print]
5) Chan WM, Lai TY, Liu DT, Lam DS. Intravitreal Bevacizumab (Avastin) for Choroidal Neovascularization Secondary to Central Serous Chorioretinopathy, Secondary to Punctate Inner Choroidopathy, or of Idiopathic Origin. *Am J Ophthalmol.* 2007 Apr 23; [Epub ahead of print]

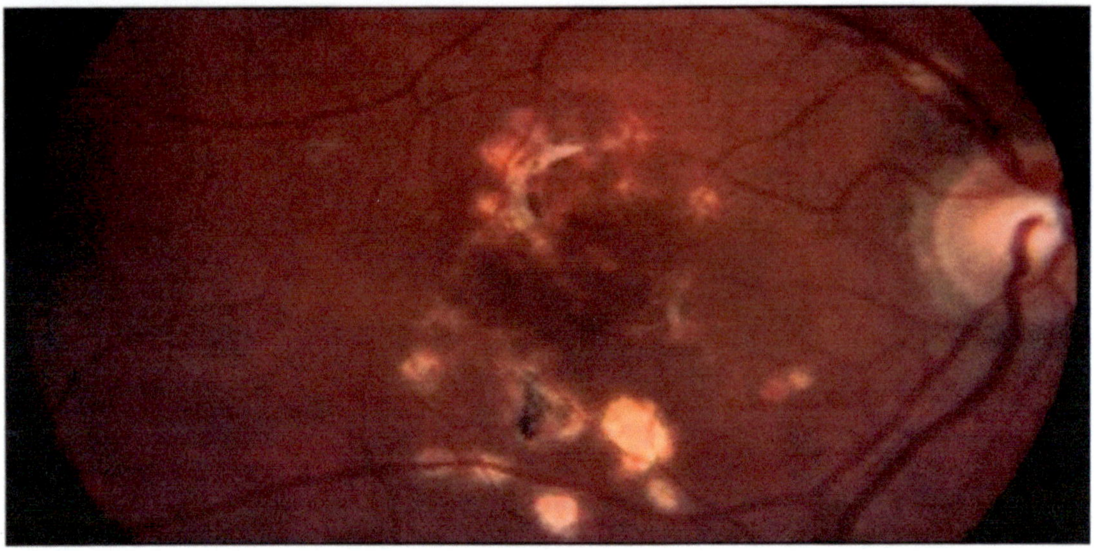

Figure 199: Multifocal areas of subretinal fibrosis in a patient with punctate inner choroidopathy.

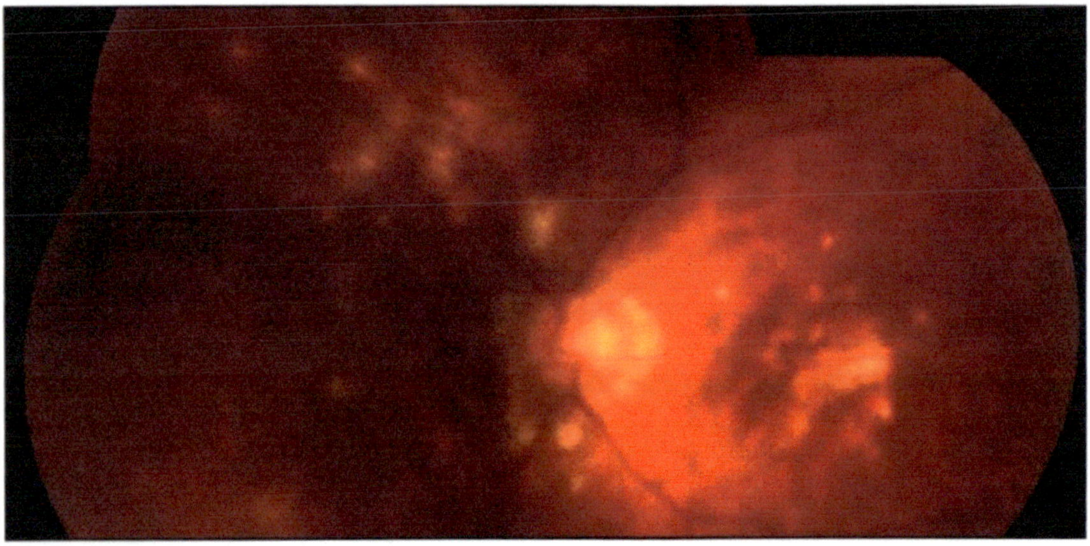

Figure 200: Montage of a patient afflicted with punctate inner choroidopathy. This appearance can be mistaken for multifocal choroiditis and panuveitis except for the lack of vitreous cells.

Serpiginous Choroiditis

Introduction: Serpiginous choroiditis is a rare, chronic, progressive, and recurrent bilateral inflammatory disease involving the retinal pigment epithelium, the choriocapillaris and the choroid. Junius described the classical clinical features of this disease in 1932.

It accounts for only 1.6% of all posterior uveitides. Most of the patients are white males with an average age of 47.5 years (range of 29- 70 years).

Pathophysiology: Maumenee suggested that serpiginous choroiditis is a degenerative disease, but the acute nature and the absence of familial cases tend to question this theory. There is an increased frequency of HLA-B7, elevation of von Willebrand factor VIII antigen and increased sensitization to retinal S-antigen in these patients.

Clinical Manifestations: Serpiginous choroiditis is a bilateral (although asymmetric), chronic, progressive inflammatory condition affecting both the choroid and retinal pigment epithelium with a high incidence of recurrence. Symptoms include blurry vision, photopsias, paracentral scotomas, metamorphopsia, and visual field loss. On examination, the anterior segment is quiet with mild vitritis. Serpiginous choroiditis mainly affects the peripapillary region and the posterior pole. Acute lesions are jigsaw puzzle-shaped lesions at the level of the choriocapillaris and retinal pigment epithelium and are commonly located adjacent to atrophic scars. Areas of retinal pigment epithelium hyperpigmentation and subretinal fibrosis are common. Choroidal neovascularization may develop, but is uncommon.

Diagnosis: The diagnosis is clinical.

Fluorescein angiography: Shows early hypofluorescence of the active lesions and late-phase hyperfluorescence of the border. In the inactive phase of the disease, the fluorescein angiogram shows a mottled hyperfluorescence as a result of pigment clumping with some late staining.

Electrophysiologic studies: Are unremarkable, but may show abnormalities in cases of extensive disease damage.

Visual field testing: May show dense scotomas that correspond to the active lesions.

Treatment: Corticosteroids alone do not appear to be effective over the long term. Alkylating agents seem to be effective for the control of the active inflammation and may help in achieving durable remission.

References:

1) Rodriguez A. Calongne M, Pedroza-Seres M, et al. Referral Patterns of uveitis in a tertiary eye care center. *Arch Ophthalmol* 1996;114:593-599
2) Gass JDM. *Stereoscopic atlas of macular diseases: a funduscopic and angiographic presentation.* St. Louis: Mosby, 1970:66.
3) Laatikainen L, Erkkila H. Serpiginous choroiditis. *Br J Ophthalmol* 1974;58:777-783.
4) Jampol LM, Orth D, Daily MJ, Rabb MF. Subretinal neovascularization with geographic (serpiginous) choroiditis. *Am J Ophthalmol* 1979;88:683-689.
5) Maumenee AE. Clinical entities in uveitis. An approach to the study of intraocular inflammation. *Am J Ophthalmol.* 1970 Jan;69 (1):1-27.
6) Broekhuyse RM, van Herck M, Pinckers AJ, et al. Immune responsiveness to retinal S antigen and opsin in serpiginous choroiditis and other retinal diseases. *Doc Ophthalmol* 1988;69:83¬93-
7) Christmas NJ, Oh KT, Oh DM, Folk JC. Long-term follow-up of patients with serpiginous choroiditis. *Retina* 2002;22:550-556.
8) Akpek EK, Jabs DA, Tessler HH, Joondeph BC, Foster CS. Successful treatment of serpiginous choroiditis with alkylating agents. *Ophthalmology.* 2002 Aug;109(8):1506-13.

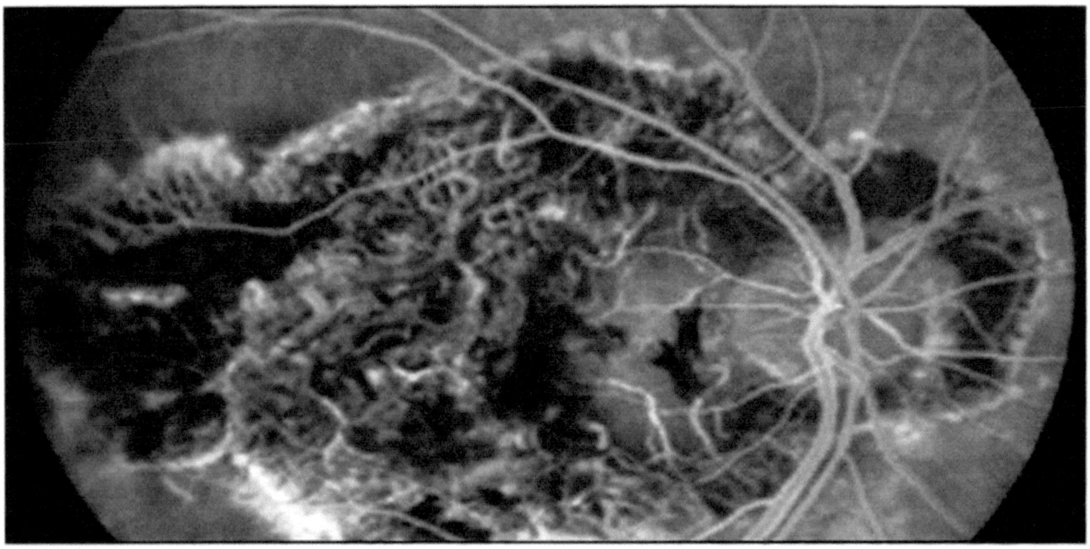

Figure 201: Visualization of the deep choroidal vasculature due to chorioretinal scarring and atrophy in a patient with serpiginous choroiditis.

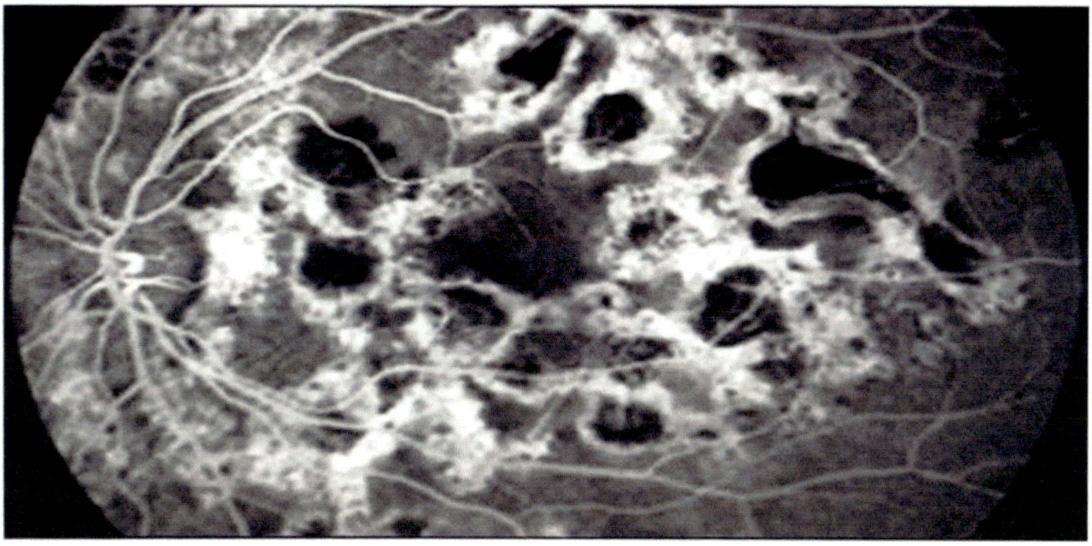

Figure 202: Serpiginous choroiditis in a patient with a Snellen visual acuity of 20/20

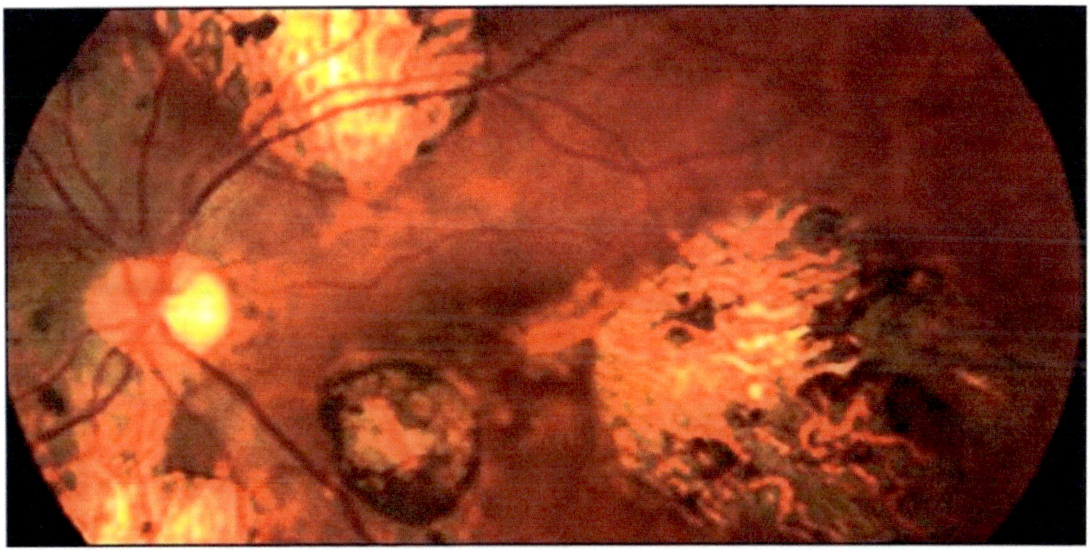

Figure 203: Multifocal chorioretinal scars in the macular and peripheral regions in a patient afflicted with serpiginous choroiditis.

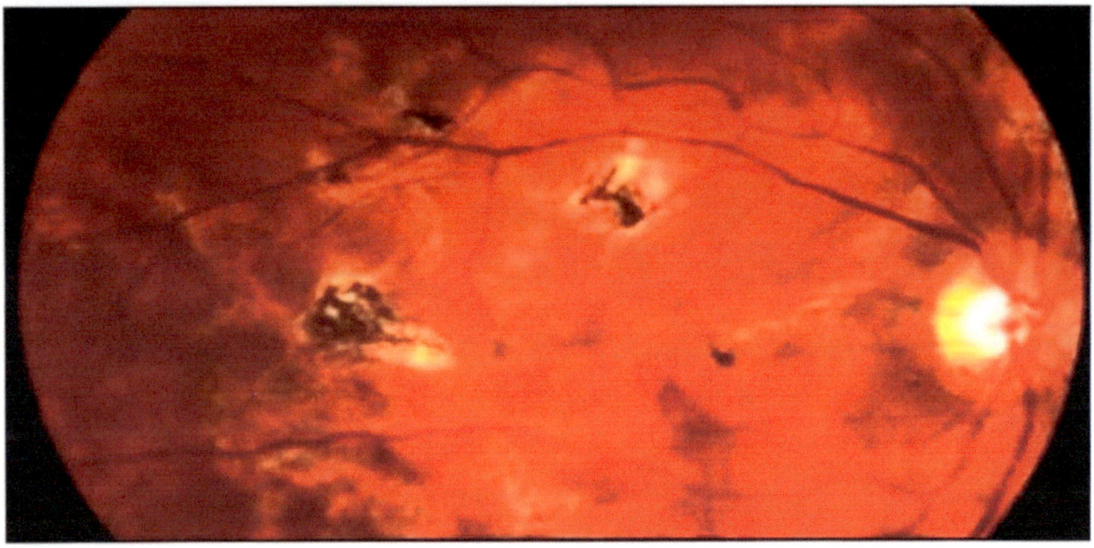

Figure 204: Twenty-four year-old female serpiginous choroiditis patient with extensive chorioretinal scarring.

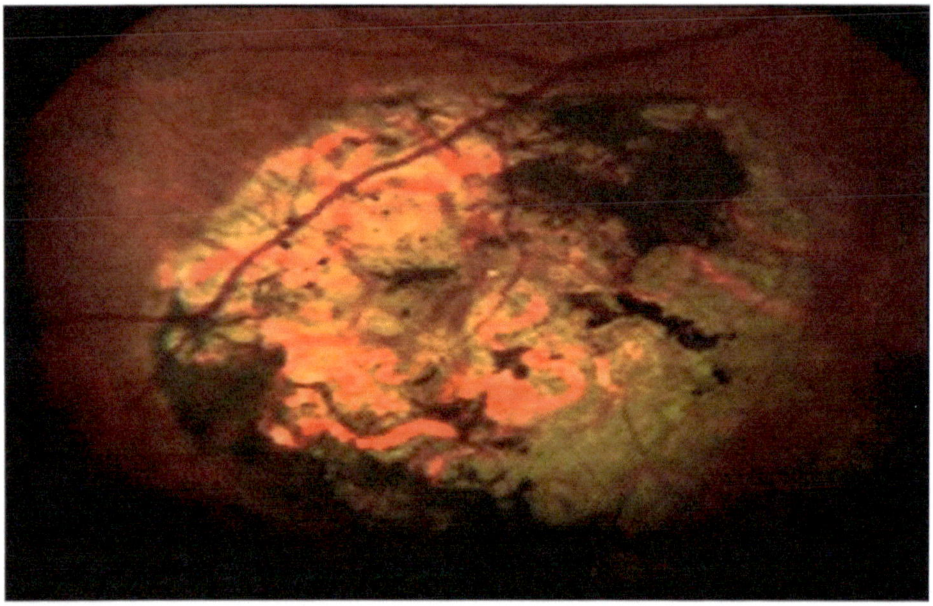

Figure 205: Large chorioretinal scar with visible choroidal vessels and overlying pigment.

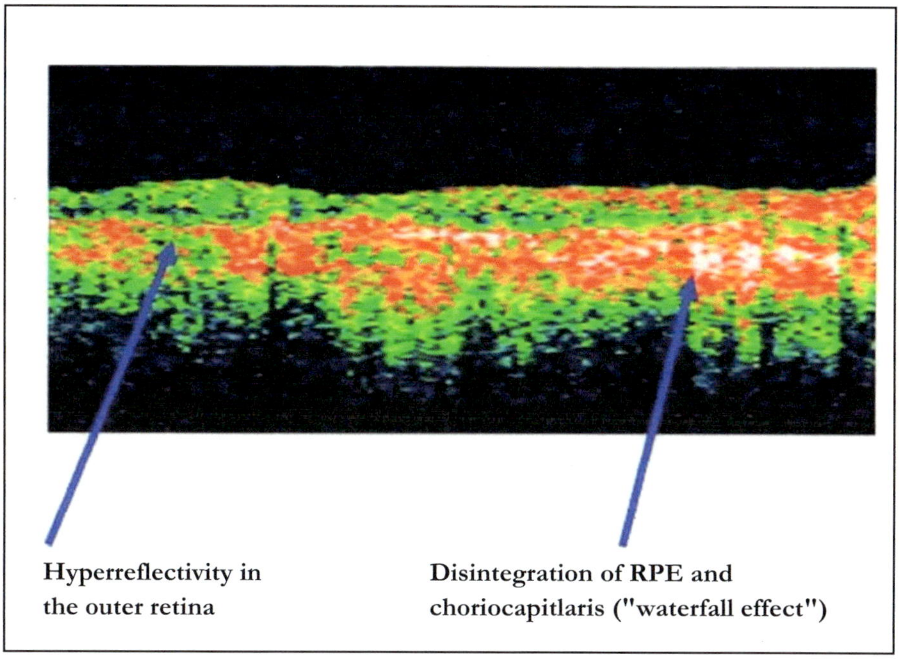

Figure 206: Active serpiginous chorioretinitis lesion

Part Four:

Infectious Diseases

Aspergillosis

Definition: Aspergillosis is characterized by an infection due to various species of the Aspergillus fungus. It is a disease most commonly seen in immunocompromised patients, but has been reported in patients afflicted with lung disease, transplant patients, and in otherwise healthy individuals.

History: In 1847, Sluyter reported the first well-documented case of human pulmonary aspergillosis.

Epidemiology: There is no race, gender, or age predilection.

Pathology/Pathogenesis: Out of the several species of *Aspergillus* that exist, *A fumigatus* is the most common cause of infection in humans. Macrophage and neutrophil phagocytosis is inhibited by the Aspergillus-produced toxic metabolites.

Clinical Features:

Systemic Manifestations: Aspergillosis is commonly known to affect the lungs and sinuses. Chest pain, pain, and fever are symptoms of infection by this particular fungus.

Ocular Manifestations: The main ocular complication associated with Aspergillus is endogenous endophthalmitis. This form of endophthalmitis is seen most frequently in transplant patients receiving intense immunosuppressive agents. Aspergillus was the second leading cause of fungal keratitis in a study done by Xie and co-workers whereby 72 eyes (12.1%) were affected. Bilateral optic neuritis, conjunctival aspergilloma, orbital apex syndrome, and scleritis have also been described. Orbital aspergillosis may also masquerade as an orbital pseudotumor.

Diagnosis: A culture for the Aspergillus fungus is a confirmatory test for ocular diagnosis. A chest X-ray is performed to rule out the presence of pulmonary aspergillomas. Magnetic resonance imaging and computed tomorgraphy scans are also used to establish the diagnosis of aspergillosis.

Treatment: Pars plana vitrectomy, intravitreal amphotericin B, systemic amphotericin B, and oral antifungal agents are commonly used to treat systemic and endogenous Aspergillus endophthalmitis with maximal effect.

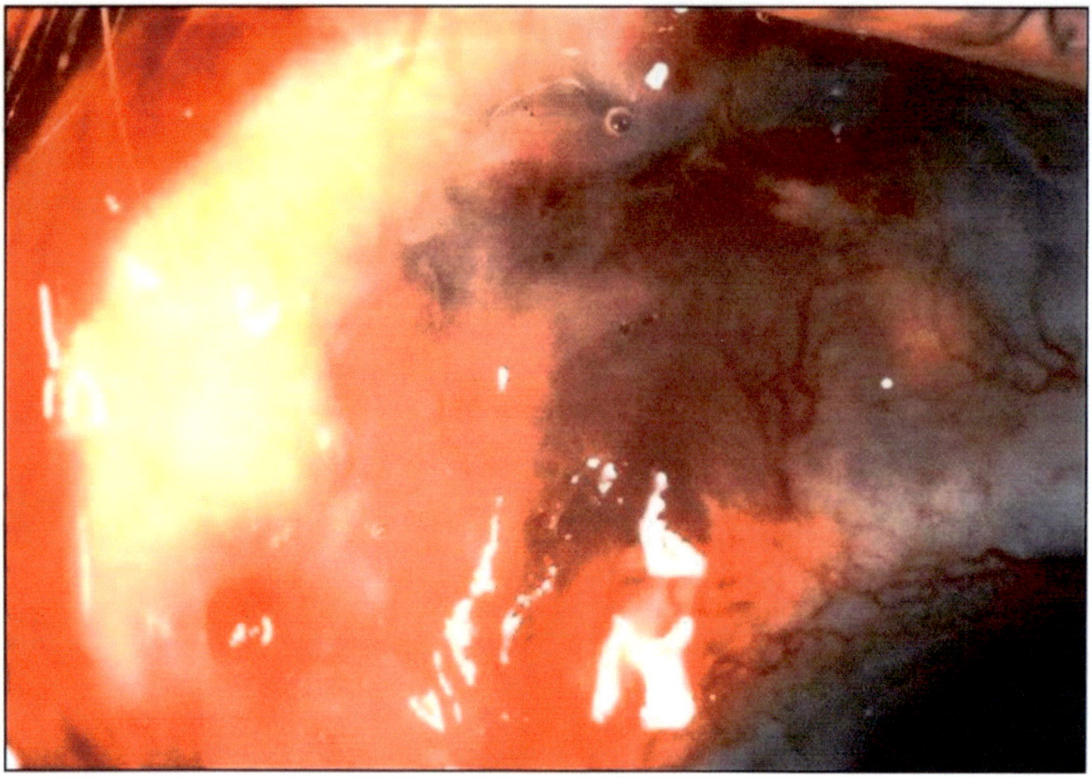

Figure 207: Aspergillus-associated necrotizing scleritis secondary to an excisional biopsy.

References:

1.) Maalouf T, Schmitt C, Crance J, et al. Endogenous Aspergillus endophthalmitis: a case report. J Fr *Ophthalmol* 2000;23:170 -3.

2) Kramer M, Kramer MR, Blau H, Bishara J, Axer-Siegel R, Weinberger D. Intravitreal Voriconazole for the Treatment of Endogenous Aspergillus Endophthalmitis. *Ophthalmology* 2006;113:1184-1186

3) Xie L, Zhong W, Shi W, Sun S. Spectrum of Fungal Keratitis in North China. *Ophthalmology* 2006;113:1943-1948.

4) Matsuo T, Notohara K, Yamadori I. Aspergillosis Causing Bilateral Optic Neuritis and Later Orbital Apex Syndrome *Jpn J Ophthalmol* 2005;Vol 49: 423-433.

Bartonella

Definition: *Bartonella henselae*, one of the four human species of *Bartonella*, has been implicated as the cause of cat-scratch disease (CSD). This species predominantly causes neuroretinitis while the 3 others causes endocarditis (B. elizabethae), Carrion's disease (B. bacilliformis), and trench fever (B. quintana).

History: Barton described the first human Bartonella infection in 1909. Foshay created the term cat scratch fever in 1932. Sweeny and Drance made the correlation between intraocular inflammation and CSD in 1970.

Epidemiology: CSD is the leading cause of regional lymphadenopathy in children and young adults worldwide. Prevalence of neuroretinitis in the context of CSD is approximately between 1% and 2%. The infection is not known to be transmitted from human to human.

Pathology/Pathogenesis: Previous work done by Regenery showed that 86% of patients with CSD had *B. henselae* antibodies as compared to 6% of those who were healthy patients. Polymerase chain reaction assays have shown that infected cats harbor fleas infected by B. henselae.

Clinical Features:

Systemic Manifestations: Systemic manifestations include myalgia, malaise, fatigue, low-grade fever, and lymphadenopathy.

Ocular Manifestations: The condition is typically unilateral and can present in both immunocompetent and immunocompromised patients. Numerous ophthalmic manifestations occur like chorioretinitis, serous macular detachments, intraretinal hemorrhages, cotton-wool spots, Parinaud's oculoglandular syndrome, conjunctivitis, anterior and posterior uveitis, and vascular lesions of the optic nerve, while the foremost ocular manifestation is neuroretinitis. Typically, the first signs will be optic disc edema and a macular star.

Diagnosis: The diagnosis of CSD is primarily based on laboratory testing with detection of genetic material of B. henselae or the host organisms' antibodies to B. henselae.

Treatment: There are no formalized guidelines to treat the ocular complications associated with B. henselae. Despite this, several groups have used oral ciprofloxacin, prednisone, and doxycycline with favorable responses. Elevated IgM or IgG titers for Bartonella henselae can be suggestive of current or past infection.

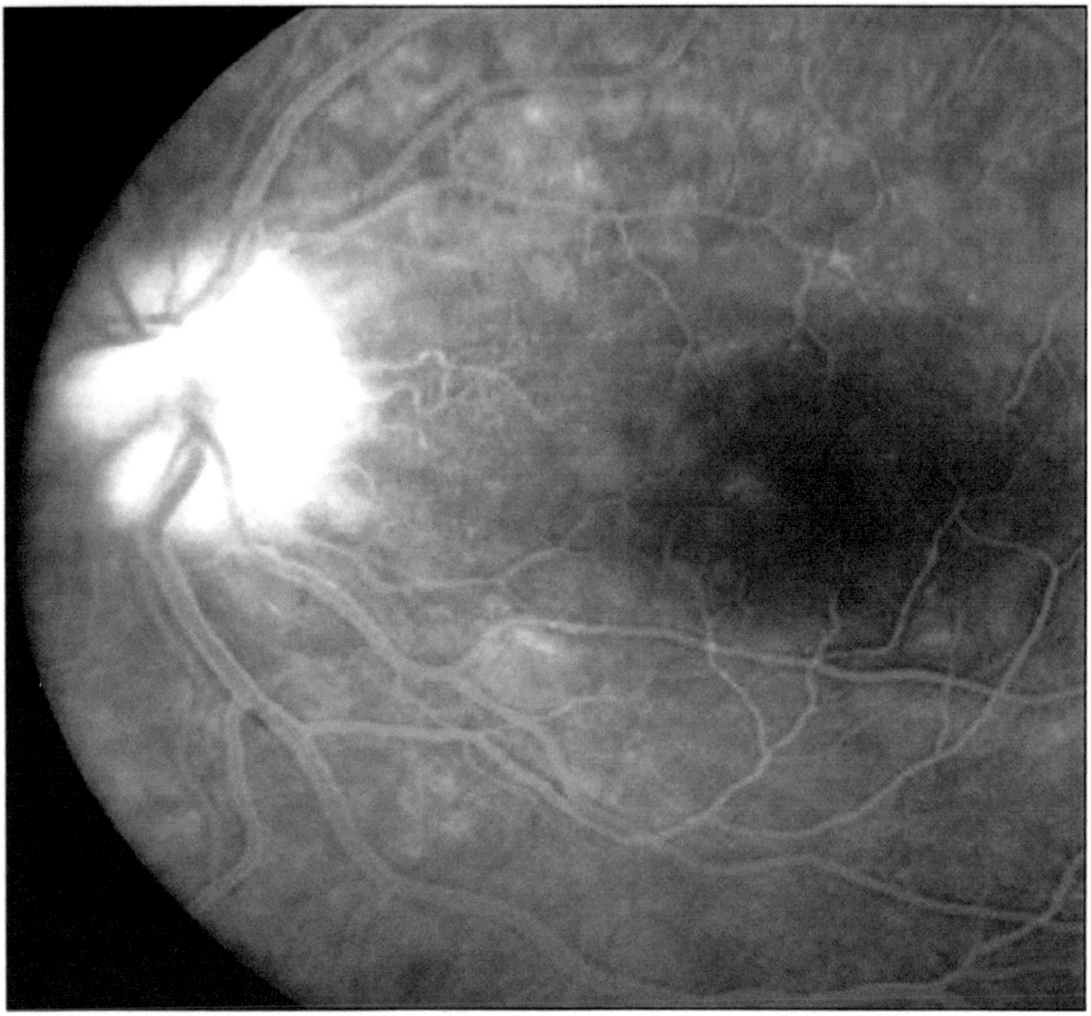

Figure 208: Mid-phase fluorescein angiogram of a 20-year-old white female with Bartonella-associated panuveitis. Note the disc hyperfluorescence and faint cystoid macular edema.

References:

1.) Henry M: Leptothricosis conjunctivae (Parinaud's conjunctivitis). *Trans Pacific Coast Oto-ophthalmol Soc* 1952;33:173-196.

2) Suhler EB, Lauer AK, Rosenbaum JT. Prevalence of serologic evidence of cat scratch disease in patients with neuroretinitis. *Ophthalmology*. 2000;107: 871-876.

3) Huang MC, Dreyer E. Parinaud's oculoglandular conjunctivitis and cat-scratch disease. *Int Ophthalmol Clin* 1996;36:29-36.

4) Regenery RJ, Olson JG, Perkins BA, Bibb W: Serological response to Rochalimaea henselae antigen in suspected cat scratch disease. *Lancet* 1992;339:1443-1445.

5) Golnik KC, Marotto ME, Maher ME, et al: Ophthalmic manifestations of Rochalimaea species. *Am J Ophthalmol* 1994;118:145-151.

Candidiasis

Definition: Ocular candidiasis commonly occurs as a chorioretinitis/endophthalmitis. The most common species is *Candida albicans*. The disease is characterized as endogenous (hematogenous dissemination) or exogenous (during ocular surgery or trauma).

History: In 1943, Miale reported the initial pathologic description of endogenous ocular candidiasis in humans. Candida chorioretinitis was first reported by Van Buren in 1958.

Epidemiology: Candida endophthalmitis represents one of the most serious and increasingly common ocular complications of intravenous drug abuse. Ocular trauma and surgery pose the highest risk for Candida infection, in particular cataract extraction with intraocular lens implantation and penetrating keratoplasty. Though seen mostly in immunocompromised patients, Candida endophthalmitis has also been reported in the immunocompetent individuals.

Pathology/Pathogenesis: 20 to 40% of health individuals harbor C. albicans in the intestines. Candida has been shown to spread hematogenously to the choroid and retina. Candida colonies may be identified by the typical budding pseudohyphae in the Bruch's membrane, choroid, and retinal pigment epithelium on histopathology.

Clinical Features:

***Systemic manifestations*:**Approximately 10% with candidemia can develop endophthalmitis. Oral thrush, oral mucosal involvement with blister formation and chronic vaginitis are also characteristic features of this disease.

Ocular manifestations: Candida endophthalmitis is of grave concern for patients with disseminated candidiasis. Prognosis is unpredictable as visual acuity varies from 20/25 to no light perception with resultant phthisis. A positive history of intravenous drug abuse is helpful in diagnosis. Patients present with a gradual decline in visual acuity, floaters, and mild ocular discomfort. Candida chorioretinitis with fluffy white lesions resembling puff balls may be joined by opaque vitreous strands, which gives this entity the characteristic "string of pearls" appearance. Anterior uveitis ,vitreous involvement and retinal hemorrhages are common.

Diagnosis: A clinical examination is key in diagnosing ocular candidiasis most effectively. A pars plana vitrectomy with an intravitreal injection of amphotericin B may help confirm the diagnosis while reducing the fungal mass and eradicating inflammatory debris in the eye. Henderson and coworkers have shown that vitreous aspiration aids in the diagnosis of *C. albicans* infection in 62% of eyes; whereas an anterior chamber tap has poor outcomes. A culture with blood agar or Sabaraud's glucose (which will reveal large, whitish mucoid colonies) in addition to a vaginal smear is useful in determination of systemic propagation. Antibody and antigen testing can be useful in early detection of disseminated candidiasis.

Treatment: The medical treatment of choice for Candida endophthalmitis is a combination of systemic and intravitreal amphotericin B with or without a pars plana vitrectomy. Flucytosine and imidazole derivatives have been described in the treatment of Candida endophthalmitis with variable success. The role of corticosteroids remains controversial as they may potentiate systemic candidiasis.

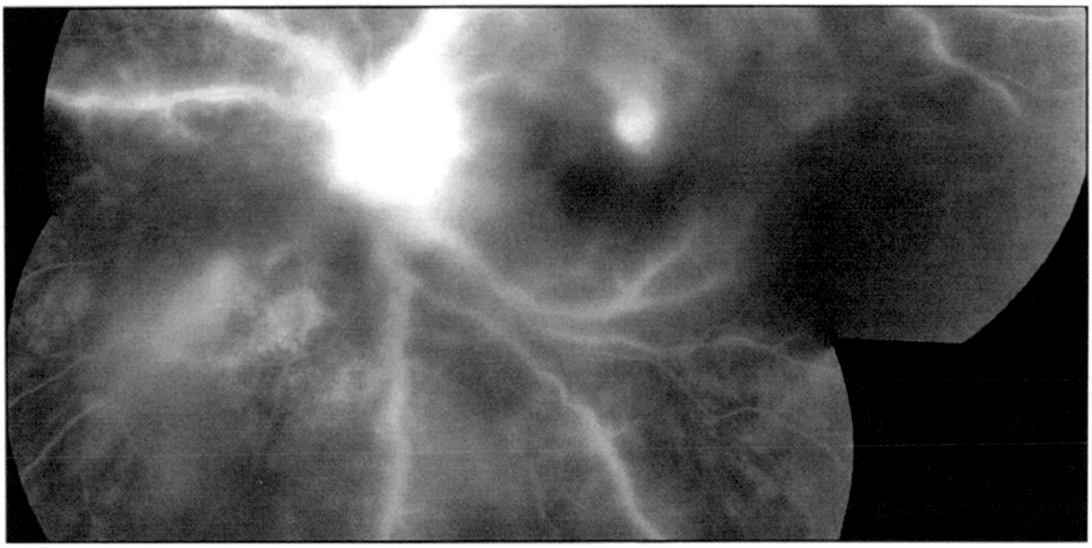

Figure 209: Papillitis with diffuse retinal vasculitis and focal areas of leakage in the superior paramacular area are seen during the fluorescein angiogram study.

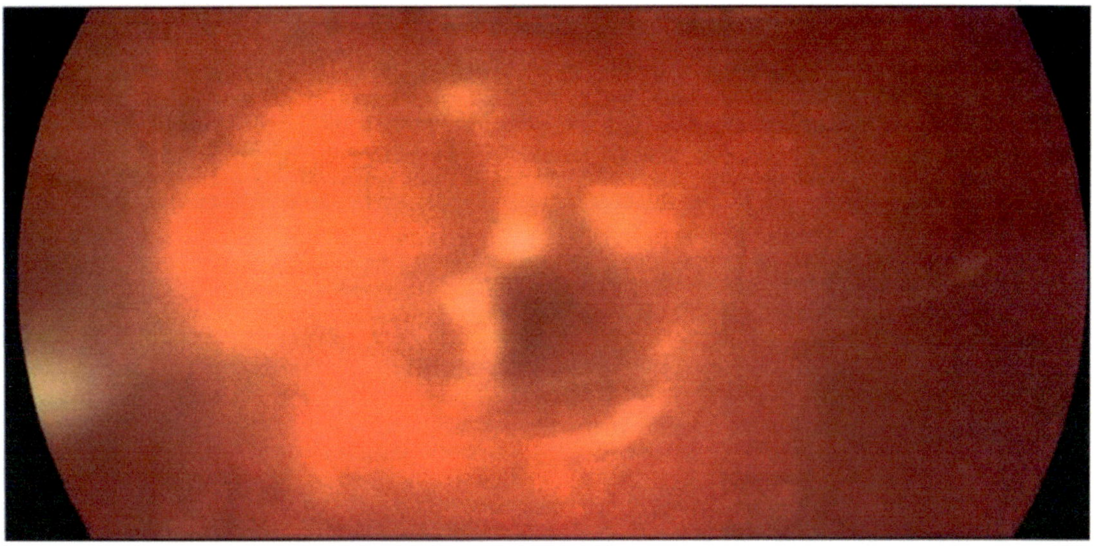

Figure 210: Classic "string of pearls" appearance of Candida albicans endophthalmitis. This is representative of fungal spore deposition in the vitreous cavity. Note that the patient had a positive history for Hepatitis C positivity and IV drug abuse.

References:

1.) Donahue SP, Greven CM, Zuravleff JJ, et al: Intraocular candidiasis in patients with candidemia. Clinical implications derived from a prospective multicenter study. *Ophthalmology* 1994;101:1302-1309.

2) Henderson DK, Edwards JE, Montogomerie JZ: Hematogenous Candida endophthalmitis in patients receiving parenteral hyperalimentation fluids. *J Infect Dis* 1981;143:655-661.

Diffuse Unilateral Subacute Neuroretinitis

Definition: Diffuse unilateral subacute neuroretinitis (DUSN) is a clinical syndrome characterized by early visual loss, vitritis, papillitis, and recurrent crops of gray-white retinal lesions. In later stages, progressive visual loss, optic atrophy, retinal vessel narrowing, and diffuse pigment epithelial degeneration are seen. DUSN is usually unilateral and is thought to be caused by a small number of different nematode larvae migrating within the subretinal space.

History: The term DUSN was first used by Gass and colleagues in 1978 to describe a distinct clinical entity seen in a short number of patients.

Epidemiology: DUSN is a rare disease. Approximately 60 cases have been reported in the United States, and a smaller number worldwide. The age range in the largest series by Gass is reported as 5 to 22 years, but older patients with DUSN have also been reported. Two main nematodes have been related with the disease: (1) *Baylisascaris procyonis* (1500-2000 microns) which predominates in Northern Midwest US and Canada, and (2) *Ancylostoma canium* (400-1000 microns) found in Southeast US, Caribbean, and Brazil.

Pathogenesis: DUSN is probably the result of the toxic effect on the outer retina by the worm in addition to an inflammatory reaction against the causative agent.

Clinical Features: The most characteristic ocular finding in the early stage is a motile subretinal worm. However, the worm is very difficult to observe, so we also need to know other frequently reported findings of these patients.

A) Early stage: Anterior segment is usually unaffected in that only a few patients may present with keratic precipitates or anterior chamber cellularity. Vitritis is present in all patients and may obscure the fundus view. Blurred margins of the optic nerve are present in half of the patients. The retina has multiple focal gray-white to yellow lesions in the deep or outer retinal layer which are often located in the peripapillary and/or juxtamacular regions. These lesions (evanescent themselves) vary in size from 1000 to 1500 μm and commonly resolve with a mild change in color of the underlying retinal pigment epithelium. Mild retinal vessel (arteriole) narrowing may also be seen in some patients.

B) Late stage: Optic atrophy and severe arteriole narrowing and sheathing seem to define the late stage most accurately. Vitritis is much less common than in early stages. Retinal pigment epithelial changes (atrophy and mottling) are also found. Choroidal neovascular membrane formation is infrequent and with a peripheral location.

Diagnosis: This is based on the characteristic clinical appearance in conjunction with the presence of an intraocular worm. Fluorescein angiography findings are especially helpful in the early stage of the disease with early blockage and late staining of the lesions. Electroretinogram often shows mild to moderate, decreased rod and cone responses (b>a wave), and electro-oculogram is abnormal in one half of the patients, especially in the late stage of the disease.

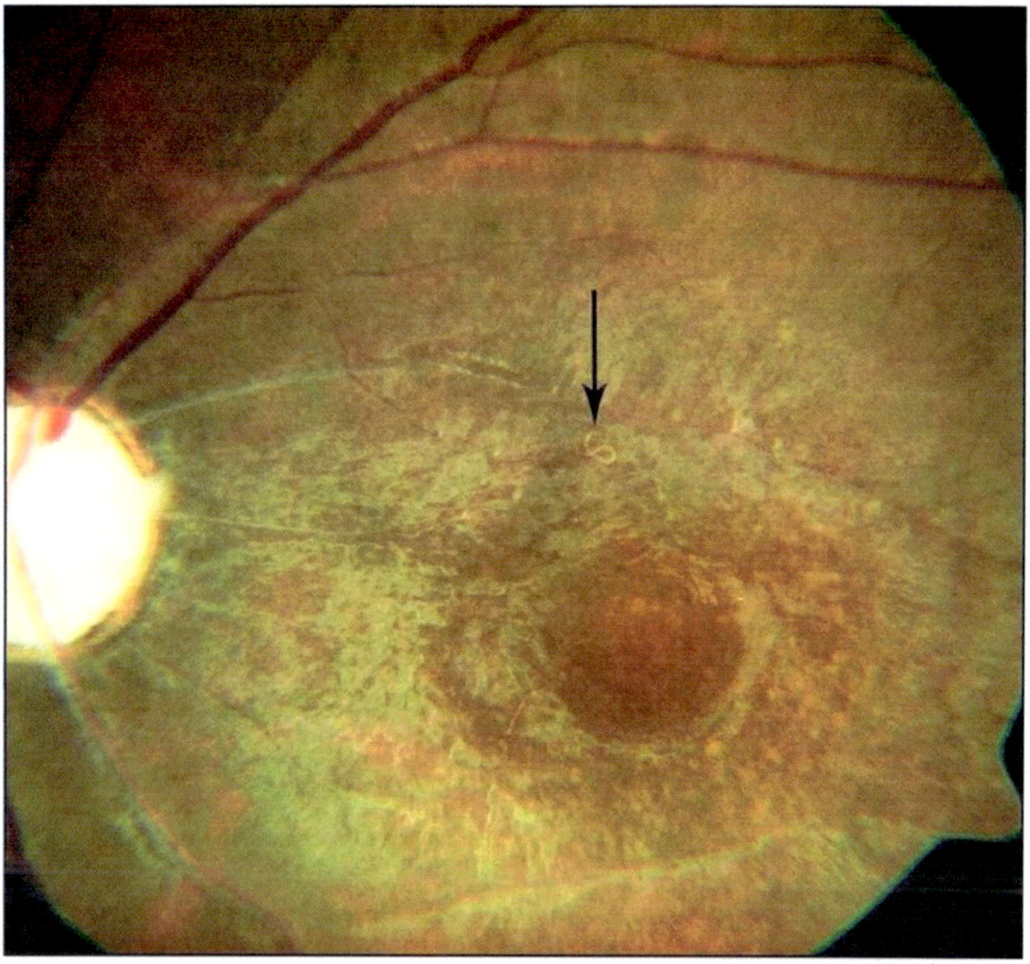

Figure 211: Diffuse Unilateral Subacute Neuroretinitis courtesy of Rafael T. Cortez MD. Centro de Cirugia Oftalmologia (CECOF). Caracas. Venezuela. The nematode is visible superior to the fovea.

Treatment: At present, direct laser photocoagulation of a visible worm is probably the best modality. Destruction of worm at the early stage seems to aid in the absence of recurrence or progression of the disease. Thiabendazole and Ivermectin are other reported therapies. It is crucial to emphasize that DUSN requires prompt treatment because it carries a poor final visual acuity if not treated in the early phase.

References:

1) Barney NP. Diffuse unilateral subacute neuroretinitis; in: Foster CS, Vitale AT. *Diagnosis and treatment of Uveitis*. Saunders. Philadelphia 2002:475-9.
2) Gass JD, Gilbert WR Jr, Guerry R, et al. Diffuse unilateral subacute neuroretinitis. *Ophthalmology* 1978; 85521.

Free-Living Amebas and Amebiasis

Definition: Free-living amebae (*Acanthamoeba* and *Naegleria*) and *Entamoeba histolytica* can cause swift and devastating ocular disease. The intestinal protozoan *E. histolytica* causes amebiasis.

History: Jones and coworkers were the first to document Acanthamoeba infection of the eye in 1973. Walker and Sellards initially reported the cyst form of E. histolytica as the infective portion of the parasite.

Epidemiology: Contact lens wearers carry the highest risk of developing Acanthamoeba keratitis. Exposure to contaminated water increases the risk of further ocular complications. Those living in tropical climates carry a much greater chance of developing amebiasis because of greater risk of fecal-ocular infections and trauma.

Pathology/Pathogenesis: Free-living amebae are spread by contaminated contact lens, water, or trauma. *Acanthamoeba* adhesion to the corneal surface involves interactions between the mannose-binding protein of *Acanthamoeba* and mannose gylcoproteins on the surface of corneal epithelium. E. histolytica transmission usually occurs through food-borne exposure. Eye adnexa show necrosis when infected by *E. histolytica.*

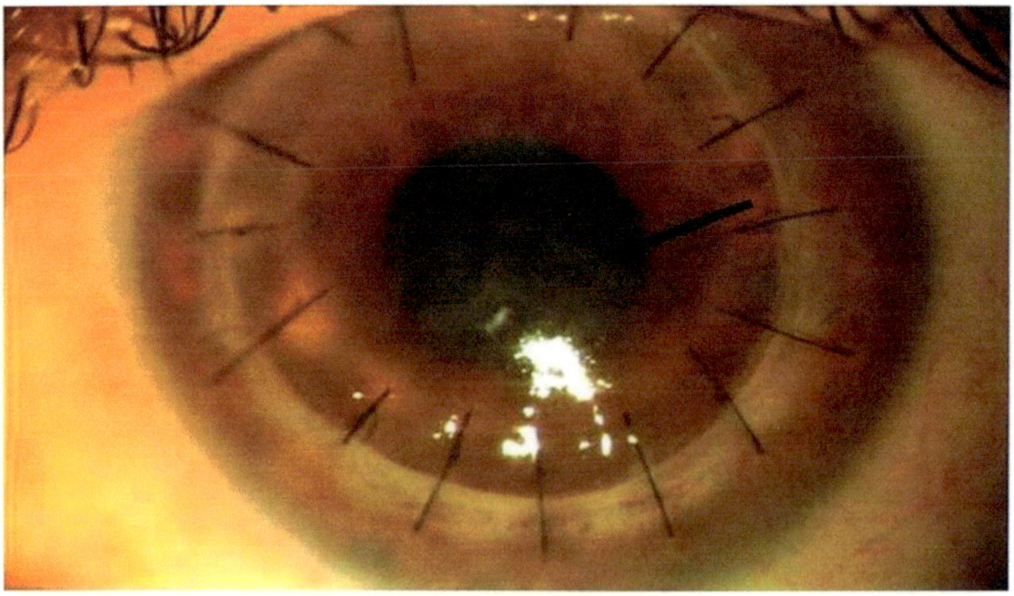

Figure 212: Khodadoust's line as seen in failing graft of a patient with Acanthamoeba keratitis.

Clinical Features:

Systemic Manifestations: Only 10% of those afflicted with amebiasis demonstrate the clinical signs of amebic colitis and liver abscesses.

Ocular Manifestations: Classically, Acanthamoeba is known to affect the cornea, but is reported to cause chorioretinitis, scleritis, glaucoma, increased intraocular pressure, and anterior chamber inflammation. Acanthamoeba keratitis can progress slowly and rapidly. Patients may be mistakenly diagnosed with herpes simplex keratitis. In amebiasis, intermediate uveitis, central serous chorioretinitis, and cutaneous infection of the eyelid have been reported.

Diagnosis: *Acanthamoeba* should be suspected in patients who have persistent chronic keratitis without any response to therapy. Proper inspection of contact lens solution and lenses, polymerasse chain reaction, in vivo confocal microscopy, stains, and corneal scrapings are some of the diagnostic tests.

Treatment: The aim of treatment is to eliminate the parasite, photophobia, pain, and inflammatory reaction caused by an Acanthamoeba infection. A combination of a biguanide and a diamidine is the medical recipe of choice according to studies done at Moorfields Eye Hospital. Corticosteroids are used in an effort to control the inflammatory response. Non-steroidal anti-inflammatory drugs are efficacious in lessening the amount of scleritis and limbal inflammation. Unfortunately, the cyst form of Acanthamoeba can be very recalcitrant to standard treatment. In such cases, surgical intervention may be necessary. In patients with corneal scarring, penetrating keratoplasty is indicated. Luminal agents, such as iodoquinol and doloxanide, along with metronidazole are effective in treating amebiasis.

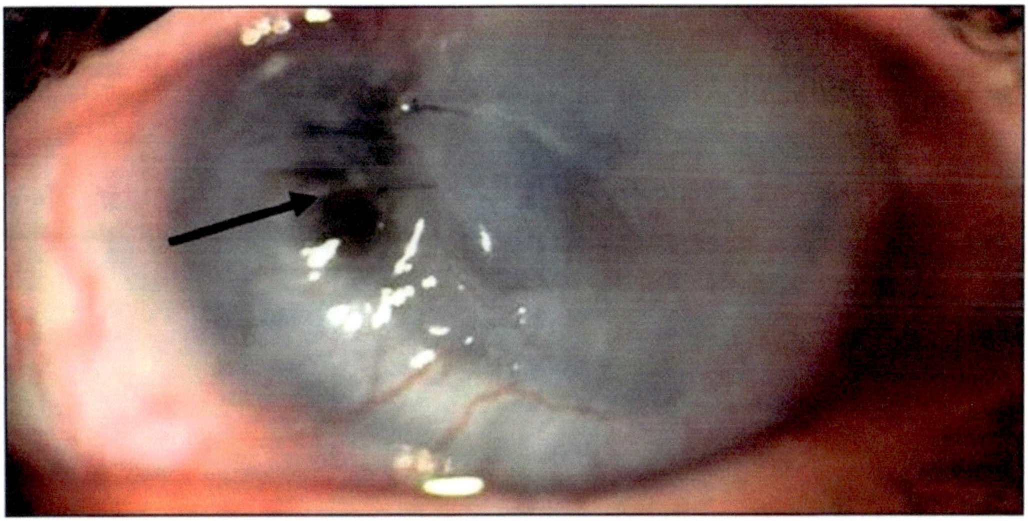

Figure 213: Descemetocele, stromal edema, and temporal stromal melt in a patient with Acanthamoeba keratitis.

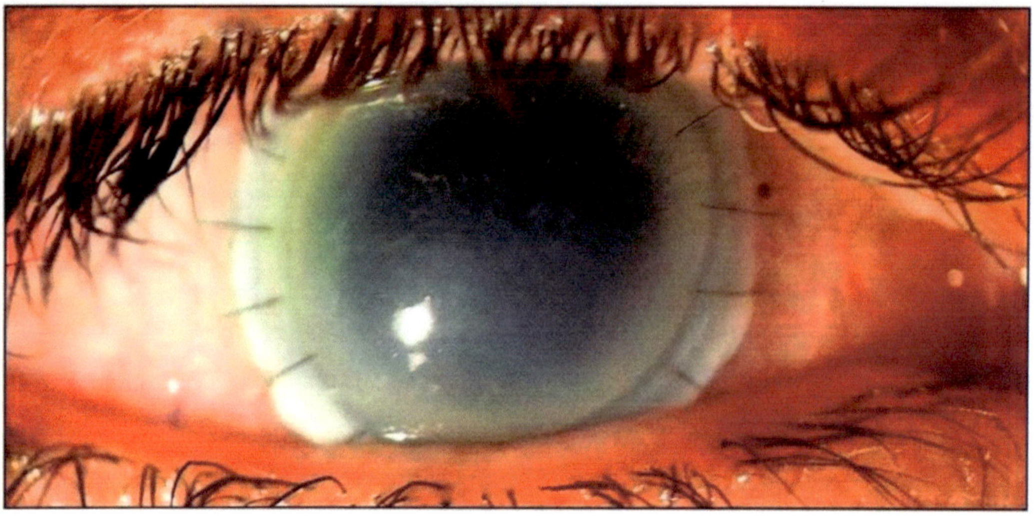

Figure 214: Same eye after tectonic corneoscleral graft.

References:

1) Sainz de la Maza M, Hemady RK, Foster CS. Infectious scleritis: report of four cases. *Doc Ophthalmol.* 1993 ; 83 (1):33-41.
2) Moshari A, McLean IW, Dodds MT, Damiano RE, McEvoy PL. Chorioretinitis after keratitis caused by Acanthamoeba: case report and review of the literature. *Ophthalmology*. 2001 Dec;108 (12):2232-6.
3) Osato MS: Parasitic keratitis and conjunctivitis. In: Smolin G, Thoft RA, eds: *The Cornea.* Boston, Little, Brown, 1994, p 253.
4) Frangie JP, Moore MB: Parasitic infections including Acanthamoeba. In: Leibowitz HM, Waring III GO, eds: *Corneal Disorders. Clinical Diagnosis and Management.* Philadelphia, W.B. Saunders, 1998, p 719.
5) Yang ZT, Cao ZY, Panjwani N. Pathogenicity of Acanthamoeba keratitis carbohydrate-mediated host parasite interactions. *Infect Immun* 1997;65: 439.
6) Fulcer T, Dart JKG: Queratitis por acatomoeba. In: Duran de las Colina J, ed: Complicaciones de las Lentes de Contacto. Madrid, *Tecnimedia* Editorial, 1998, p 263.

Acute Retinal Necrosis

Definition: Urayama and associates first described acute retinal necrosis (ARN) in 1971. It is characterized by focal, well-demarcated areas of peripheral retinal necrosis (full thickness retinitis) and can be accompanied by anterior uveitis, vitritis, and occlusive retinal arteritis. The viruses that have been implicated are: varicella zoster virus (VZV), herpes simplex virus-1 (HSV-1), HSV-2, cytomegalovirus virus (CMV), and Epstein- Barr virus (EBV).

Epidemiology: Any age, gender, or race can be affected by this disease. VZV is the most common cause of ARN. VZV or HSV-1 can cause ARN in patients older than 25 years while HSV-2 causes ARN in patients younger than 25 years. ARN (caused by HSV) can be seen in healthy and immunocompromised patients.

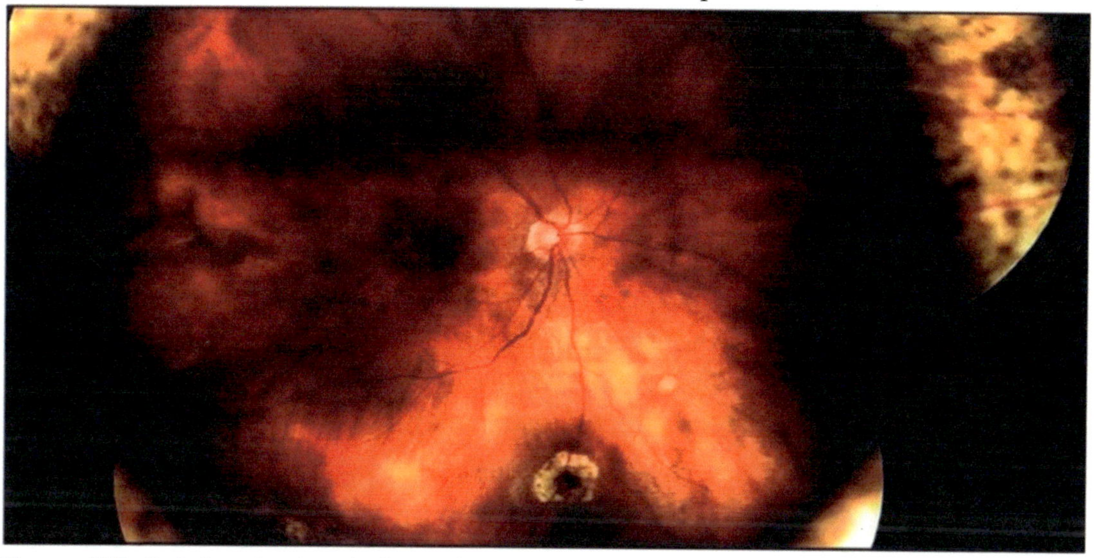

Figure 215: Inferior chorioretinal scar in a patient with ARN. A scleral buckle was required for an ensuing retinal detachment, a common sequela of ARN.

Pathogenesis: In a study done by Tran et al., raised levels of IFN γ in the vitreous gave a strong indication of visual prognosis. However, patients with the most severe forms of VZV-associated ARN had absent delayed-type hypersensitivity responses against VZV antigens in addition to low IFN γ levels.

Clinical Features: Typically, symptoms include decrease in visual acuity, irritation, reddening of the eye, and photophobia. If left untreated, retinal detachment with occlusive vasculitis may lead to further visual deterioration.

Anterior segment: Anterior and vitreous cells are present in the active state. Iris hyperemia, trabeculitis, endotheliitis, iris atrophy, and keratic precipitates may be seen on anterior segment examination.

Posterior segment: ARN typically affects the peripheral retina by forming a "swiss-cheese" pattern of creamy and confluent retinitis, which can spread rapidly. There is also an occlusive retinopathy with arteriolar involvement. Rhegmatogenous retinal detachments occur 75% of the time.

Diagnosis: The diagnosis of ARN is predominantly based on the clinical examination of the patient, yet the differentiation between CMV, VZV, or HSV retinitis is difficult due to the similar fundus appearance. In some cases, a positive history of HSV keratitis may help implicate the virus as the etiologic agent.

Polymerase Chain Reaction (PCR) and Enzyme-linked Immunosorbent Assay: Detection of viral DNA samples of the aqueous humor using ELISA and PCR is helpful, but not confirmatory.

Fluorescein angiogram (FA): There is dye leakage from the small vessels of the retina in the acute stage. Cystoid macular edema, hemorrhages, and vascular occlusions may also be seen on FA.

Treatment: Institution of intravenous acyclovir (1500 mg/m^2) per day in three divided doses over 10 to 14 days) is indicated in patients with ARN. The patient is then switched to oral acyclovir for maintenance. Immediate treatment to the affected eye reduces the overall risk of developing the disease in the fellow eye by 57%. Corticosteroids may also be used. Other forms of antiviral agents proven to have efficacy include ganciclovir, foscarnet, brivudine, valganiclovir, and famcyclovir. To prevent a retinal detachment, argon laser photocoagulation may be indicated.

References:

1) Tran THC, Stanescu D, Caspers-Velu L, et.al. Clinical characteristics of acute HSV-2 retinal necrosis. *Am J Ophthalmol* 2004;137:872-8.
2) Van Gelder RN, Willig JL, Holland GN, Kaplan HJ. Herpes simplex virus type 2 as a cause of acute retinal necrosis syndrome in young patients. *Ophthalmology* 2001;108:869-76.
3) Paylay DA, Sternberg P, Davis J, et al: Decrease in the risk of bilateral acute retinal necrosis by acyclovir therapy. *Am J Ophthalmol* 1991;112 : 250 .

Figure 216: Multiple areas of retinal whitening and hemorrhage in a patient with acute retinal necrosis syndrome.

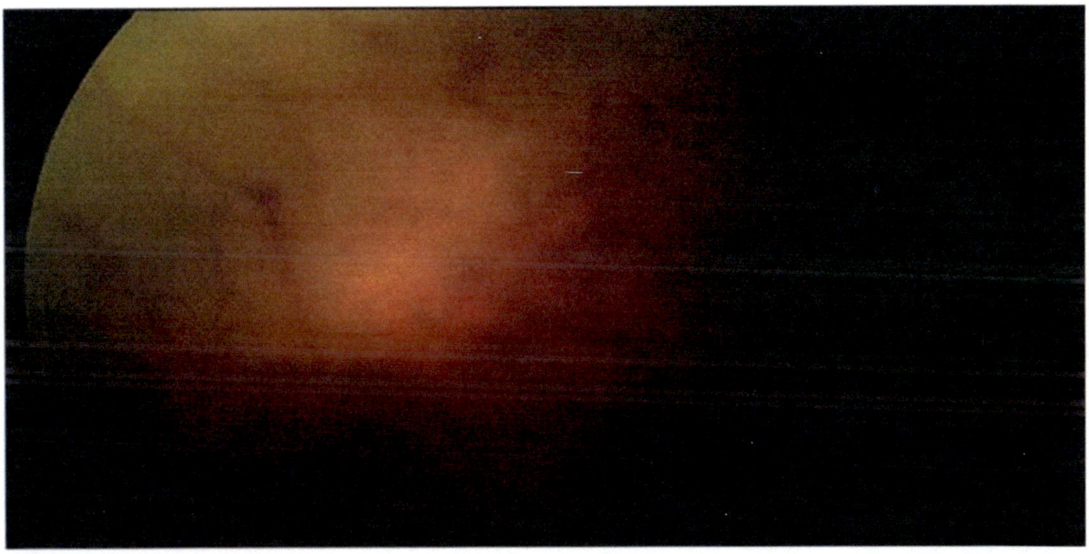

Figure 217: Superior creamy lesion with accompanying hemorrhages in a 29 year-old female with acute retinal necrosis syndrome. Note the hazy view of the fundus, a common finding in ARN.

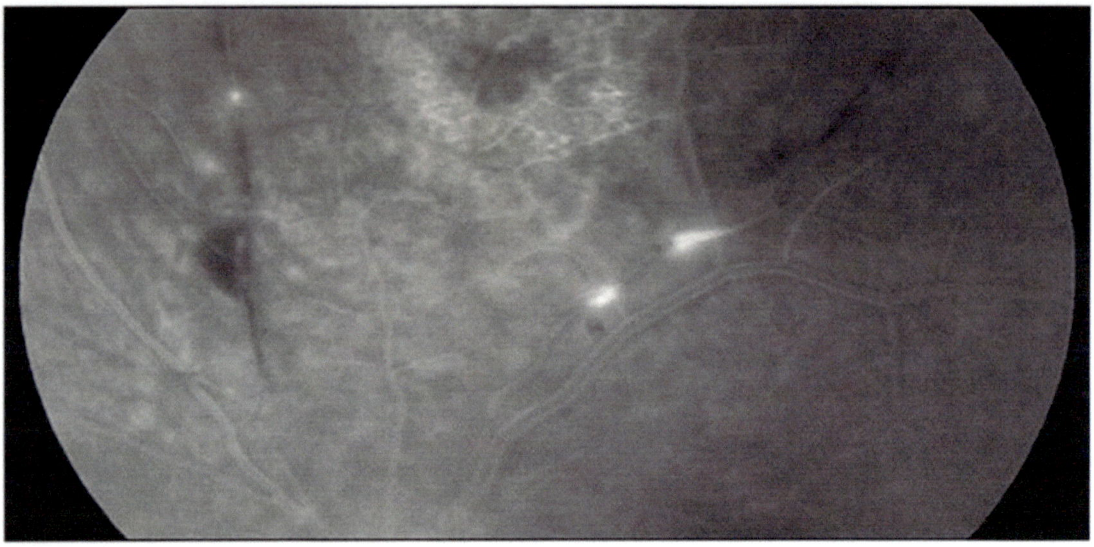

Figure 218: During the mid-phase of the fluorescein angiogram, the area of retinitis (located superiorly) can be clearly demarcated. There are also focal areas of vasculitis with multiple hemorrhages.

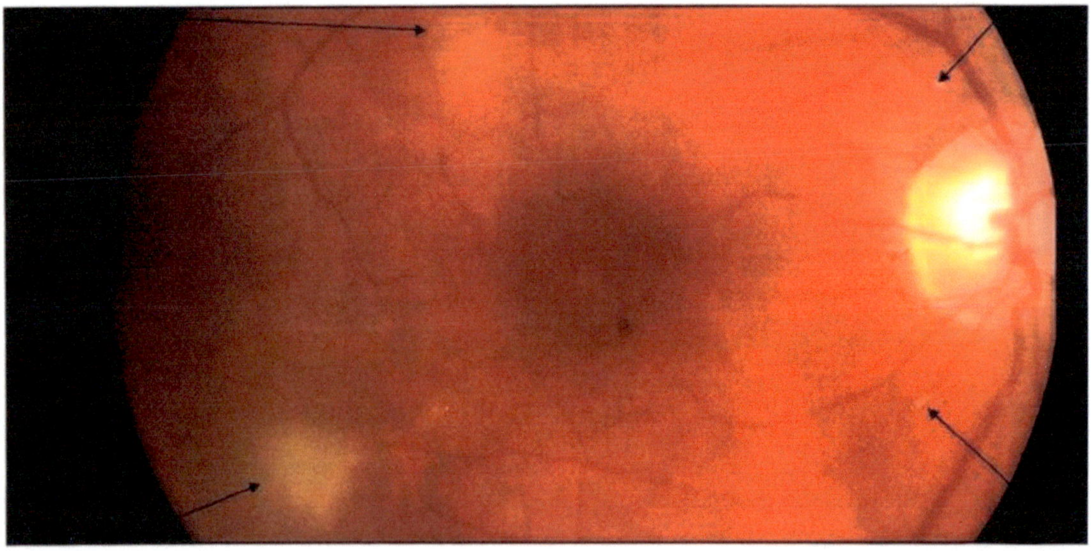

Figure 219: Two foci of retinitis in a patient with acute retinal necrosis. Note the perivascular infiltrates along the arteries, which denote an active vasculitic process.

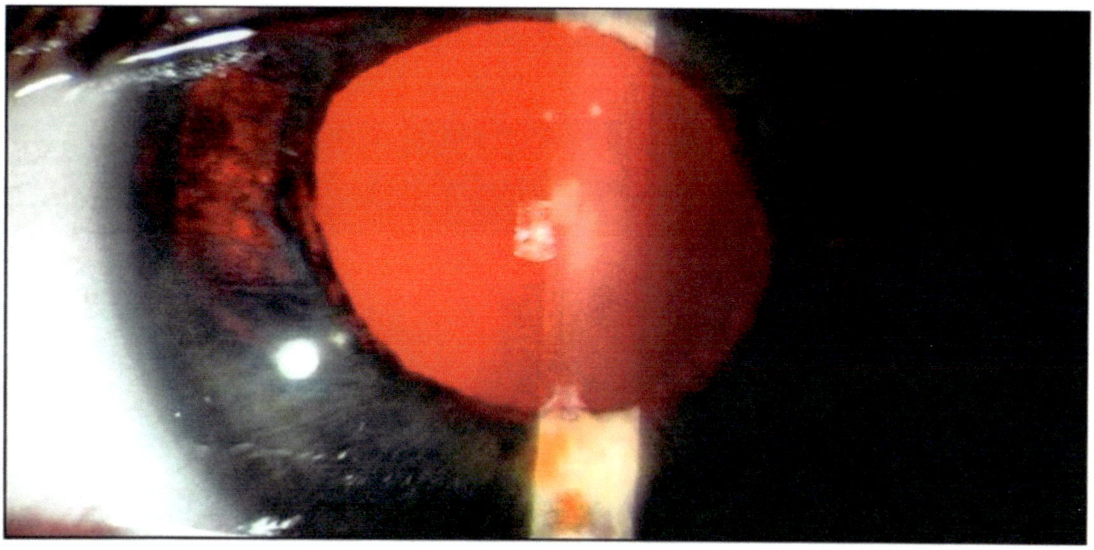

Figure 220: Slit-lamp photograph of a 23-year old male with HSV-related transillumination defects and iris atrophy spreading from 9 o'clock to 5 o'clock.

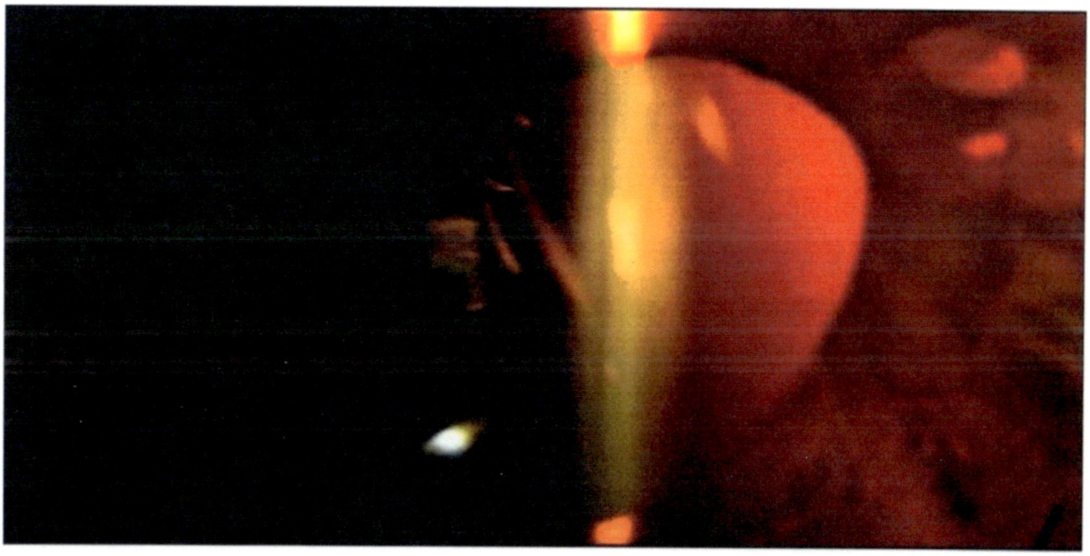

Figure 221: Large patches of iris atrophy in a patient with herpes simplex virus-related uveitis. Note the transillumination defects.

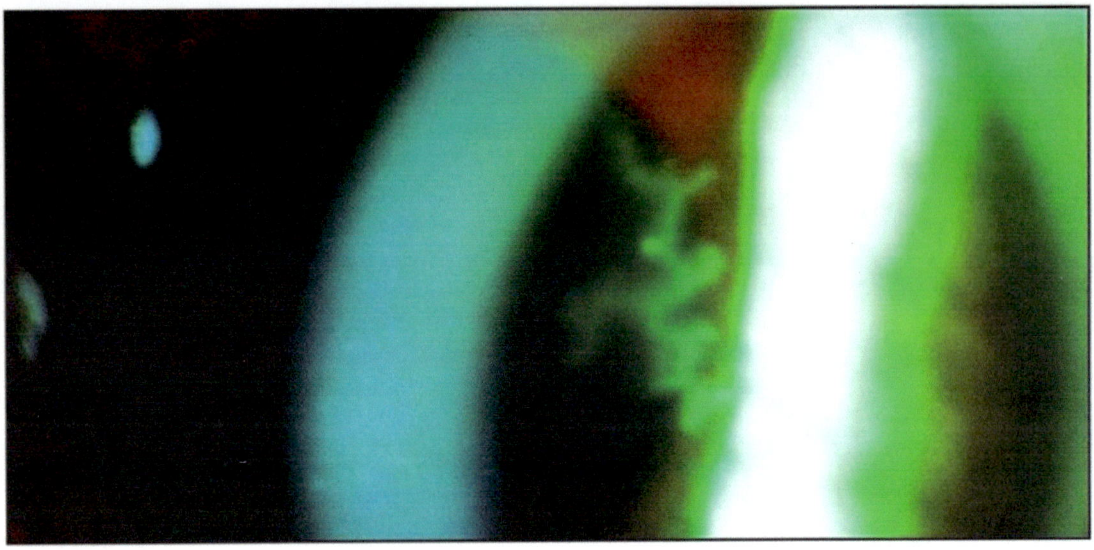

Figure 222: Dendrite with anterior stromal haze as seen in a patient with HSV-associated keratouveitis.

Epstein-Barr Virus

Definition: Epstein-Barr virus (EBV) belongs to the gamma herpes virus family. The role of EBV in ocular diseases is not completely understood because approximately 90% of the adult population is seroconverted and only a few from ocular disease. EBV may affect the eye in many different ways, usually as conjunctivitis or uveitis.

History: EBV was first isolated in 1964 from a cultured Burkitt's lymphoma cell line. During recent decades, EBV has been implicated in a broad spectrum of human diseases like infectious mononucleosis, anaplastic nasopharyngeal carcinoma, and B-cell lymphomas.

Epidemiology: EBV infection is distributed worldwide. Antibodies against EBV can be detected in approximately 90% of the population. Transmission requires contact with body fluids (primarily saliva, but also through blood transfusions). Primary infection is usually subclinical or leads to mild symptoms typical of a nonspecific viral illness, but in some cases it takes the clinical picture of infectious mononucleosis (especially when it affects adolescents).

Pathogenesis: EBV shows B-cell tropism. However, the precise role of this virus in the aforementioned associated diseases is not well understood, but defective immunosurveillance against the virus may permit an uncontrolled proliferation of EBV-infected cells.

Clinical Features: EBV may affect the eye in many different ways, usually as conjunctivitis or uveitis, and often occurs in primary infections in the context of infectious mononucleosis. Follicular conjunctivitis is the most frequent ocular feature. Severe bilateral iritis and iridocyclitis have also been reported. Retinitis, multifocal choroiditis, and other posterior segment pathologies are uncommon complications that have been described in patients with infectious mononucleosis and, more recently, in patients suffering from X-linked lymphoproliferative disorder, AIDS, or even in otherwise healthy individuals.

Diagnosis: This is principally based on clinical findings. Serum antibody titers against EBV may be helpful, especially if the initial high levels are followed by a subsequent decrease coinciding with the resolution of the acute phase. Other techniques like polymerase chain reaction (PCR) or biopsy of the affected tissues may also be helpful in selected cases.

Treatment: Ocular disease is commonly self-limiting and no treatment is indicated. Uveitis sometimes requires corticosteroid therapy. Severe cases, especially those rare instances where the posterior segment is affected, may require antiviral agents.

References:

1) Heilingenhaus A, Helbig H, Fiedler M. Herpesviruses; in: Foster CS, Vitale AT. *Diagnosis and treatment of Uveitis*. Saunders. Philadelphia 2002:315-32.
2) Cordero Coma M, Anzaar F, Yilmaz T, Foster CS. Herpetic retinitis. *Herpes* 2007. Accepted for publication. Ahead of print

CMV Retinitis

Definition: Cytomegalovirus (CMV), a β Human herpes virus, is an omnipresent pathogen in the general population, but seldom causes clinically apparent disease in an immunocompetent individual. Neonates and immunocompromised patients are the main groups at risk for CMV retinitis (CMVR), which is the most frequent cause of blindness among patients with AIDS.

History: CMV eye disease was first reported in 1947. In the 1980s, with the AIDS pandemic, CMV became a frequent form of posterior uveitis. In the mid-1990s, before the introduction of the highly active antiretroviral therapy (HAART), about 30% of patients with AIDS developed CMVR during their lifetime. However, the introduction of HAART achieved a 75% reduction in the incidence of CMVR.

Epidemiology: About half of normal population has antibodies against CMV. However, CMV infection in immunocompetent hosts does not usually produce symptomatic disease. The mode of transmission is not totally clear and probably requires close contact with body fluids containing the virus. Most of the CMVR cases result from reactivation of previously acquired disease. In patients with AIDS, CMV is one of the most common opportunistic infections. CMVR usually presents in an advanced disease stage and is strongly associated with a low CD4+ T cell count (almost all cases below 50 cells/mm3).

Pathogenesis: After primary infection, CMV remains in its host, establishing a latent infection typical for all herpes viruses. In most cases, the retina is infected via hematogenous spread. Damage of capillary endothelial cells caused by HIV infection probably facilitates the passage of CMV-infected cells through the blood-retinal barrier.

Clinical Features: CMVR is a slowly expanding lesion, usually beginning as a small, white, retinal infiltrate. Initially, it may be difficult to diagnose because it can simulate a cotton-wool spot, commonly present in HIV-retinopathy. The clinical features, representing distinct manifestations (or perhaps only different stages related with the quickness of dissemination and the defenses from the host) of the same entity, are mainly:

1) Granular, white, multifocal satellite lesions of patchy retinitis (may represent infection of a terminal vessel) with limited or no retinal hemorrhage. This variant often shows a central atrophic zone.

2) Arc-shaped solitary expanding patch of retinitis, usually concurrent with multiple retinal hemorrhages and no atrophic zone in the center of the lesion. This variant is normally referred to as "fulminant" retinitis and is probably caused by infection of the major vascular arcades.

3) Sometimes, in CMVR, the perivasculitis may be predominant with some retinal necrosis. This variant is called "Frosted branch angiitis".The degree of vitritis in these patients is typically low because of the extreme immunosuppression.

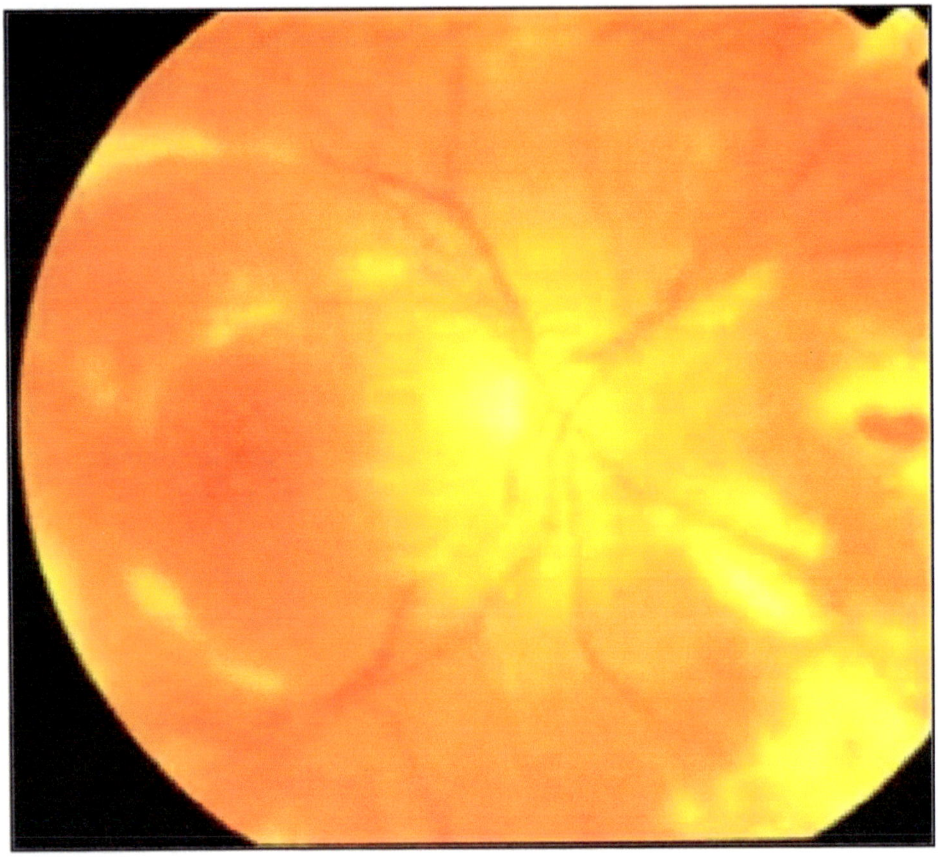

Figure 223: Right eye afflicted by extensive perivascular retinitis with areas of retinal whitening secondary to cytomegalovirus infection

Diagnosis: This diagnosis is principally based on clinical criteria: the typical clinical features in an immunocompromised patient. Detection of antibody levels from the vitreous and/or aqueous humor (and comparing it with the serum levels using the Goldmann-Witmer coefficient) can be helpful in selected cases. Viral culture and PCR from ocular tissue (if other malignant entities are suspected) or fluid can demonstrate the existence of viral DNA, but it is important to remember that this does not directly give the diagnosis of CMVR, because CMV can persist in the tissue without causing disease.

Treatment:. In AIDS, HAART therapy has demonstrated improvement of the immune system (immune reconstruction) and is beneficial not only for prevention, but also for treating CMVR. The most common are ganciclovir, foscarnet and cidofovir. Others approved for treatment include fomivirsen and valganciclovir. These drugs are usually administered systemically (W and/or orally), but in patients who show progression despite high dose of therapy, intravitreal (injections or implants) ganciclovir or foscarnet can also be considered. The size of the lesion will be the main sign to evaluate the response to the treatment. In chronic immunocompromised patients, the anti-CMV therapy will need to be maintained indefinitely.

References:

1) Heilingenhaus A, Helbig H, Fiedler M. Herpes viruses; in: Foster CS, Vitale AT. *Diagnosis and treatment of Uveitis*. Saunders. Philadelphia 2002:315-32.
2) Jabs DA, Van Natta ML, Thorne JE et at Course of cytomegalovirus retinitis in the era of highly active antiretroviral therapy:2. Second eye involvement and retinal detachment. *Ophthalmology* 2004; 111(12):2232-9.
3) Cordero Coma M, Anzaar F, Yilmaz T, Foster CS. Herpetic retinitis. *Herpes*.2007.

Progressive Outer Retinal Necrosis

Definition: Progressive outer retinal necrosis (PORN) is a necrotizing chorioretinitis and is almost exclusively found in patients with advanced stages of AIDS, being the second most common cause of blindness in such patients. Others have reported cases of PORN in patients otherwise immunocompromised, such as those with idiopathic thrombocytopenic purpura, cutaneous non-Hodgkin's lymphoma, renal transplantation and allogenic stem cell transplantation. It is most commonly caused by the varicella zoster virus.

History: PORN was first reported in 1990 by Forster.

Epidemiology: The incidence of PORN is much less than that of ARN.

Pathology/Pathogenesis: Varicella zoster virus remains latent in the cerebral or posterior root ganglia. In AIDS patients, the virus often becomes active and leads to PORN.

Clinical Features: The typical clinical symptoms of PORN are decreased vision (20/20 to no light perception), floaters, and loss of peripheral vision. Rarely, an afferent pupillary defect is present. Optic nerve involvement can also masquerade as papillitis or neuroretinitis. On slit-lamp biomicroscopy, there is usually very little vitritis, minimal vasculitis, cotton-wool spots, multifocal areas of retinal whitening with confluent necrosis, and rare intraretinal hemorrhages. A "cracked mud" appearance can also be seen. 74% of patients have unilateral disease at presentation, but can become bilateral in 70% of patients. The multifocal, peripheral lesions coalesce and rapidly progress despite treatment. The disease generally advances rapidly, leading to bilateral, complete visual loss despite treatment with antiviral gents. The majority of patients with PORN have generalized herpes zoster infection prior to or coincident with its development, and hematogenous dissemination of the virus has been suggested as a risk factor, as has the resistance of VZV to acyclovir (as a result of mutations in VZV TK genes). Complications include rhegmatogenous retinal detachment (occurring in 90% of cases), secondary to an atrophic and thinned retina with multiple holes.

Diagnosis: Using the polymerase chain reaction is helpful in ruling out entities, such as herpes simplex virus, toxoplasmosis, varicella zoster virus, Epstein-Barr virus, and cytomegalovirus using polymerase chain reaction.

Treatment: The combination of foscarnet and ganciclovir are used to treat PORN. However, many patients respond very poorly antivirals. As a result, 67% of individual become no light perception within 4 weeks.

Figure 224: Multifocal areas of retinal whitening and necrosis.

References:

1) Engstrom RE Jr, Holland GN, Margolis TP, Muccioli C, Lindley JI, Belfort R Jr, Holland SP, Johnston WH, Wolitz RA, Kreiger AE. The progressive outer retinal necrosis syndrome. A variant of necrotizing herpetic retinopathy in patients with AIDS. *Ophthalmology*. 1994 Sep; 101(9):1488-502.
2) Lim WK, Chee SP, Nussenblatt RB. Progression of varicella-zoster virus necrotizing retinopathy in an HIV-negative patient with transient immune deviation. Graefes *Arch Clin Exp Ophthalmol*. 2005 Jun ; 243 (6) : 607-9.

Varicella Zoster Virus

Definition: Primary infection with the varicella zoster virus (VZV) causes varicella disease, and reactivation of the virus leads to zoster.

History: Giovanni Filippo provided the first description of the varicella virus.

Epidemiology: Ninety-percent of the population demonstrates serologic evidence of exposure to VZV by age 60, but only 20% will have experienced an episode of zoster reactivation.

Pathogenesis: VZV establishes its latent phase in the satellite cells of sensory ganglia; the thoracic and lumbar dermatomes are most frequently involved clinically. The trigeminal ganglion is often also infected.

Clinical features:

Systemic Manifestations: Initially, there is a general malaise, fever, and headache. Subsequently, characteristic papules, macules, vesicles, and, later, crusting occur with VZV.

Ocular Manifestations: The typical clinical features of intraocular inflammation caused by VZV include trabeculitis, iridocyclitis, acute retinal necrosis and variants of necrotizing herpetic retinopathy. Inflammation of the endothelium occurs relatively early in the course of disease and leads to stromal and epithelial edema. Endotheliitis is typically accompanied by signs of mild anterior chamber inflammation. Keratic precipitates often appear under affected regions of the cornea and they can be either small or large (mutton fat). Iridocyclitis tends to occur within 1 to 2 weeks of disease onset, but can appear many months later. Later inflammation is mediated by an immune reaction against persistent viral antigen presence in the corneal stroma. Sectoral occlusion of the iris vasculature leads to atrophic sectoral patches in approximately 20% of cases and can produce hypopigmentation or, infrequently, hyperpigmentation, and iris sphincter damage.

Treatment: Systemic antivirals are the mainstay management of VZV-uveitis. Oral acyclovir is usually given in doses of 800 mg two times a day for an indefinite period of time. Alternative antiviral medications are famciclovir and valacyclovir (a prodrug of acyclovir). Topical corticosteroids also are useful and effective in controlling iridocyclitis and the inflammatory manifestations of corneal disease, including disciform keratitis, endotheliitis, and keratouveitis. In the acute stages, cycloplegic agents also should be used to relieve the discomfort of photophobia and prevent the formation of synechiae.

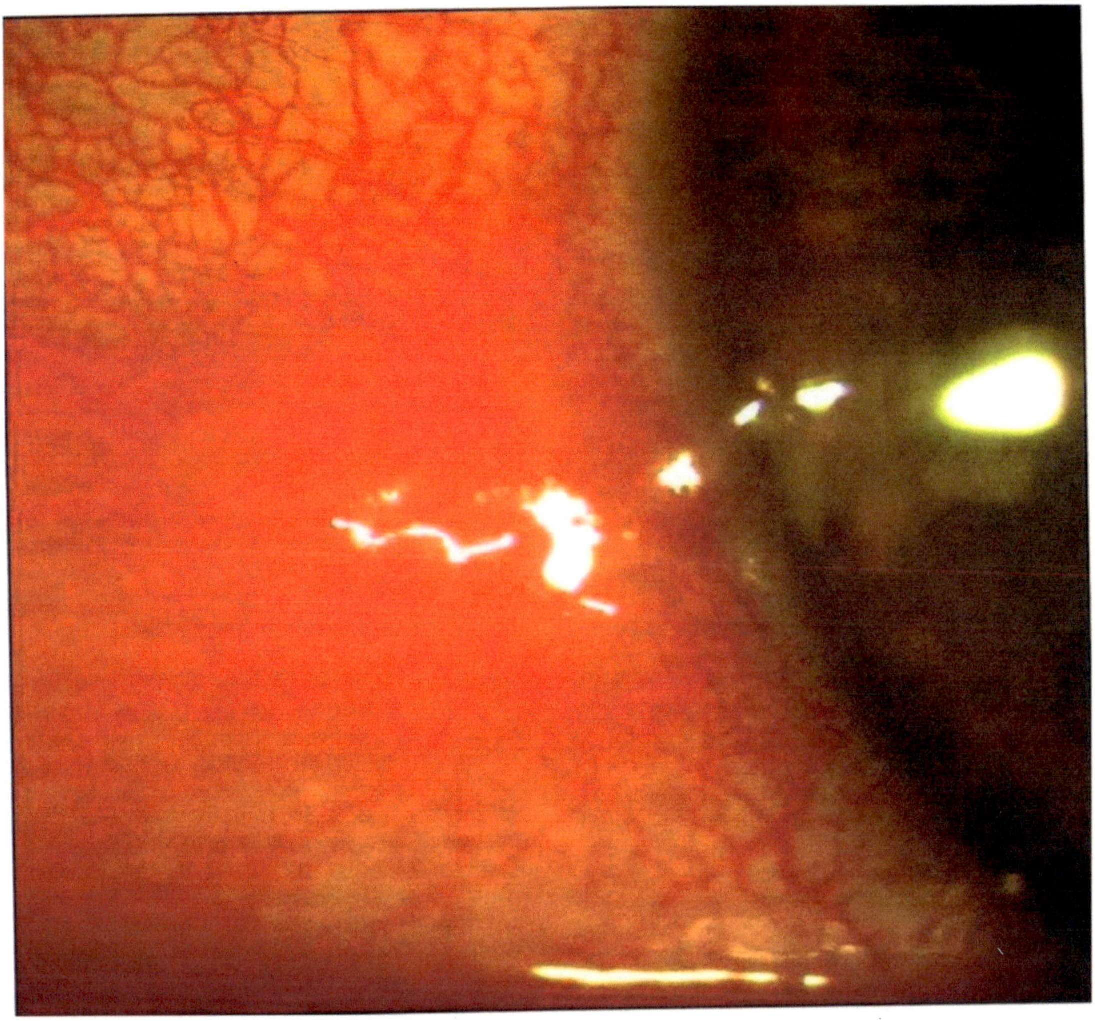

Figure 225: Nodular scleritis as seen in a patient with VZV-associated uveitis

References:

1) Gershon AA, Steinberg SP: Antibody responses to varicella-zoster virus and the role of antibody in host defense. *Am J Med Sci* 282:12, 1981.
2) Liesegang TJ: Diagnosis and therapy of herpes zoster ophthalmicus. *Ophthalmology* 98: 1216, 1991
3) Cobo M, Foulks GN, Liesegang T et al: Observations on the natural history of herpes zoster ophthalmicus. *Curr Eye Res* 6:195, 1987.
4) Womack LW, Liesegang TJ: Complications of herpes zoster ophthalmicus. *Arch Ophthalmol* 101:42, 1983.
5) Naumann G, Gass JDM, Font RL: Histopathology of herpes zoster ophthalmicus. *Am J Ophthalmol* 533:65, 1968.

HIV-associated Uveitis

Definition: There are several possible ocular manifestations of human immunodeficiency virus (HIV) infection which may involve almost all parts of the globes, ocular adnexa, and nerves. Ocular manifestations have been reported in up to 70% of persons infected with HIV, and it has become evident that the ocular manifestations almost invariably reflect systemic disease and may be the first sign of disseminated systemic infection. The most frequent ocular manifestation of AIDS is HIV-associated retinopathy. However, the main retinal opportunistic infection is CMV retinitis.

History: The acquired immunodeficiency syndrome (AIDS) was first recognized in 1981, being the first pandemic since the first half of the 20th century. HW was identified as the etiologic agent in 1984.

Epidemiology: HIV is transmitted by sexual contact, by blood, and from mother to child. In industrialized countries, the main groups at risk were promiscuous homosexuals, and intravenous drug users, but heterosexual transmission is on the increase and now represents the most important form of infection. It is estimated that more than 50 million people are infected worldwide. The absolute cumulative number of cases is highest in Africa, followed by the Americas, Asia, and Europe.

Pathogenesis: HIV retinopathy is probably the result of both an underlying microvasculopathy and hematologic abnormalities, such as increased leukocyte activation and rigidity. Cidofovir-related uveitis may be associated with a direct toxic effect of cidofovir on the ciliary body. The pathogenesis of Rifabutin-related uveitis remains unclear.

Clinical Features: In HIV infection, ophthalmic involvement is often a sign of a disseminated opportunistic disease, and requires special monitoring and therapy to preserve visual function.

HIV has been isolated from the cornea, vitreous, and retina. The presence of HIV in the endothelium of the retinal vasculature induces HIV retinopathy, which is the most common ocular finding in patients with AIDS, occurring in about 50-70% of the cases. It is characterized by cotton-wool spots (representing focal areas of retinal ischemia in the nerve fiber layer), retinal hemorrhages, and microaneurysms. Although rare, anterior or posterior uveitis can be related to FIW infection.

The other two main causes of uveitis in AIDS patients are:

Opportunistic infections (visual morbidity occurs primarily with posterior segment involvement, particularly retinitis): The most important agent is cytomegalovirus, but there are more involved microbes, such as Toxoplasma, varicella zoster virus, Pneumocystis carinii, miliary tuberculosis, Cryptococcus and others. Chorioretinitis is a very serious ocular consequence caused by these pathogens.

Drug-related uueitis: Rifabutin was the first medication reported to induce drug-related uveitis. Other reported medication which may cause uveitis is cidofovir, an anti-Cytomegalovirus nucleoside analogue.

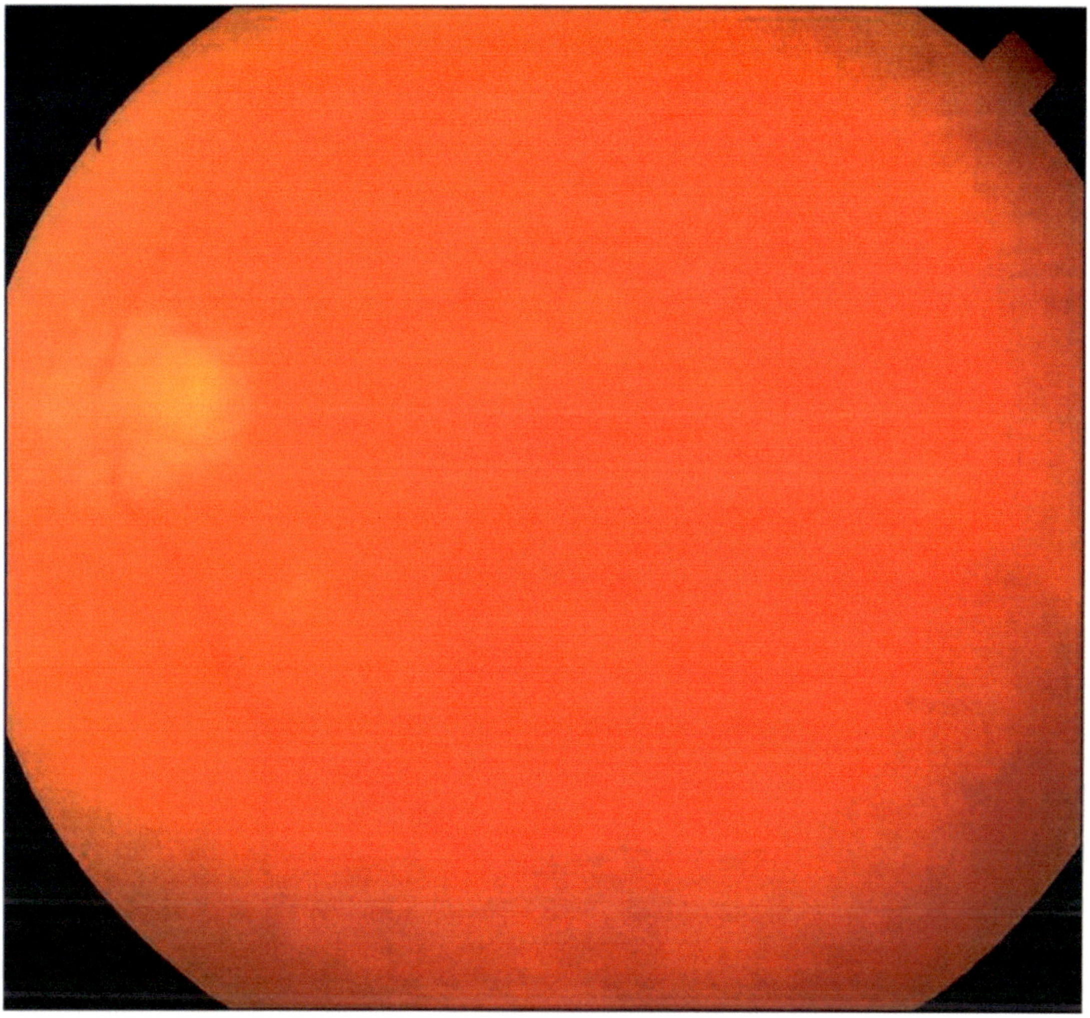

Figure 226: Characteristic cotton wool spots and scattered hemorrhages in a patient with HIV retinopathy.

Diagnosis: Laboratory work-up is essential to establish the diagnosis of HIV infection, which depends on demonstration of virus-specific antibodies by enzyme-linked immunosorbent assay and Western blot. Other helpful tests to make this diagnosis are polymerase chain reaction (PCR), which detects HIV nucleic acids, or direct isolation of HIV from the blood by culture (less used). Diagnosis of AIDS is based on clinical criteria in addition to previous demonstration of HIV infection.

Treatment: Early disease detection, immunization (hepatitis B and other vaccines), and prophylactic antimicrobial agents when needed, are essential to prevent complications Systemic antiretroviral drugs have demonstrated improvement of the immune system (immune reconstruction) being the main therapy against HIV-associated ocular manifestations. Opportunistic chorioretinal infections require prompt diagnosis and aggressive therapy, which differs among the aforementioned pathogens.

References:

1) Cochereau I, Hoang-Xuan T.Human Immunodeficiency Virus-associated uveitis; in: Foster CS, Vitale AT. *Diagnosis and treatment of uveitis.* Saunders. Philadelphia 2002:493-502.
2) Cunningham ET Jr, Belfort R. *HIV/AIDS and the Eye: A Global Perspective.* Ophthalmology Monograph 15. San Francisco. American Academy of Ophthalmology; 2002.
3) Cunningham ET Jr, Margolis TP. Ocular manifestations of HIV infection. *N Engl J Med* 1998; 339:236-44.

Leprosy

Definition: Leprosy, also known as Hansen's disease, is caused by the bacillus *Mycobacterium leprae*. Classification of this chronic, granulomatous disease is separated into two main forms of leprosy: paucibacillary or multibacillary.

History: Systemic leprosy has been described as early as 600 B.C. Bull and Hansen, in 1873, reported ocular complications associated with leprosy, which may present in 100% of the population after a protracted course.

Epidemiology: Leprosy is highly prevalent in many countries of Africa, particularly Madagascar, Mozambique, and Ethiopia, which share the common public health problem of leprosy. The disease is also widespread in the Middle East and Southeast Asia. Leprosy generally affects those between those in their early teens and late thirties, male gender, and indigent.

Pathology/Pathogenesis: The chief mode of transmission is from infected nasal secretions. Close contact with others leaves an individual the most vulnerable to leprosy. The incubation period can be from as early as 6 months to 40 years or longer.

Clinical Features:

Systemic Manifestations: The effects of leprosy range from asymptomatic and self-limiting disease to progressive, unrelenting disease. In general, leprosy includes hypopigmented or reddish skin lesions with anesthetic patches, enlarged peripheral nerves, and mucous membrane involvement.

Ocular Manifestations: Early signs of ocular involvement can be recognized by diminished pupillary reactions and reduced accommodation. In type I reactions of leprosy, patients can experience keratitis, scleritis, and uveitis whereas in type II reactions superficial punctuate keratitis, acute, diffuse, plastic iridocyclitis, and episcleritis/scleritis may ensue. Lepromas can exist in two forms: miliary (iris pearls) or nodular. Miliary lepromas are pathognomic for leprosy. Madarosis and brow hair loss is frequent. Retinal vasculitis, corneal edema, fibrovascular membrane formation, posterior synechiae, and cystoid macular edema have also been reported. At least half of all blindness that occurs in leprosy is due to cataract formation. Ocular hypotony is commonly found in patients with iridocyclitis whereas glaucoma typically occurs in chronic cases.

Diagnosis: The diagnosis is based mainly on clinical signs and symptoms. Sites of peripheral nerve involvement and skin manifestations help the clinician make the diagnosis of leprosy. A skin-smear positive test for acid-fast bacilli is also a confirmatory test for leprosy.

Treatment: The treatment regimen for leprosy consists of multidrug therapy (dapsone, rifampicin, and clofazimine). Other drugs that have been used to treat leprosy include ofloxacin, sparfloxacin, minocycline, and clarithromycin.

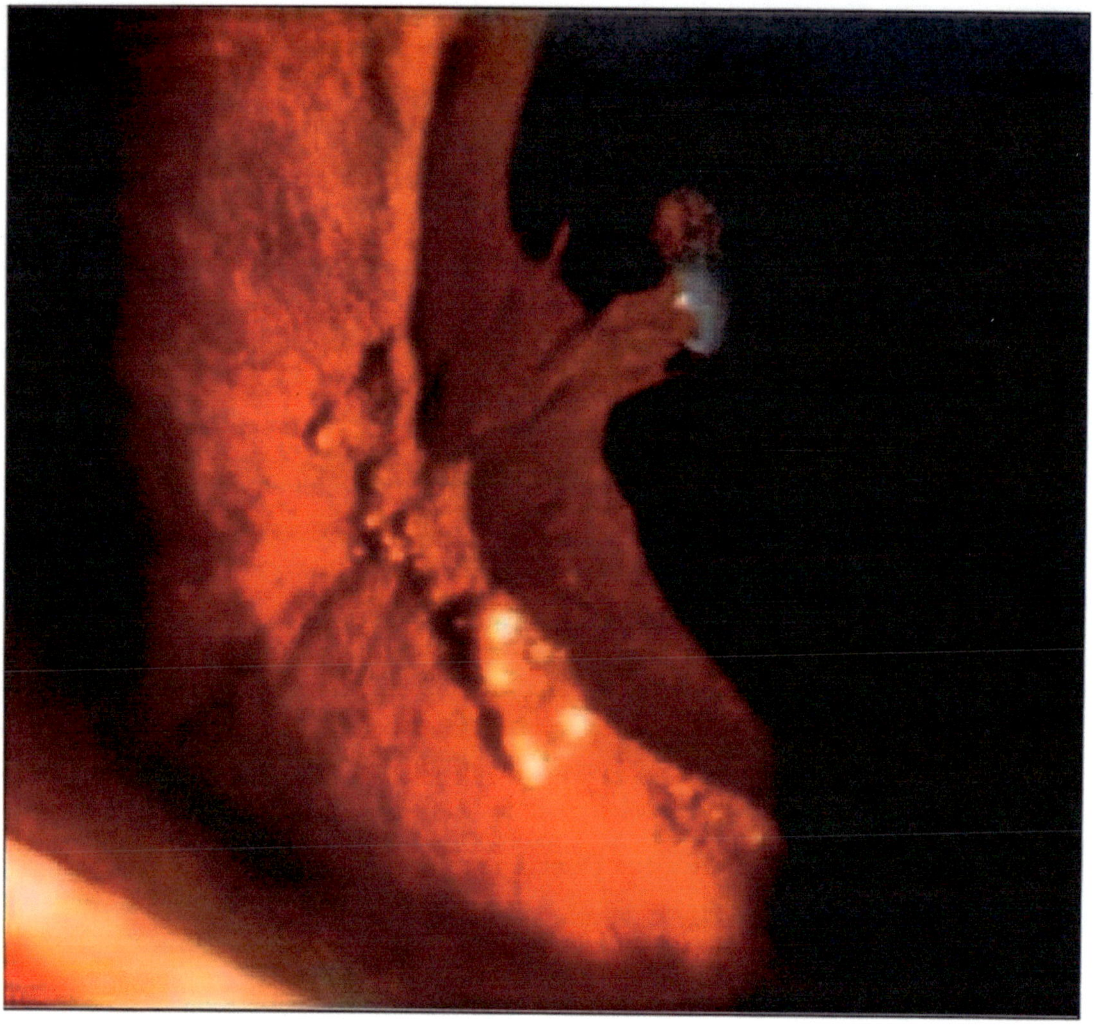

Figure 227: Iris granuloma formation (iris pearls) in lepromatous uveitis.

References:

1) Messmer EM, Raizman MB, Foster CS. Lepromatous uveitis diagnosed by iris biopsy. Graefe's *Arch Clin Exp Ophthalmol* 1998;236: 717-719.
2) Mpyet C, Solomon AW. Prevalence and causes of blindness and low vision in leprosy villages of north eastern Nigeria. *Br J Ophthalmol* 2005; 89:417-419.

POHS (Presumed Ocular Histoplasmosis Syndrome)

Definition: An ocular syndrome characterized by peripheral punched-out chorioretinal lesions , maculopathy, and peripapillary pigment changes with clear vitreous was originally presumed to be associated with the fungus Histoplasma capsulatum because of case clusters in areas endemic for that organism and because of skin test positivity to H. capsulatum skin test antigen in some patients with the ocular problem, and thus its name, presumed ocular histoplasmosis syndrome (POHS). Epidemiologic and immunologic data have supported the connection of these ocular manifestations with systemic infection by the yeast form of this fungus. However, the definite pathogenesis has eluded scientists. POHS is a distinct entity, distinguished from the exudative infection of ocular tissues by H. capsulatum which is part of disseminated histoplasmosis typically associated with immunologic disorders.

History: In 1959 Woods and Wahlen were the first to describe a distinct ocular syndrome in otherwise healthy people which was linked with a benign histoplasmosis. In 1966, Schlaegel and Kenney gave a more accurate description of the syndrome and were the first to name it POHS.

Epidemiology: Systemic histoplasmosis has a worldwide distribution. The mycelial form of this fungus grows in the soil, fertilized by droppings of birds, chicken, and bats. POHS is frequently found (with a prevalence of up to 2%) in endemic areas of the U.S. such as the Ohio-Mississippi River valleys, San Joaquin Valley of California and also in Central and South America, Asia, Mediterranean countries, and Australia. However, sporadic cases are seen in other areas as well. POHS usually affects middle aged adults, with no sex or race predilection. There is a high prevalence of histocompatibility antigens HLA-B7 and HLA-DRw2 among cases of POHS.

Pathogenesis: Ocular histoplasmosis does not become apparent until 10 to 30 years later to the primary infection. Hematogenous spread of H. capsulatum to the eye could explain its frequent bilaterality and the number, distribution, and changes over time of the histo spots. Inflammatory injury caused by H. capsulatum-induced chorioretinitis would lead to damage to Bruch's membrane, RPE, and chriocapillaris. However this model does not explain all the cases.

Clinical Features: Primary infection occurs early in life after inhalation of the fungal spores into the lungs. Dissemination to the spleen, liver, and choroid follows the initial pulmonary infection. Acquired histoplasmosis is usually asymptomatic or may result in a benign illness.

Ocular features:

1) Disseminated choroiditis ("histo spots") first appear in the eye during adolescence and are usually asymptomatic. The condition manifests as mild choroidal inflammation which is self-limiting, and as it heals it leaves behind histo spots, which are small, circular, depigmented, and atrophic chorioretinal scars. Linear equatorial streaks can be seen in 5 % of the patients.

2) Peripapillary chorioretinal degeneration and pigment changes, presumably caused by an underlying choroiditis, are frequently seen in patients with POHS, and produce blind spot enlargement on perimetry. Sometimes these lesions can harbor subretinal neovascular membranes.

3) Macular lesions, which are usually a benign syndrome although POHS often becomes symptomatic because of their recurrence or reactivation. They may be an atrophic punched-out pigmented scar similar to those seen at the peripheral retina, or more commonly a raised fibrovascular scar (disciform scar) which develops as a result of an underlying choroidal neovascular membrane.

Clear vitreous is an important part of the clinical appearance of POHS.

Diagnosis: This is based on the classic clinical triad previously described. Other hclpful test that may support the diagnosis of POHS are chest X-ray examination (showing calcified lesions), and HLA typing (HLA-B7 and HLA-DRw2 are more frequent in POHS). Fluorescein angiogram may help determine the activity of the lesions showing dye blockade in the early stages if there is active choroiditis. In later frames, the choroidal lesions stain and become hyperfluorescent. Indocyanine green angiogram may also assist in cases of occult choroidal neovascular (CNV) lesions.

Treatment: Laser photocoagulation for choroidal neovascularization has been the main modality during the last 20 years. This is essentially indicated when it lies in the disc-macula area to prevent further loss of vision. Photodynamic therapy has recently played an important role in the management of these neovascular lesions. Intravitreal anti-vascular endothelial growth factor agents have recently shown encouraging results when used for treatment of other causes of CNV (such as age-related macular degeneration). Other choices such as submacular surgery (with removal of the membrane) may also be considered. Oral or regional corticosteroids may be useful if there are symptomatic areas of active choroiditis.

References:

1) Singh G. Presumed ocular histoplasmosis syndrome; in: Foster CS, Vitale AT. *Diagnosis and treatment of uveitis*. Saunders. Philadelphia 2002:348-63.
2) Prasad AG, Van Helder RN. Presumed ocular histoplasmosis syndrome. *Curr Opin Ophthalmol.* 2005;16(6):364-8.
3) Oliver A, Ciulla TA, Comer GM. New and classic insights into presumed ocular histoplasmosis syndrome and its treatment. *Curr Opin Ophthalmol.* 2005 Jun;16(3):1643-5.

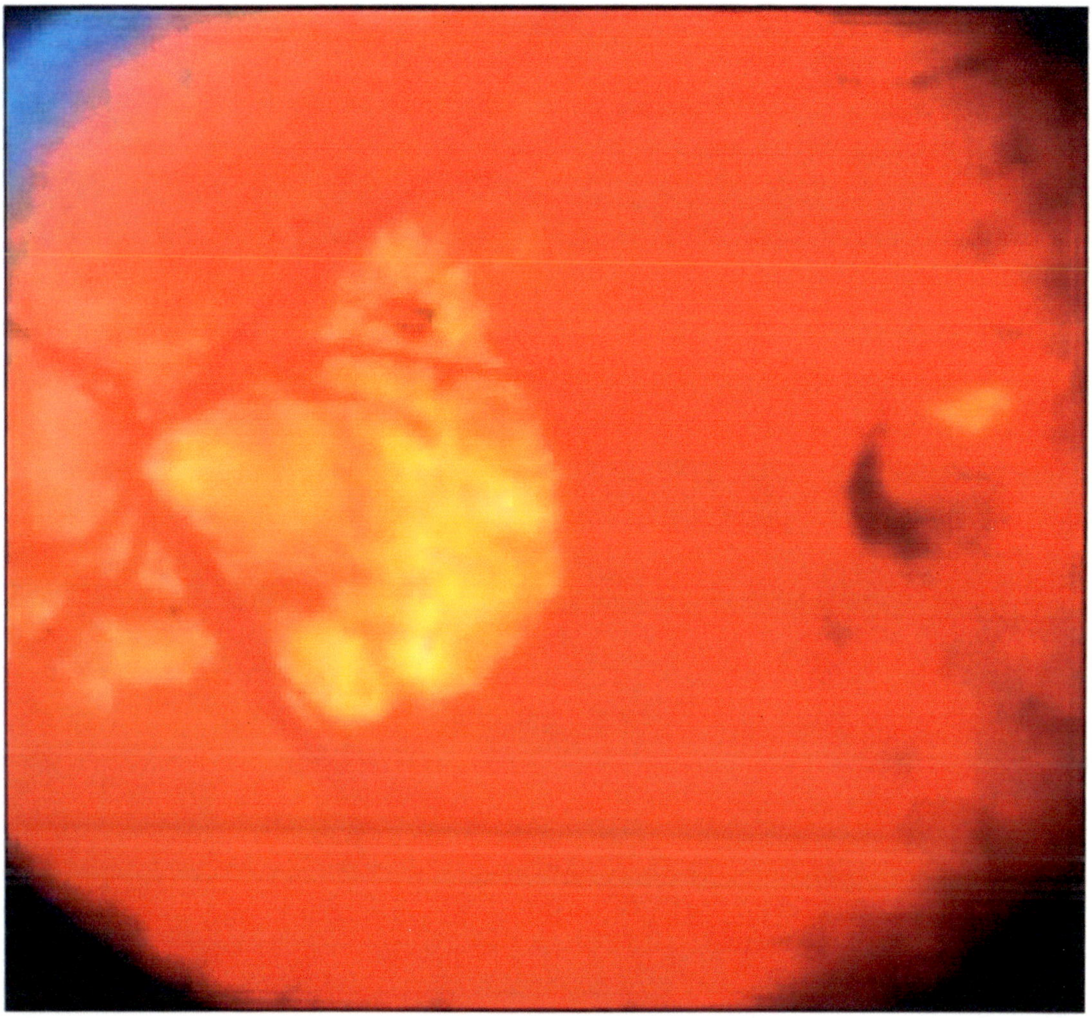

Figure 228: A subretinal neovascular membrane in a patient with presumed ocular histoplasmosis syndrome. Note the peripapillary atrophy.

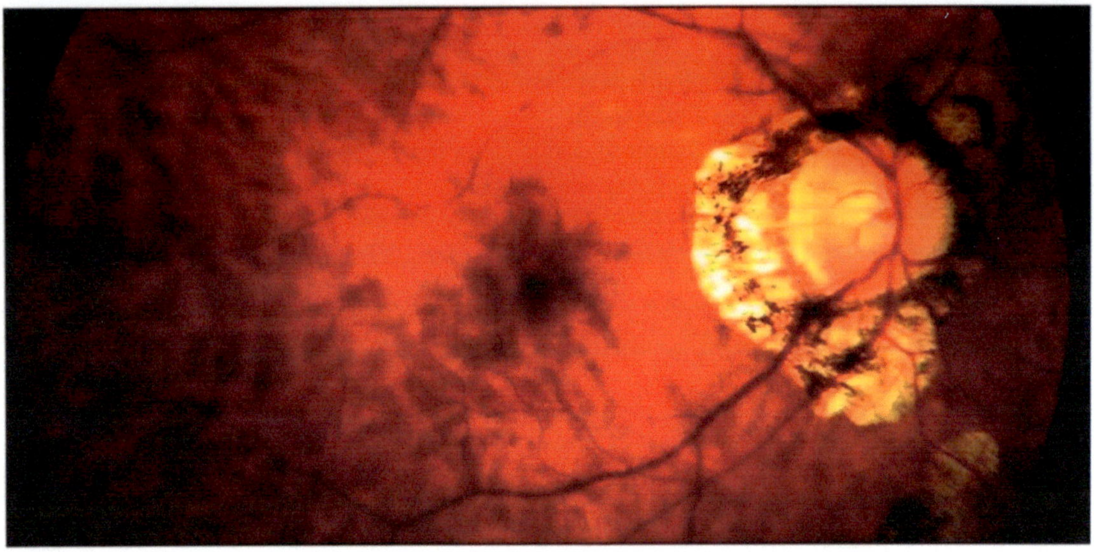

Figure 229: Peripapillary atrophy in a patient with presumed ocular histoplasmosis.

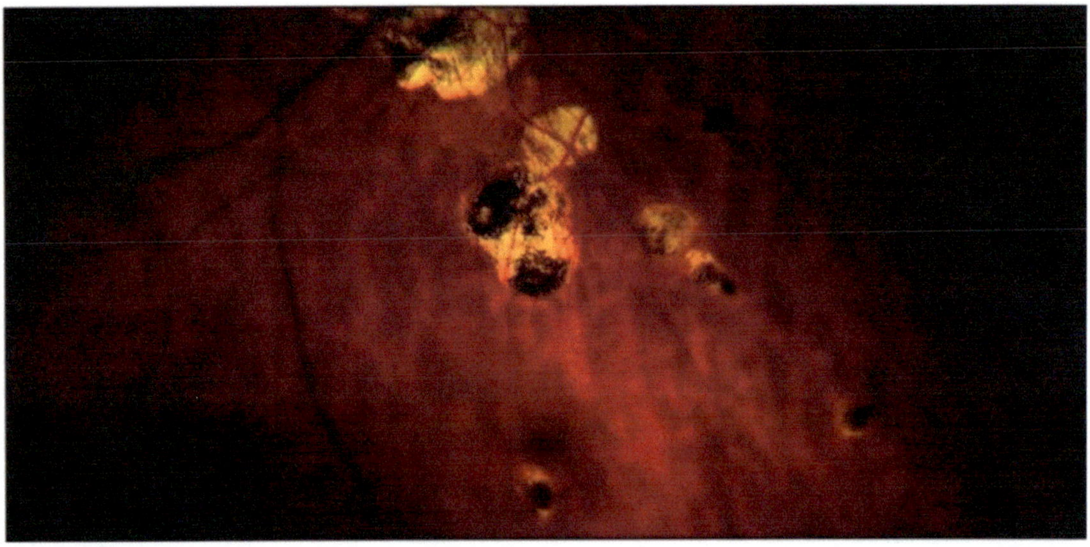

Figure 230: Peripheral punched-out chorioretinal scars ("histo spots").

Rubella

Introduction: Rubella is an exanthematous and contagious disease caused by the rubella virus, which may cause stillbirth, abortion, or congenital defects. The disease may be congenital or acquired.

History: In 1941, Gregg described the initial case of a congenital cataract secondary to rubella infection. Mitchell was the first to report a case of retinopathy associated with rubella infection.

Epidemiology: The highest risk of congenital rubella syndrome occurs during the first weeks of pregnancy. There is a 20% to 78% chance of ocular abnormalities in congenital rubella infection. After the introduction of the rubella vaccine in the U.S., rubella epidemics ceased to occur. Nevertheless, sporadic infections occur during the year in urban settings.

Pathology/Pathogenesis: Defects caused by congenital rubella arise from the inability of cellular proliferation and function with a marked reduction in the number of cells in organs. Since there is a paucity of an inflammatory response, changes may occur prior to the development of the immune system in the fetus. Acquired rubella infection is disseminated via a respiratory route. IgA, IgG, and IgM antibodies may appear in the sera of affected patients.

Clinical Features:

Systemic Manifestations: Congenital rubella syndrome (CRS) is known for its characteristic ocular, cardiac, and hearing involvement. Common manifestations include general malaise, fever, headache, rhinitis, and fine pinkish macules. Encephalitis is rarely seen in this disease. With acquired rubella, a rash on the skin is the initial sign of infection in children. Lympadenoapthy is also present in a large majority of those affected by rubella infection.

Ocular Manifestations: Pigmentary retinopathy with characteristic "salt and pepper" appearance is the most common ocular complication secondary to CRS. Subretinal neovascular membrane formation is of great concern in patients with pigmentary retinopathy. In CRS, cataracts and microphthalmia are the main culprits of poor visual acuity. Cases of strabismus, nystagmus, iris atrophy, and amblyopia have been reported. Conjunctivitis is present in 70% of patients with acquired ruibella. Retinitis and epithelial keratitis are common findings of acquired rubella.

Diagnosis: The coexistent presence of maternal rubella infection and neonatal abnormalities suggests the diagnosis of congenital rubella. Elevated IgM antibodies to rubella are an important serologic marker in uneventful pregnancies. Fluorescein angiography reveals both patterns of hyperfluorescence and hypofluorescence, which is predominantly caused by the diffuse mottling of retinal pigment epithelium. Active subretinal membranes will hyperfluoresce in late phase of the angiogram. Retinitis in acquired rubella infection reveals areas of hyperfluorescence without dye leakage from the retinal vasculature.

Treatment: Vaccination against the virus is the mainstay of treatment. Mothers susceptible to the disease or exposure to the rubella virus can be treated with intravenous immunoglobulins. Neonates should be kept in isolation if they are believed to be infected. Rubella retinitis and optic neuritis has been shown to respond favorably to systemic corticosteroids.

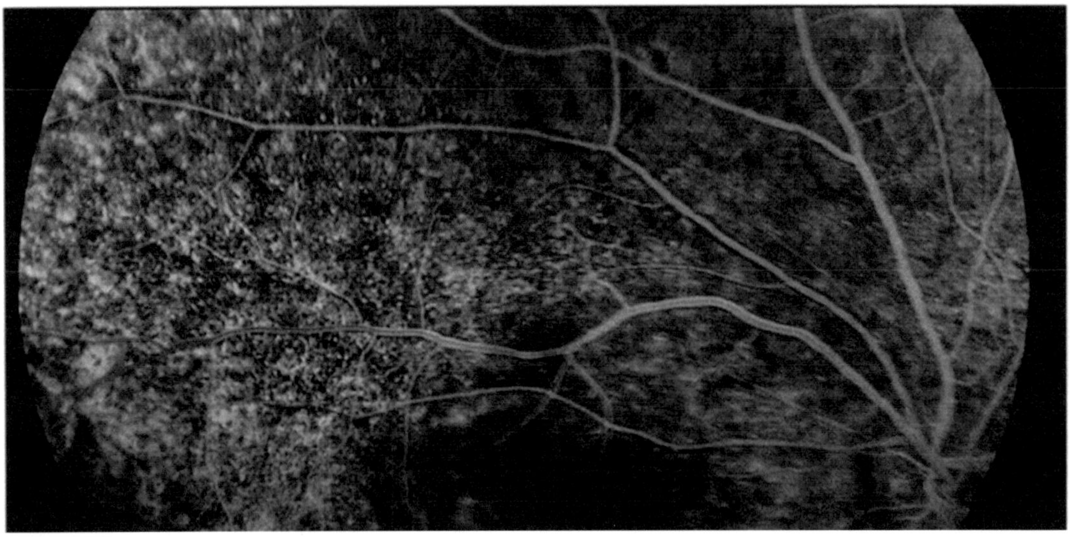

Figure 231: Diffuse pigmentary retinopathy seen in patients afflicted by rubella virus.

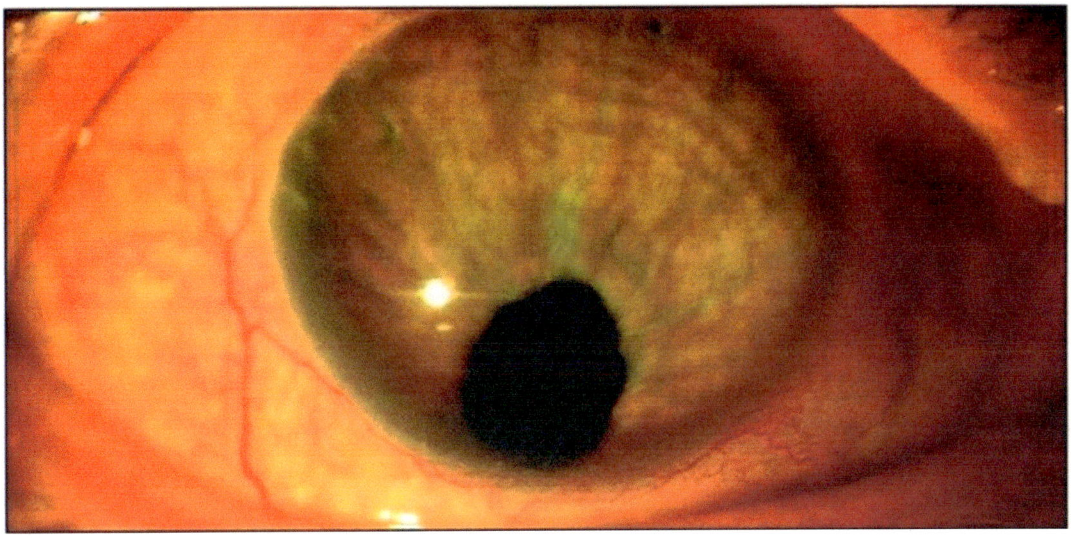

Figure 232: Corectopia secondary to congenital rubella syndrome.

References:

1) Collis WJ, Cohen DN: Rubella retinopathy: A progressive disorder. *Arch Ophthalmol* 1970;84: 33-35-
2) Kazarian EL, Gager WE: Optic neuritis complicating measles, mumps, and rubella vaccination. *Am J Ophthalmol* 1978;86:544-547

Syphilis

Definition: Syphilis is caused by the spirochete *Treponema pallidum*. It can mimic many different diseases throughout its course for which is has been called the "Great Imitator." It can persist in the affected person for a lifetime, and if left untreated can progress through four stages. It is a sexually transmitted disease, which enters the body through the genitals, mouth, or skin breaks.

History: Schaudin and Hoffman isolated the spirochete in 1905 from the skin lesions of infected patients.

Epidemiology: Although it was the second leading cause of uveitis before the 1940s, currently it comprises about 1-2% of all uveitis cases.

Pathology/Pathogenesis: The inflammatory response against the spirochete causes the damage and destruction of ocular tissue. The host immune response role in syphilitic infection is being investigated. The difficulty in culturing *T. pallidum* in vivo has been an impediment in the study of its pathogenic mechanisms.

Clinical Features:

Systemic Manifestations: Primary syphilis is characterized by a chancre at the inoculation site that appears 2-6 weeks after infection and resolves about 4 weeks after its appearance. If untreated, the disease progresses to secondary syphilis, with generalized maculopapular rash and lymphadenopathy. The rash typically affects the palms and soles, and can be accompanied by fever, malaise, headache, nausea, hair loss, mouth ulcers, and joint pain. At this stage, the eyes are affected in 10% of the cases. Then, during the latent stage, there are no evident systemic disease manifestations, and the infection is not contagious. This stage can last for the lifetime of the patient. Tertiary syphilis can affect any system, but mainly the cardiovascular (aortitis, aortic aneurysm, aortic valve insufficiency) and neurologic system (meningovascular syphilis, tabes dorsalis). The typical lesion in this stage is the gumma, which is a granuloma, and can be found anywhere in the body.

Ocular manifestations: Most patients that develop syphilitic uveitis develop it during the latent stage of the infection. Anterior uveitis may be unilateral or bilateral, granulomatous or nongranulomatous. It can present with iris nodules or atrophy, anterior cells with or without anterior vitritis, dilated iris vessels, interstitial keratitis, and lens dislocation. Syphilis can affect the posterior segment, most commonly causing chorioretinitis. The fundus lesions are usually grayish yellow in color. Other manifestations include: disc edema, arterial or venous vasculitis, vitritis, intermediate uveitis, serous retinal detachment, neuroretinitis, necrotizing retinitis. Complications include glaucoma, cataracts, macular edema, and choroidal neovascular membranes.

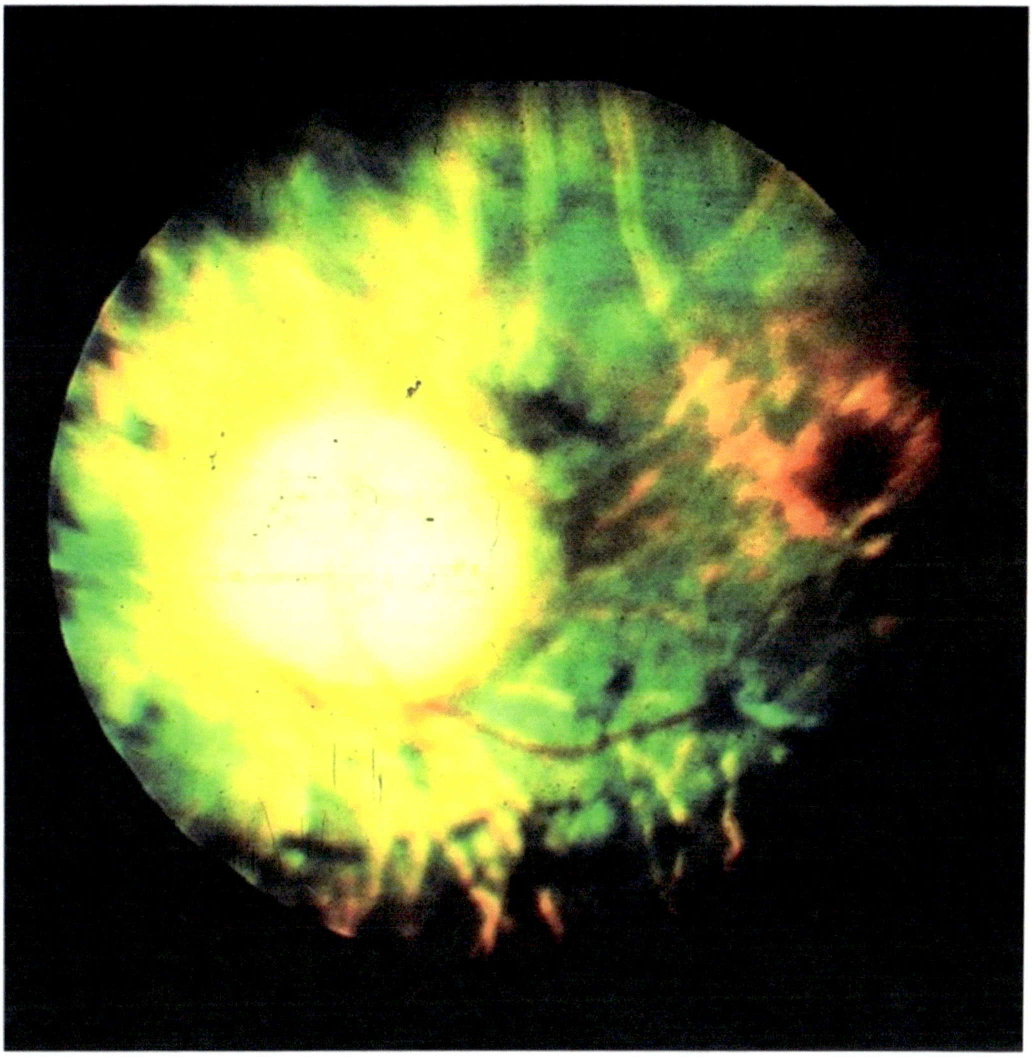

Figure 233: Neororetinitis with delayed diagnosis of Syphilis and total destruction of the retina

Diagnosis: Diagnosis is based on serologic tests and clinical characteristics. Available nonspecific serological tests quantify the amount of serum anticardiolipin antibody are the rapid plasma reagin (RPR), and the Venereal Disease Research Laboratory (VDRL). Specific tests measure the amount of serum antibody against treponemal antigens. The fluorescent treponemal antigen absorption test (FTA-ABS) is the one mostly used. This test becomes positive during the secondary stage of Syphilis and remains positive for the patient's lifetime. With the microhemagglutination assay for T. pallidum (MHA-TP) test, treponemes can be visualized by incubating infected body fluid (from chancre or skin pustule) with fluorescent-tagged antibody and visualizing it under darkfield microscopy. The T. pallidum particle agglutination test (TP-PA) is used to confirm a positive FTA-ABS. Patients with uveitis who are diagnosed with syphilis must have examination of the cerebrospinal fluid (CSF).

Treatment: Penicillin is the treatment of choice in syphilis. Two recommended regimens for syphilitic uveitis are: intramuscular Penicillin injection once weekly for 3 weeks, or intravenous daily penicillin G for 10-14 days. As syphilitic uveitis is considered a form of neurosyphilis, the intravenous regimen is favored. Alternative treatments for penicillin allergic patients include doxycycline or tetracycline. Penicillin desensitization is another option for these patients.

Reference

1) Samson CM. Syphilis; in: Foster CS, Vitale AT. *Diagnosis and treatment of uveitis*. Saunders. Philadelphia 2002:237-244.

Toxocariasis

Definition: Toxocariasis is an important zoonotic disease caused by the invasion of tissue by the second-stage larvae of *Toxocara canis* or *Toxocara cati*, which are nematode parasites commonly present in the small intestine of dogs or cats, respectively. *Toxocara* larva in the eye can especially induce uveitis, retinal granuloma, endophthalmitis, and other ocular lesions, collectively known as ocular toxocariasis.

History: In 1937, Calhoun described the invasion of the eye by a nematode larva for the first time. Histopathology of the lesions of ocular toxocariasis was described before the recognition of its classic clinical appearance by Wilder in 1950.

Epidemiology: Contact with dogs (especially puppies) and cats are well-known risk factors for ocular toxocariasis. However, it is important to emphasize that the most common route of infection is the ingestion of soil contaminated with *Toxocara* larvae.

Pathology/Pathogenesis: The larvae reach the eye via the blood-stream and become encysted in the ocular tissues. Definitive diagnosis of ocular toxocariasis requires the identification of the larva, though in most specimens the organism has been entirely destroyed. The presence of inflammation in the absence of the larvae or their remnants has suggested that secreted antigens may be implicated.

Clinical Features: The most commonly affected tissue is the retina. The disease has been commonly classified into three clinical types: peripheral inflammatory mass type, posterior pole granuloma type, and diffuse nematode endophthalmitis. The course of the disease is usually asymptomatic and impairment of visual acuity (VA) is the most common manifestation when symptoms are present. The youngest children do not complain about visual changes even if VA is tremendously affected, and other clinical manifestations, such as strabismus or leukocoria must lead to suspect this entity.

Systemic manifestations: Approximately 10% of the patients have mild eosinophilia. Liver abscesses or cystic lesions located in other areas are uncommon findings.

Anterior segment: Low-grade anterior uveitis and posterior synechiae are seen in cases of chronic endophthalmitis. Recurrent nodular sderitis or keratitis are only occasional findings.

Posterior segment: A granulomatous reaction located in the posterior pole or in the periphery is the typical finding. Commonly posterior pole toxocariasis lesions are white or gray, round, and elevated. The diameter is generally one or two disc diameters in size, and may be centered anywhere in the posterior pole. The predominance of peripheral granuloma, usually hazy-white and elevated, is frequently associated with retinal folds that may extend from the peripheral mass to the optic nerve head (see figure 234).

Another common manifestation of ocular toxocariasis is chronic endophthalmitis, which are usually associated with retinal detachment, cyclitic membranes between the detached retina and the lens. Papillitis, macular edema, vitreous exudates, and (rarely) retrolental masses are possible associated findings.

The spectrum of ocular inflammatory diseases caused by Toxocara is now thought to be much wider than previously described and may include cases previously diagnosed as pars planitis and panuveitis.

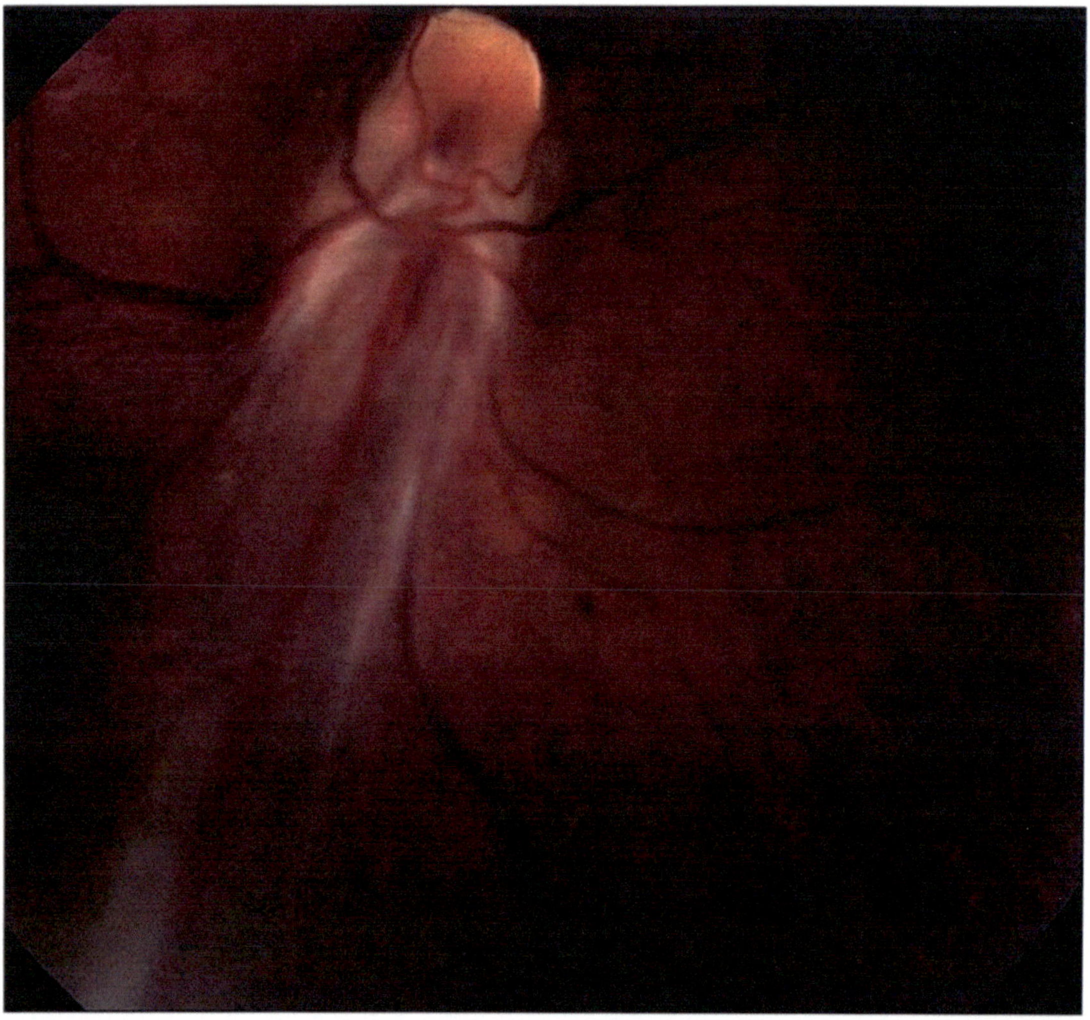

Figure 234: 9 year-old white female affected by ocular toxocariasis. Retinal fold that extends from the peripheral mass (toxocara granuloma) to the optic nerve head.

Diagnosis: The disease is usually diagnosed by characteristic clinical findings and a positive result in an enzyme—linked immunosorbent assay (ELISA) for anti-*T.canis* antibody in serum or in intraocular fluid. More important than serum titer is the detection of antibodies in aqueous humor and the use of the Goldmann-Witmer coefficient to ensure that the positive result is due to local production of antibodies and not as a consequence of the blood-eye barrier breakdown.

Treatment: The strategy is principally based on the local and systemic administration of corticosteroids toward the inflammatory response that may produce structural damage to the eye and visual impairment. Some authors have reported clinical improvement using systemic larvicides, such as thiabendazole. Surgical procedures, such as a pars plana vitrectomy (with or without cryopexy or photocoagulation) must be considered in those cases in which the response to medical treatment has been poor or for those who have marked vitreous fibrosis and tractional complications.

Reference:

Romero-Rangel T, Foster CS. Toxocariasis; in: Foster CS, Vitale AT. *Diagnosis and treatment of uveitis.* Saunders. Philadelphia 2002:428-436.

Toxoplasmosis

Definition: Toxoplasmosis is the leading cause of posterior uveitis in the world in otherwise healthy individuals. *Toxoplasma gondii* is an intracellular obligate protozoan, which causes ocular toxoplasmosis by the release of actively proliferating tachyzoites. It is transmitted to humans via ingestion of tissue cysts in raw or undercooked meat or through contact with the fecal matter of cats, which contains *T. gondii* oocysts. Ocular toxoplasmosis is characterized predominantly by focal retinitis in the active form and large, pigmented scars in the inactivated state. It is characterized by four different forms: acquired, congenital, in the immunocompromised individual, and ocular.

History: In 1940, Pinkerton and Weinman described the first case of acquired toxoplasmosis with ocular manifestations. However, the initial case of congenital toxoplasmosis was reported by Jankti in 1923.

Epidemiology: Toxoplasmosis is a very widely distributed zoonosis. Seropositive individuals typically live in countries with tropical climates. In France, by the fourth decade of life, 90% of the French population is seropositive for toxoplasmosis. In the United States 70% of the population over 50 shows seropositivity. The incidence of congenital toxoplasmosis in the United States is approximately 0.2%-1%.

Pathology/Pathogenesis: *T. gondii* is found in the host's saliva, urine, semen, and peritoneal fluid. The organism presents in three forms: tachyzoite, bradyzoite, and sporozoite. Tachyzoites are responsible for the acute form of the disease. Tachyzoites stain with Giemsa and have a bluish cytoplasm and a reddish ovoid nucleus. Cysts have eosinophilic walls with the bradyzoites inside and are PAS-positive.

Clinical Features: Typically, the patient complains of floaters and decreased visual acuity.

Systemic manifestations: Congenital toxoplasmosis may present several months or even years after the infection with characteristic features, such as paralysis, encephalomyelitis, seizures, hydrocephalus, microcephaly, and intracranial calcifications. In the acquired form of the infection, lymphadenopathy is the most common finding. However, the disease is typically self-limiting in the immunocompetent patient.

Ocular manifestations: In the congenital form of the disease, the most common finding is retinochoroiditis occurring 70% to 90% of the cases. Associated ocular sequelae include cataracts, nystagmus, optic atrophy, and strabismus. Retinochoroidal scars are typically found in both the acquired and congenital forms and can be solitary or multiple. Focal retinitis is seen in the active form .

Anterior segment: Mutton-fat keratic precipitates, anterior chamber reaction, and posterior synechiae may be present in the active part of the disease.

Posterior segment: T. gondii has a strong predilection for invading the macula and optic nerve with a tendency to recur. A yellow, elevated, fluffy lesion is seen in the hallmark "headlight in the fog" appearance of the active Toxoplasma lesion. In the active form of the disease, vitritis is almost always present in all cases. Vasculitis, choroiditis, neuroretinitis, papillitis and necrotizing retinitis may present as well.

Diagnosis: Some other tests may be helpful:

Polymerase Chain Reaction (PCR): With samples of the aqueous and vitreous humor, one can definitively confirm the presence of T. gondii with high specificity and selectivity.

Fluorescein angiogram (FA) and indocyanine green angiography (ICGA): During the early phase of the FA study, there is hypofluorescence of the lesion which then leaks dye in late phase. In ICGA, active retinochoroiditis may reveal areas of hypofluorescence or hyperfluorescence in the early phases and, in the later phase, hyperfluorescence predominates.

Other tests: The Sabin and Feldman dye, hemagglutination, enzyme-linked immunosorbent assay (ELISA), complement fixation, and immunofluorescence antibody tests may be used to detect for presence of toxoplasmosis.

Treatment: The use of pyrimethamine, sulfadiazine, and corticosteroids is the gold standard since Eyles and Coleman advocated this triad of treatment in 1953. Folinic acid is used as adjuvant therapy to pyrimethamine, which has antifolate properties. Other agents used include, clindamycin, spiramycin, atovaquone, tetracycline, minocycline, clarithromycin, azithromycin, trimethoprim, and sulfamethoxazole. Laser photocoagulation and pars plana vitrectomy have had limited success. If the central macula and optic nerve are spared, prognosis is generally good because the disease will be self-limiting in the immunocompetent patient.

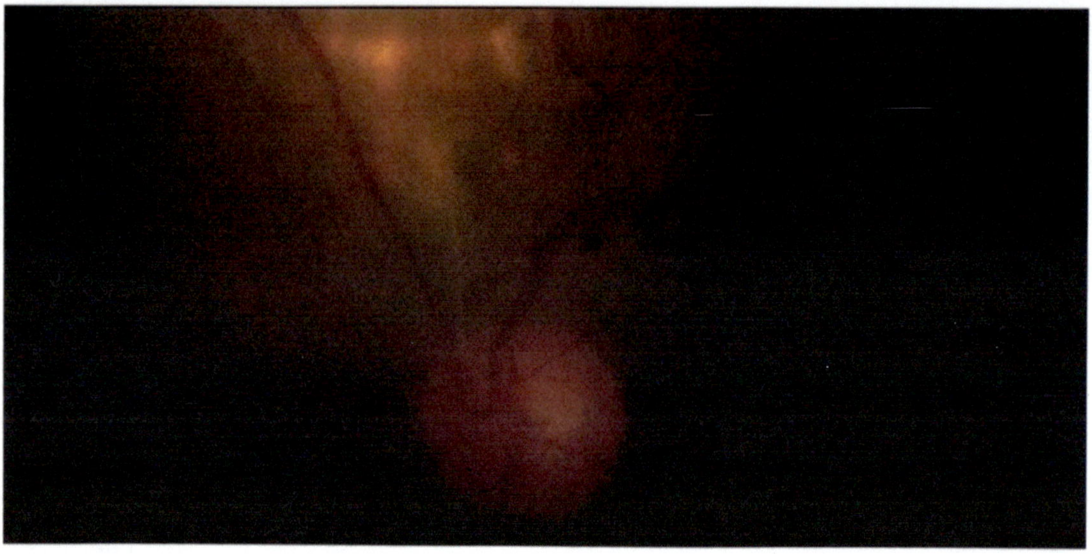

Figure 235: Inactive toxoplasmosis scar located superior to the optic disc. It is crucial to monitor these scars for reactivation.

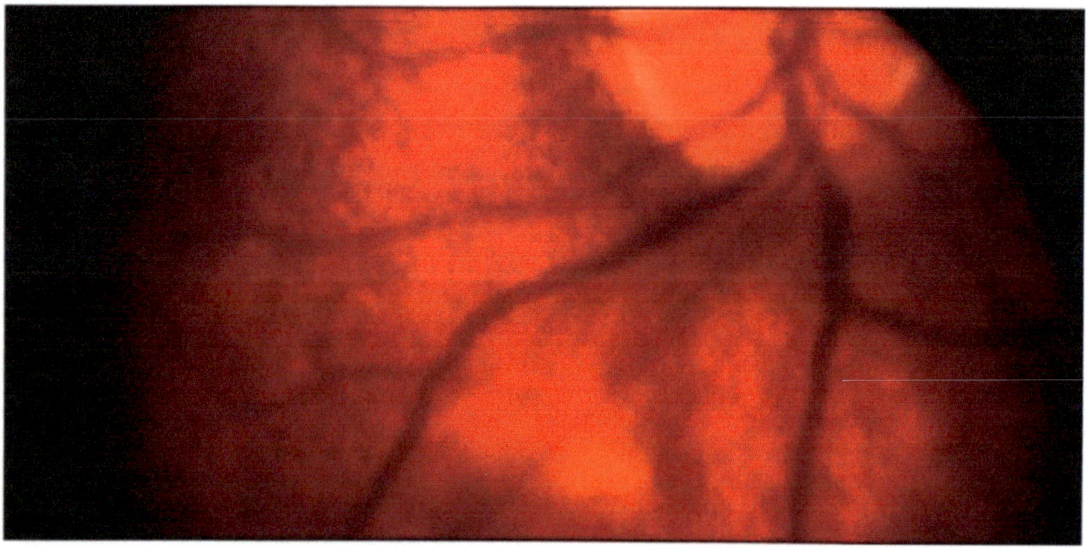

Figure 236: Active toxoplasmosis lesion located along the inferior arcade (artery) of the right eye. The lesion is elevated with indistinct borders.

<u>Figure 237:</u> Active toxoplasmosis lesion spreading along the inferior arcade. Note the fuzzy borders

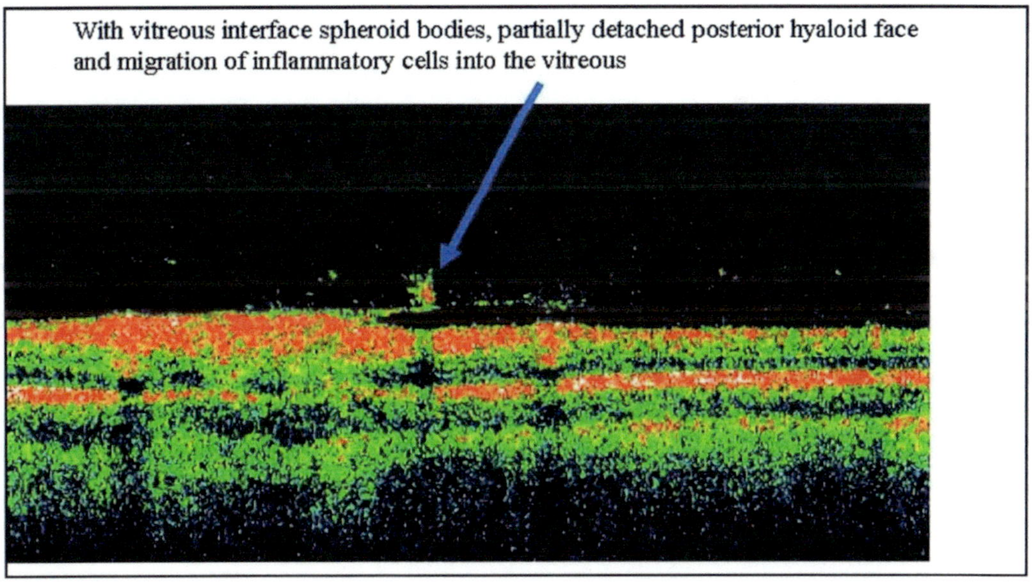

<u>Figure 238:</u> Active Toxoplasma chorioretinitis lesion.

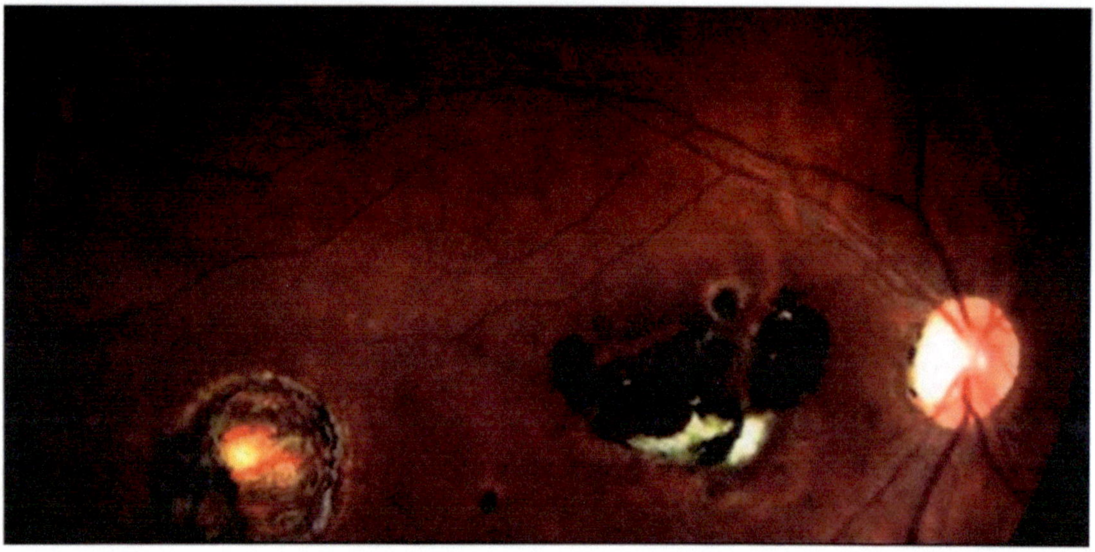

Figure 239: Central macular toxoplasmosis scar with overlying fibrotic tissue. Note the temporal scar with prominent choroidal vasculature.

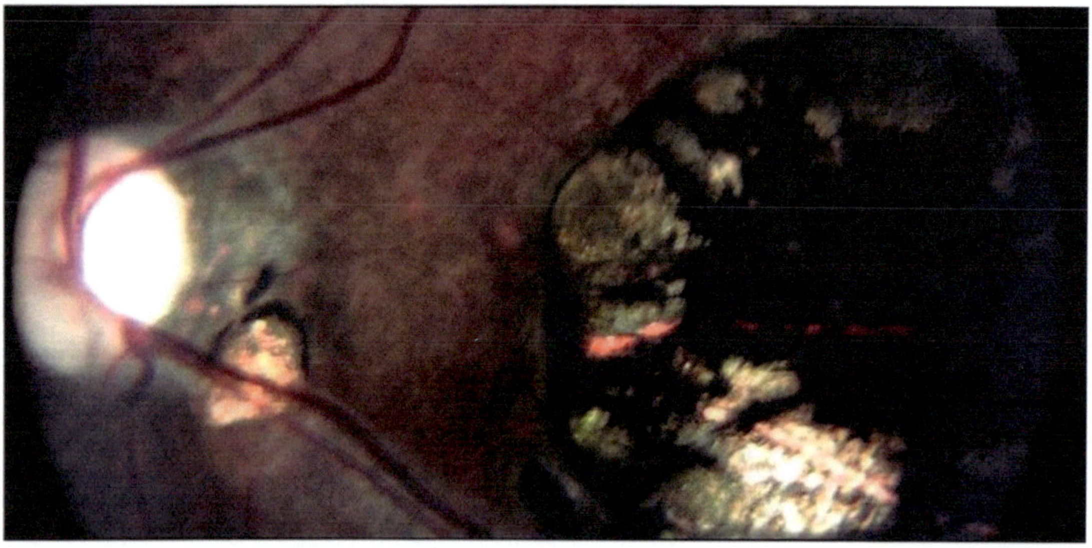

Figure 240: Typical pigmented, wagon wheel appearance of congenital toxoplasmosis scar spreading temporally. Note the temporal excavation and atrophy of the optic nerve with accompanying juxtapapillary scar along the inferior arcade.

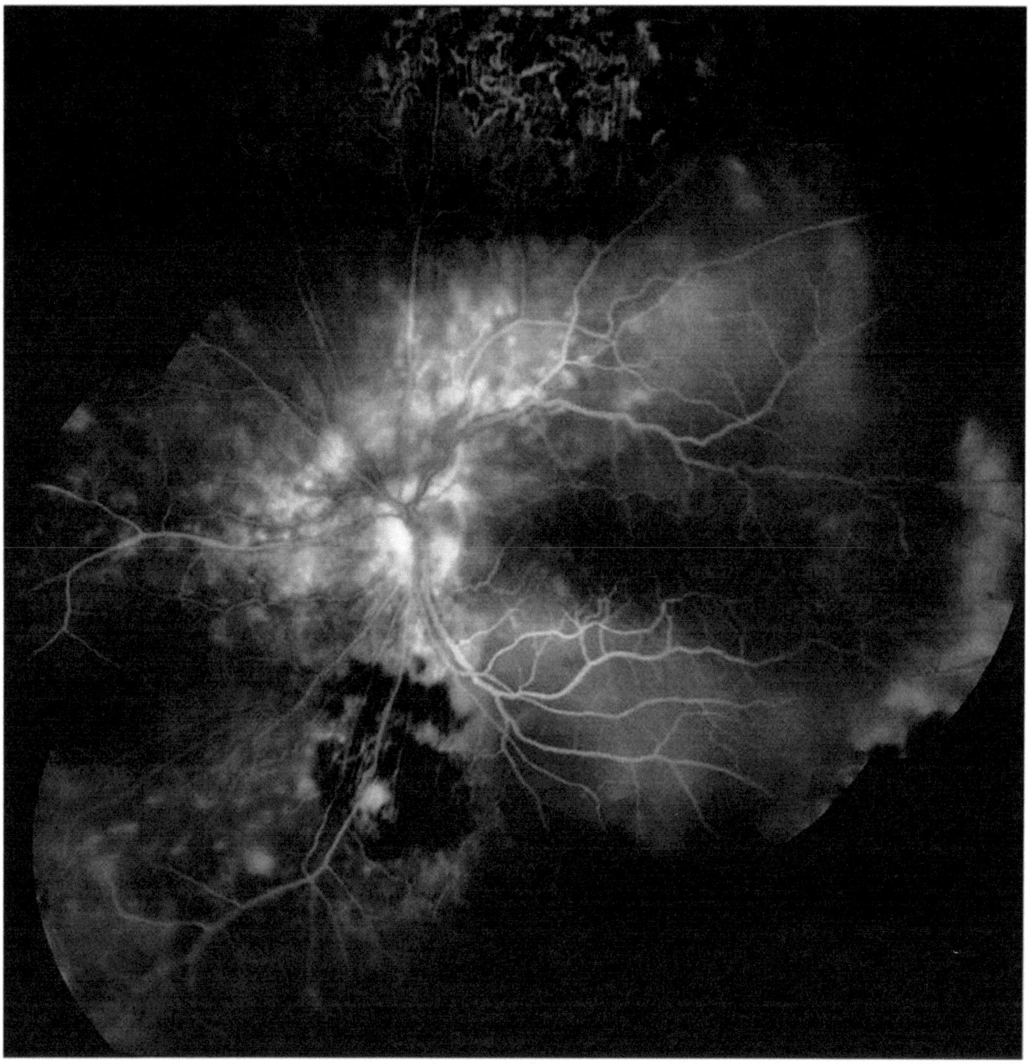

Figure 241: Fluorescein angiography in a 43 year-old Brazilian male with a history of toxoplasmosis. The inactivated scar blocks the fluorescein dye whereas the areas of surrounding the arcades accumulate the dye due to a serous retinal detachment.

References:

1) Sabin AB, Feldman HA: Dyes as microchemical indicators of a new immunity phenomenon affecting a protozoan parasite (Toxoplasma). *Science* 1948;108:660-663.
2) Pinkerton H, Weinman D: Toxoplasma infections in man *Arch Pathol* 1940;30:374-392.
3) Kasper LH: Toxoplasma infection. In: Brauwald E, Fauci AS, Isselbacher KJ, et al, eds: *Harrison's Principles of Internal Medicine Online.* New York: McGraw-Hill, 1999.
4) Park SS, To KW, Friedman AH, Jakobiec FA: Infectious causes of posterior uveitis. In: Albert DM, Jakobiec FA, eds: *Principles and Practice of Ophthalmology, Vol 1.* Philadelphia, W.B. Saunders, 1994, PP 460-461.
5) Roberts T, Frenkel JK: Estimating income losses and other preventable costs caused by congenital toxoplasmosis in people in the United States. *JAMA* 1990;2:249-256.
6) Indocyanine Green Angiography. Yilmaz T, Foster CS. *Contemporary Ophthalmology.* Vol. 5 #19 2006.
7) Eyles DE, Coleman N: Synergistic effect of sulphadiazine and daraprim against experimental toxoplasmosis in the mouse. *Antibiot Chemother* 1953;3:483-490.

Tuberculosis

Definition: Tuberculosis (TB) is an airborne communicable disease caused by a bacterium called Mycobacterium tuberculosis or by one of three other closely related species M. bovis, M. africanum, and M. microti. Ocular tuberculosis encompasses any infection by M. tuberculosis in the eye and has been classically divided into two types: primary and secondary. Primary ocular TB implies that the eye is the initial port of entry; this type includes conjunctival, corneal, and scleral disease. Secondary disease implies that organisms spread to the eye hematogenously; this type includes tuberculous uveitis.

History: This disease has been called by many names since ancient times (phthisis, "white plague"). In 1882, Robert Koch proved that the bacilli which he had previously discovered and named as M. tuberculosis, were the cause of the various TB lesions in animal experiments. Years later, Von Pirquet, and soon after Mantoux, developed scratch tests crucial in the diagnosis of the disease.

Epidemiology: Known risk factors for TB infection include close contact with infected individuals and HIV infection. In addition, individuals from countries in which TB is endemic are at risk (for example China, India or Mexico).

Pathology/Pathogenesis: Caseating necrosis is specific, but not always present. Lymphocytes, plasma cells, and giant cells accompany the essential epithelioid cells as the major infiltrating inflammatory cells. The pathogenesis is attributable to the reaction of the immune system to *M. Tuberculosis*, which serves as the model for what is now known as type IV hypersensitivity reaction (from the model proposed by Gell, Coombs, and Lackman) and is the basis for the tuberculin skin test.

Clinical Features: Uveitis is the most common ocular_manifestation of TB.

Anterior segment: Lid masses or orbital involvement is infrequent. Anterior tuberculous uveitis is typically granulomatous with extensive granulomatous keratic precipitates. Iris nodules can also be seen. Other less frequent associated findings are elevated intraocular pressure or an exudative mass in the anterior chamber. Almost all primary ocular infections are limited to conjunctival and corneal diseases that present as ulceration, a tumor mass, phlyctenulosis, or interstitial keratitis.

Posterior segment: The most common presentation is of disseminated choroiditis. The lesions may vary in size and elevation within the same eye. They are deep in the choroid, appear yellow, white or gray, fairly well-circumscribed, and, in the vast majority of cases, located in the posterior pole. After uveitis, the next most frequent clinical presentation is focal choroiditis. Disc edema with nerve fiber layer hemorrhages can also be seen. Associated anterior uveitis is not always present.

Diagnosis: The diagnosis of ocular TB is complicated by the difficulties associated with ocular sampling for microbiologic examination. A presumptive diagnosis is frequently based on microscopic observation (using the acid-fast bacilli technique) of a diagnostic specimen (vitreous and/or aqueous humor in cases of uveitis). A definitive diagnosis is dependent on a positive culture for the organism from the specimen. The tuberculin skin test is of limited value because of its low sensitivity and specificity. One of the most promising diagnostic techniques, the amplification and detection of DNA by polymerase chain reaction, is being used frequently in hospitals worldwide.

Fluorescein angiogram testing may also be helpful, especially in cases of focal chorioretinitis. Typically, the choroidal mass exhibits diffuse fluorescence in the early frames, which evolves into intense diffuse hyperfluorescence by the venous phase. Large vessels are typically not seen within the choroidal lesion.

Treatment: The treatment of TB is relatively effective and cost-efficient. Systemic therapy should always be given as the primary treatment for ocular TB, because pulmonar or other foci of disease may coexist. The drugs that make up first-line treatment of TB are isoniazid (INH), rifampicin, pyrazinamide (PZA), streptomycin, and ethambutol. A number of second-line drugs (kanamycin and amikacin) are used to treat patients who are resistant to first-line drugs. A multidrug regimen is recommended. Corticosteroids are sometimes used cautiously in conjunction with antimicrobial therapy. The response to treatment in ocular TB has to be assessed clinically. During treatment, patients must be monitored for drug toxicity.

References:

1) Samson CM, Foster CS. Tuberculosis. In: Foster CS, Vitale AT. *Diagnosis and Treatment of Uveitis.* Philadelphia: WB Saunders 2001; pp 264-71.
2) Bonfioli AA, de Miranda SS, Campos WR, et al. Tuberculosis. *Semin Ophthalmol.* 2005;20 (3):169-75.
3) Kurup SK, Buggage RR, Clarke GL, et al. Gamma interferon assay as an alternative to PPD skin testing in selected patients with granulomatous intraocular inflammatory disease. *Can J Ophthalmol.* 2006;41(6):737-40.

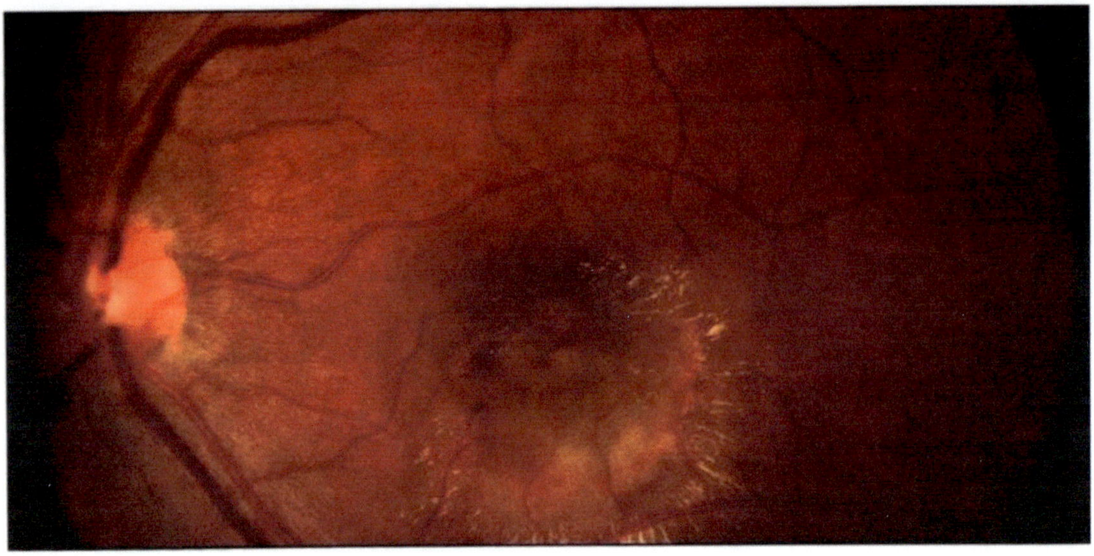

Figure 242: Tuberculosis-associated active choroidal neovascular membrane with overlying hemorrhages and exudates.

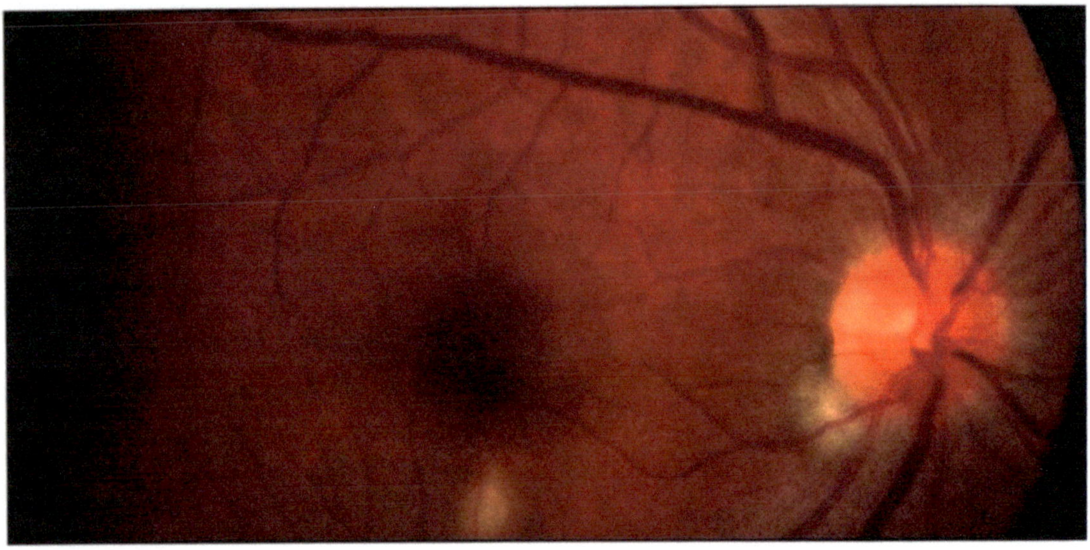

Figure 243: Single choroidal tubercle, also termed focal choroiditis, adjacent to fovea. Note the optic disc hyperemia with a prominent nerve fiber layer.

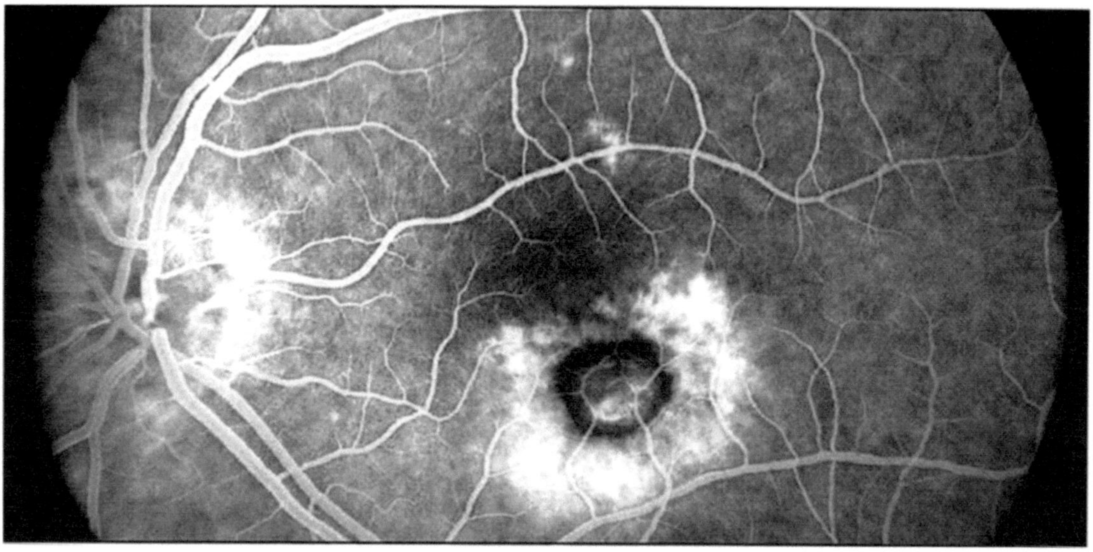

Figure 244: Active choroidal neovascular membrane in a patient with tuberculosis.

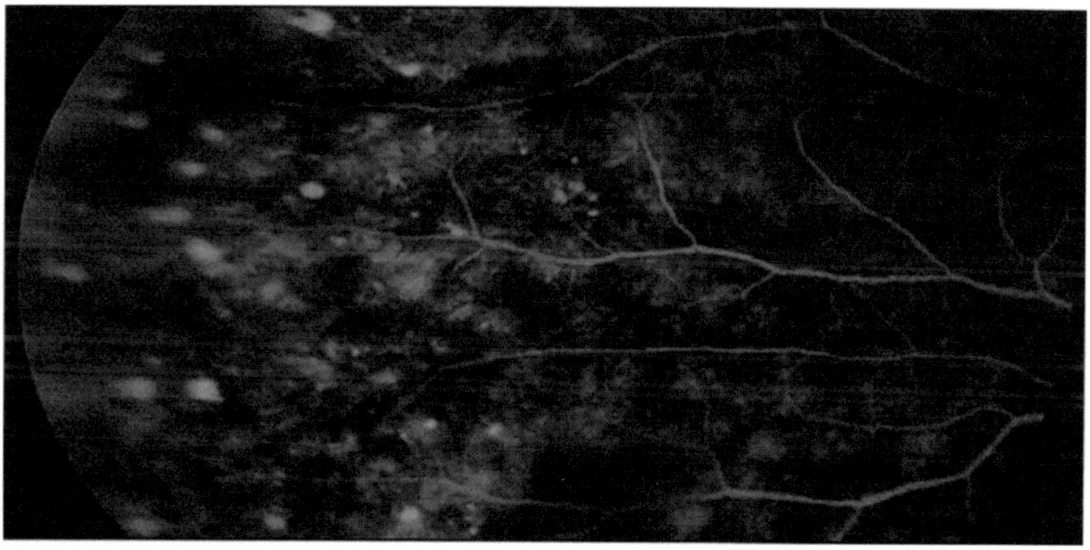

Figure 245: Late phase of FA displaying areas of RPE defects along the periphery.

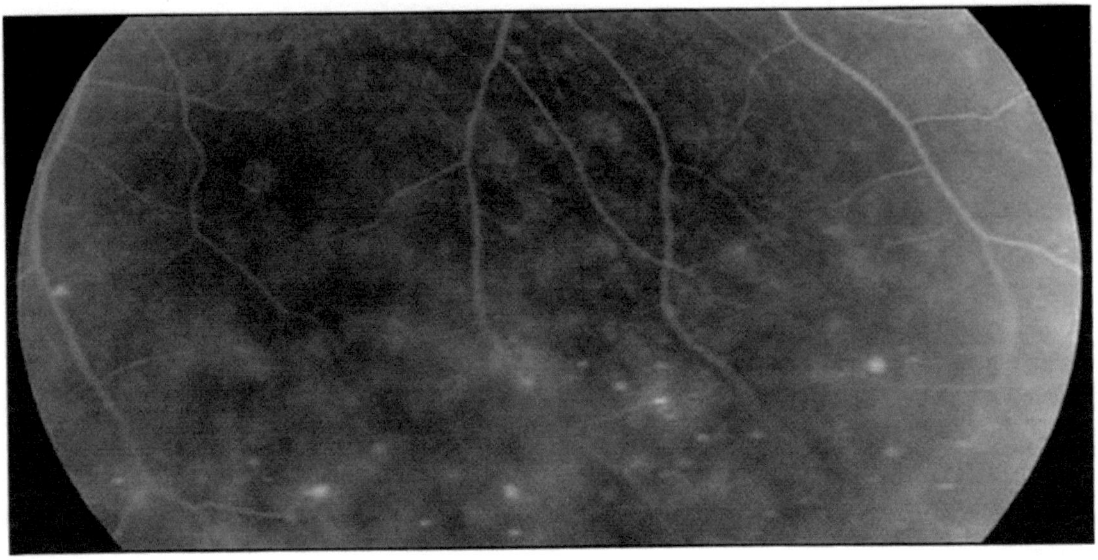

Figure 246: Observe the discrete and numerous lesions which vary in size and elevation within the same eye located inferiorly.

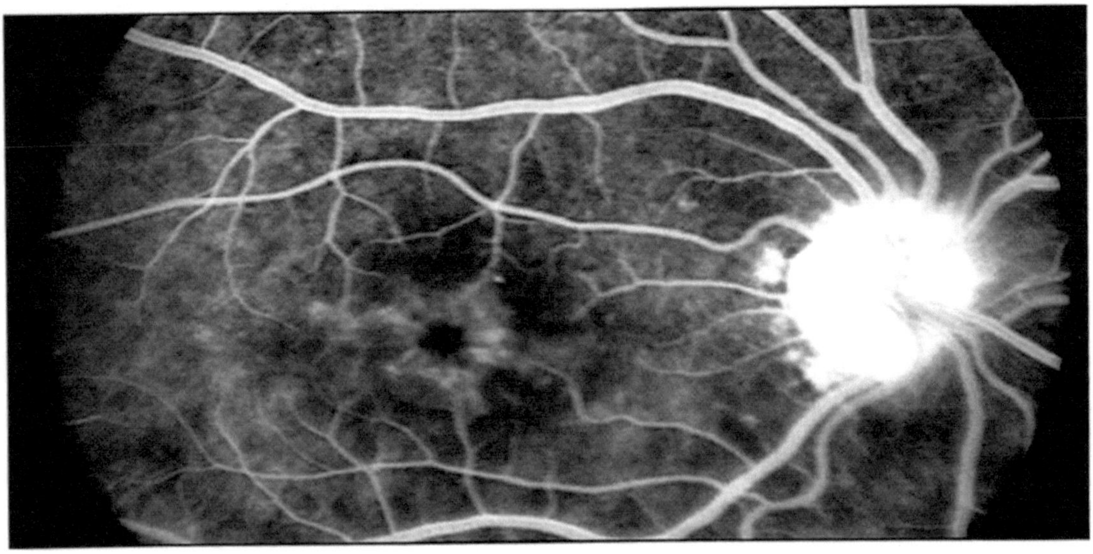

Figure 247: Note the prominent cystoid macular edema accompanied by mild optic disc leakage, secondary to inflammation.

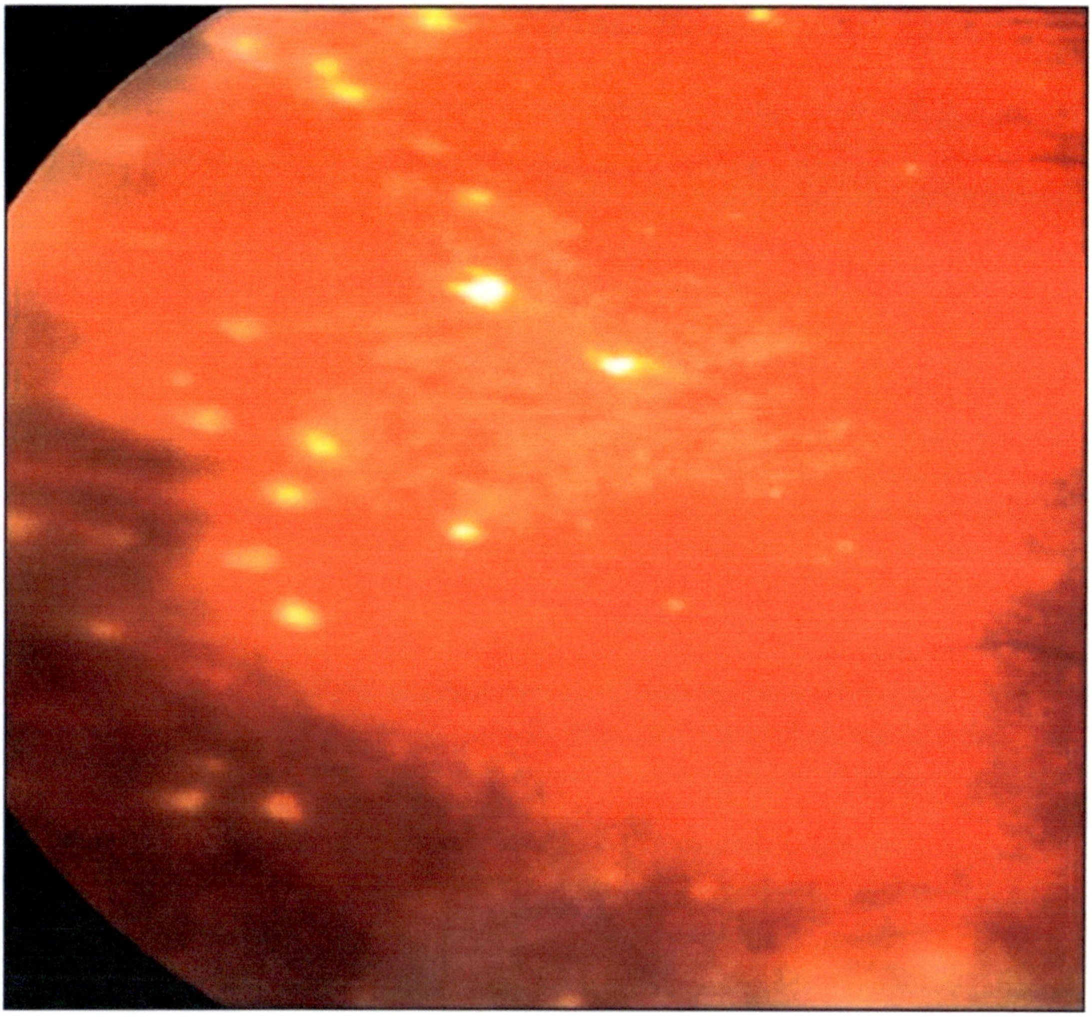

Figure 248: Disseminated choroiditis in an eye affected by miliary tuberculosis-associated intermediate uveitis in the far temporal periphery.

West Nile Virus

Definition: The West Nile virus (WNV) is an RNA arbovirus transmitted by mosquitoes (primarily the *Culex* species) to humans and other mammals. Those most susceptible are infants, young children, the elderly, and immunocompromised patients.

Pathology/Pathogenesis: The virus is injected into animals and humans from infected mosquitoes who have fed on infected birds

Clinical Features:

Systemic Manifestations: 80% of infected individuals are asymptomatic. Fever, joint pain, malaise, anorexia, lymphadenopathy, and rash are seen in symptomatic individuals. Meningoencephalitis and altered mental status may also occur. Increased risk of ocular and systemic complications is seen in diabetics and in patients greater than 50 years of age.

Ocular Manifestations: Chorioretinitis is the most common ocular manifestation associated with WNV infection with a characteristically benign clinical course (Figure 249). Other ocular findings include: optic neuritis, occlusive vasculitis, arterial narrowing, perivascular sheathing, vascular occlusion, and vitritis.

Diagnosis: Polymerase chain reaction is the most sensitive test for WNV. However, WNV-specific immunoglobulin M antibody-capture enzyme-linked immunosorbent assay, indirect fluorescent antibody assay, and plaque reduction neutralization test have shown to be useful.

Treatment: There are no known antiviral agents that have yet to be found in being effective against WNV.

References:

1) Chan CK, Limstrom SA, Tarasewicz DG, Lin SG. Ocular features of West Nile virus infection in North America: a study of 14 eyes. *Ophthalmology*. 2006 Sep;113(9):1539-46.
2) Garg S, Jampol LM. Systemic and intraocular manifestations of West Nile virus infection. *Surv Ophthalmol.* 2005 Jan-Feb ; 50 (1): 3-13.

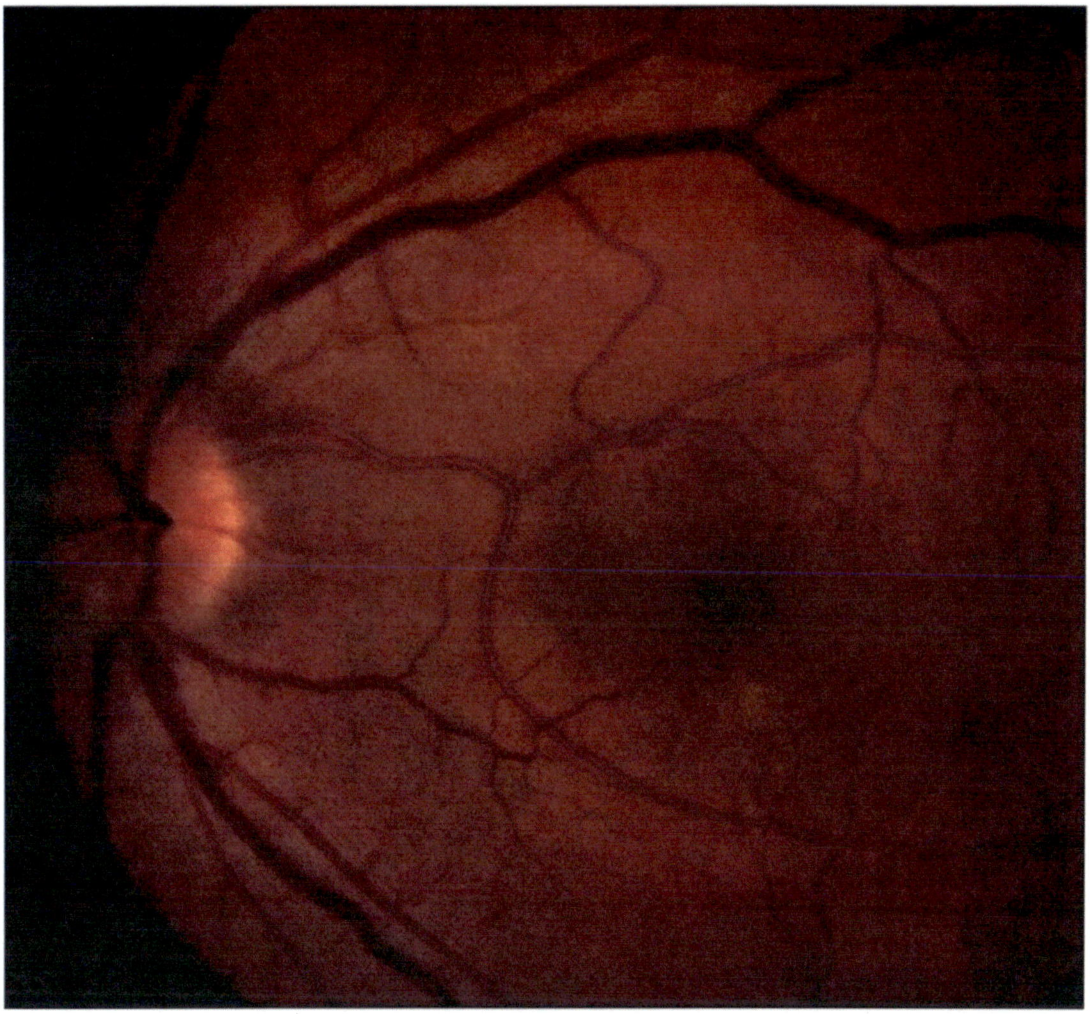

Figure 249: Chorioretinitis as seen in West Nile virus.

Part Five:

Masquerade Syndromes

Masquerade syndromes

Lymphoid Hyperplasia of the Uvea

Lymphoid hyperplasia of the uvea, also known as inflammatory pseudotumors of the uveal tract or intraocular pseudotumors, are characterized by infiltration of the uveal tract by well-differentiated small lymphocytes. This condition, which is usually unilateral, can present with anterior uveitis, vitritis, choroidal infiltrates, and iris heterochromia. Extraocular extension may present as conjunctival salmon-colored lesions, or orbital masses, which may cause proptosis and diplopia. The condition is painless unless secondary severe glaucoma develops.

Diagnosis is made through biopsy of extraocular extension or chorio-retina. Lymphoid hyperplasia of the uvea often responds to therapy with corticosteroids although some tumors require moderate dose of radiotherapy. The prognosis is favorable.

Leukemia

In leukemia, the retina is the most common ocular tissue affected clinically and choroid histopathologically. Leukemia can masquerade as uveitis both in the adult and pediatric population. Acute lymphoblastic leukemia, chronic myeloid leukemia in blast crisis, and relapsing acute myeloid leukemia have previously been reported as masquerade syndromes. Patients can present with a severe anterior segment cellular infiltration and hypopyon. Anterior chamber paracentesis with cytology can reveal the presence of malignant cells and should be considered in all cases of refractory uveitis.

Uveal Melanoma

The incidence of uveal melanoma is approximately six per million per year. 80% of cases present in the choroid, with 12% presenting in the ciliary body, and 8% in the iris. Melanomas of the Iris can produce anterior chamber cells and flare while melanomas involving the ciliary body can produce dilated episcleral vessels termed sentinel vessels, which can masquerade as an episcleritis. Primary choroidal melanomas can present as a focal choroidal mass, which may mimic sarcoidosis, a tuberculous granuloma, or posterior scleritis. Ciliary body melanomas may also present with secondary raised intraocular pressure in 17% of cases.

Choroidal Metastases

Choroidal metastases can masquerade as uveitis. In one case series by Ferry and Font, up to half of the ocular metastases are recognized before the diagnosis of a primary malignancy. Renal and lung carcinomas are most likely to manifest with ocular metastases. Breast carcinomas also frequently metastasize to the eye. The primary lesion however, is known at the time of ocular presentation in greater than 90% of cases.

Childhood Malignancies

Retinoblastoma is the most common intraocular malignant process in childhood. The initial presentation can be quite diverse, from tumor cells in the anterior chamber, masquerading as uveitis to leucokoria and strabismus. Medulloepitheliomas and benign lesions such as juvenile xanthogranuloma can also masquerade as idiopathic uveitis.

Paraneoplastic syndromes

Cancer-Associated Retinopathy (CAR)

This condition was first described in 1976 in three patients with oat cell carcinomas of the lung. It has now been reported in association with a number of malignant conditions. Patients often present with loss of vision. The fundus can appear normal early in the course of the disease. There may be however, eventual vascular sheathing, disturbances of the RPE, and optic disc pallor.

Retinal autoantibodies have been identified in patients with CAR. This finding together with the fact that the disease responds to corticosteroid therapy, suggests that the retinal destruction may be partly immune-mediated.

Bilateral Diffuse Uveal Melanocytic Proliferation

In 1966, Machemer first described bilateral diffuse melanocytic tumors in a patient with a large retro peritoneal mass thought to be pancreatic carcinoma[15]. This condition can occurs in patients with carcinomas, but underlying malignant processes are often occult. Histopathology reveals diffuse uveal tract infiltrates with benign, spindle-shaped melanocytic cells, which have foamy cytoplasm. Mitotic figures are not characteristic.

Further study by Gass and Glazer in 1991[16] demonstrated the presence of multiple subtle round and oval subretinal red patches that show early hyperfluorescence on fluorescein angiography; multiple, slightly elevated, pigmented, and non-pigmented uveal melanocytic tumors with evidence of diffuse thickening of the uveal tract. In addition, there may be episcleral injecition, vitritis, and exudative retinal detachment present.

References

1) Jakobiec FA, Sacks E, Kronish JW, et al. Multiple static creamy choroidal infiltrates: an early sign of lymphoid neoplasia. *Ophthalmol*, 94: 397-406, 1987.
2) Ryan SJ, Frank RN, Green WR. Bilateral inflammatory pseudotumors of the ciliary body. *Am J Ophthalmol*, 72: 586-591, 1971.
3) Ryan SJ, Zimmerman LE, King FM. Reactive lymphoid hyperplasia: an unusual form of intraocular pseudotumor. *Trans Am Acad Ophthalmol Otolaryngol*, 76: 652-671, 1971.
4) Jakobiec FA, Sacks E, Kronish JW, et al. Multiple static creamy choroidal infiltrates: an early sign of lymphoid neoplasia. *Ophthalmol*, 94: 397-406, 1987.

5) Yi DH, Rashid S, Cibas ES et al. Acute unilateral leukemic hypopyon in an adult with relapsing acute lymphoblastic leukemia. *Am J Ophthalmol.* 2005 Apr;139(4):719-21.

6) Ayliffe W, Foster CS, Marcoux P et al. Relapsing acute myeloid leukaemia manifesting as hypopyon uveitis. *Am J Ophthalmol* 119:361-4,1995.

7) Spalton DJ, Hitchings RA, Hunter PA. *Atlas of clinical ophthalmology.* London: Wolfe Publishing, Mosby-Yearbook, 1994: 9.11.

8) Shields CL, Shields JA, Shields MB, et al. Prevalence and mechanisms of secondary intraocular pressure elevation in eyes with intraocular tumors. *Ophthalmol*, 94: 839-846, 1987.

9) Ferry AP, Font RL. Carcinoma metastatic to the eye and orbit. A clinicopathologic study of 227 cases. *Arch Ophthalmol*, 92: 276-286, 1974.

10) Nussenblatt RB, Whitcup SM, Palestine AG. *Uveitis: Fundamentals and Clinical Practice,* Third Edition, Mosby, 2004: Chapter 29, 409¬419.

11) Croxatto JO, Fernadez MR, Malbran ES. Retinoblastoma masquerading as ocular inflammation. *Ophthalmologica*, 1986: 48-53, 1983.

12) DeBarge LR, Chan CC, Greenberg S et al; Chorioretinal, iris, and ciliary body infiltration by juvenile xanthogranuloma masquerading as uveitis, *Am J Ophthalmol* 39:65-71,1994.

13) Sawyer RA, Selhorst JB, Zimmerman LE, et al. Blindness caused by photoreceptor degeneration as a remote effect of cancer. *Am J Ophthalmol*, 81: 606-613, 1976.

14) Thirkill CE, Roth AM, Keltner JL. Cancer-associated retinopathy. *Arch Ophthalmol,* 105: 372-375, 1987.

15) Machemer R. Zur Pathogenese des flichenhaften malignen Melanoms. *Klin Monatsbl Augenheilkd*, 148: 641-652, 1966.

16) Gass JDM, Glatzer RJ. Acquired pigmentation simulating Peutz-Jeghers syndrome: initial manifestation of diffuse uveal melanocytic proliferation. *Br J Ophthalmol,* 75: 693-695, 1991.

Leukemia

Definition: Leukemias are malignant neoplasms of the hematopoietic stem cells characterized by diffuse replacement of the bone marrow by neoplastic cells.

History: Leukemic ophthalmology was first established as a clinical entity in the late 19th century by Liebreich in his paper on leukemic retinopathy and central retinal artery embolism.

Epidemiology: Estimates of ocular involvement in leukemia vary, but it is generally accepted that the eye is involved far more often in acute rather than in chronic leukemias. Ridgeway and associates report abnormalities on ocular examination in 9% of patients suffering from acute leukemias whereas Duke-Elder estimates that up to 90% of patients with leukemia demonstrate some ocular abnormality at some point in the course of the disease.

Clinical Features: (Figures 250-253) The retinal vessels can become tortuous and dilated with perivascular sheathing representing infiltration of leukemic cells. Cotton wool spots are common, but the most striking feature of leukemic involvement of the retina is the presence of retinal hemorrhages most commonly located in the posterior pole.. The classic white-centered Roth spots may occur with the white centers representing cellular debris, capillary emboli, or accumulations of leukemic cells. Nodular retinal infiltrates have also been described and peripheral retinal microaneurysms are a feature of chronic leukemias. The choroid is commonly infiltrated with leukemic cells. Secondary changes such as atrophy, hypertrophy, and hyperplasia may occur in the retinal pigment epithelium giving rise to a "leopard-spot" pattern. Although anterior segment involvement in leukemias is unusual, patients characteristically present with unilateral or bilateral symptoms of acute iridocyclitis with conjunctival injection, iritis, hypopyon, pseudohypopyon, or spontaneous hyphema. The anterior chamber may be the first presenting site of acute leukemia. Leukemic optic nerve infiltration occurs primarily in children with acute lymphocytic leukemia, and implies involvement of the central nervous system.

Pathogenesis:. A correlation between low red cell and platelet counts and retinal hemorrhages has been reported.

Diagnosis: In the case of suspected orbital involvement, a biopsy may be required for diagnosis of leukemia. In cases of iris and anterior segment involvement, diagnosis is established by anterior chamber paracentesis with cytologic examination of the aqueous humor. With vitreous involvement, a pars plana vitrectomy with cytologic examination can be diagnostic. A Gram stain and culture of the vitrectomy specimen should also be performed to exclude infection. Fluorescein angiographic changes in patients with choroidal infiltration and overlying serous retinal detachment of the retina demonstrates a multitude of retinal pigment epithelium leakage points in the early phase of the angiogram described as a "milky-way" pattern.

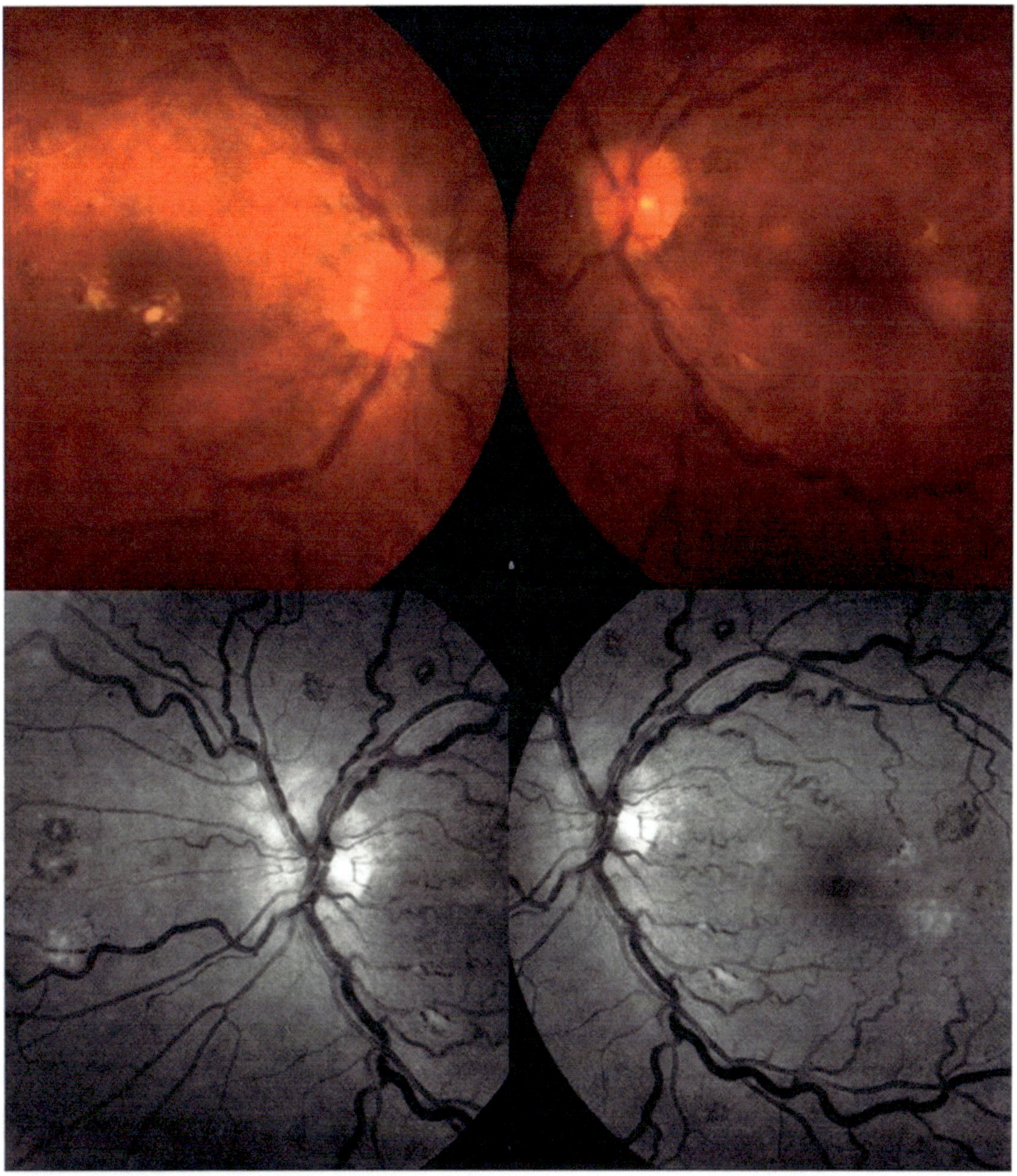

Figures 250, 251, 252 & 253: Fundus photos show evidence of bilateral vessel tortousity, scattered white-centered hemorrhages (roth spots) and cotton-wool spots, in a patient with leukemic retinopathy.

Treatment: As increasing attention is being given to the ocular manifestations, both as a sign of extramedullary disease and relapse, and in terms of vision preservation to enhance quality of life. However, even with irradiation and intrathecal methotrexate, visual outcome is not always favorable.

Reference:

Waheed NK, Foster CS. Masquerade Syndromes: Malignant; in: Foster CS, Vitale AT. *Diagnosis and treatment of uveitis*. Saunders. Philadelphia 2002:504.

Malignant Melanoma

Definition: Malignant melanoma of the choroid and ciliary body is the most common primary intraocular malignancy. It represents a malignant melanocytic stromal proliferation of the choroid, the ciliary body, or the iris.

History: Malignant melanomas were once considered to be the most common malignancy of the eye. In recent times however, with the increased survival of cancer patients, it has come to be realized that malignant melanomas, although the most common primary eye malignancy, are much less common than metastatic tumors of the eye.

Epidemiology: Posterior segment melanomas occur at a higher frequency than iris melanomas. These lesions typically present between the ages of 40 and 50 years with an equal sex predilection. They occur more often in whites and in patients with light coloured irides than in Asians and blacks. Iris melanomas which account for between 3.3% and 12.5% of all surgically excised melanomas, typically arise from the inferior portion of the iris.

Clinical Features: Iris melanomas arise from pre-existing lesions that undergo active change.. They can present in three patterns-ring, tapioca, or diffuse melanomas. Diffuse melanomas can present with unilateral acquired heterochromia and secondary glaucoma. Differentiation between malignant and benign lesions is based on clinical features. A lesion is considered malignant if it is 3mm or greater in diameter and 1mm or greater in thickness and associated with three of the following five features: secondary glaucoma, secondary cataract, photographic documentation of growth, ectropion irides, and prominent vascularity. Choroidal melanomas present with symptoms of visual loss, photopsia, and visual field defects although they can be asymptomatic.. Furthermore, in addition to these lesions presenting with inflammation, tumors of the iris and ciliary body can induce pigment dispersion in the anterior chamber and on the anterior surface of the lens and hence masquerade as uveitis

Pathology: The histopathologic classification of iris and choroidal melanomas was originally described by Callender. Uveal melanomas are assigned into the following groups based on their histopathologic features: spindle A, spindle B, fasicular, mixed, epithelioid, and necrotic.

Diagnosis: It is important to differentiate iris melanomas from primary ciliary body melanomas with iris extension as the management and prognosis of these two conditions is completely different. This can be done by indirect ophthalmoloscopy with scleral depression, scleral transillumination and gonioscopy. Ultrasonography can be performed if primary ciliary body melanoma cannot be excluded. Photographic documentation of any stromal melanocytic tumor of the iris is required. Photographic evidence of progressive growth or the presence of secondary glaucoma may point towards a malignant lesion. Fluorescein angiographic patterns may also help differentiate between a benign and malignant lesion. Benign nevi have a filigree vascular network pattern (early filling, late leaking) or they may be angiographically silent. Malignant tumors have irregular and indistinct vascular channels that fill later in the angiogram (greater than 30 seconds). Although these angiographic features are useful they are not definitively diagnostic.

The characteristic features on B scan ultrasonography are an acoustically silent zone within the melanoma, choroidal excavation and shadowing in the orbit. scan features include medium to low vitreal echoes, with smooth attenuation and vascular pulsations within the tumor. Ancillary investigations include fluorescein angiography, CT, MRI, indocyanine green angiography (ICG), and radioactive phosphorous uptake. High resolution CT is actually less accurate than ultrasonography. ICG may be useful in the diagnosis of choroidal melanomas. A radioactive phosphorus uptake test has low sensitivity and specificity and fine needle aspiration biopsy is neither generally required nor a good diagnostic measure for determining cell type differentiating melanoma from nevi or other spindle tumors. Additionally it carries with it the additional possibility of seeding of the needle tract.

Treatment: Iris melanomas generally have a good prognosis, with surgical excision indicated if tumor growth is pronounced or refractory glaucoma occurs. Since up to 50% of patients undergoing iridocyclectomy retain no useful vision, some investigators have recommended ultrasound-guided needle biopsy cytologic diagnosis before iridocyclectomy. Another surgical modality for which smaller melanomas of the ciliary body or anterior choroid may be amenable is partial lamellar sclerouvectomy.

The management of choroidal tumors is based on their size. External beam radiation has proved to be a major advance in the treatment of these tumors. The most common modality, however for treating medium-sized choroidal melanomas is radiotherapy, employing either radioactive iodine or ruthenium plaques to the sclera over the base of the tumor. Transpupillary thermotherapy is an emerging modality for the treatment of small to medium-sized tumors. Large tumors require enucleation except in the elderly, unfit, or monocular patients. Medical evaluation in patients undergoing enucleation is important not only for assessing the general health of the patient but also for detecting associated malignancies or the presence of metastases.

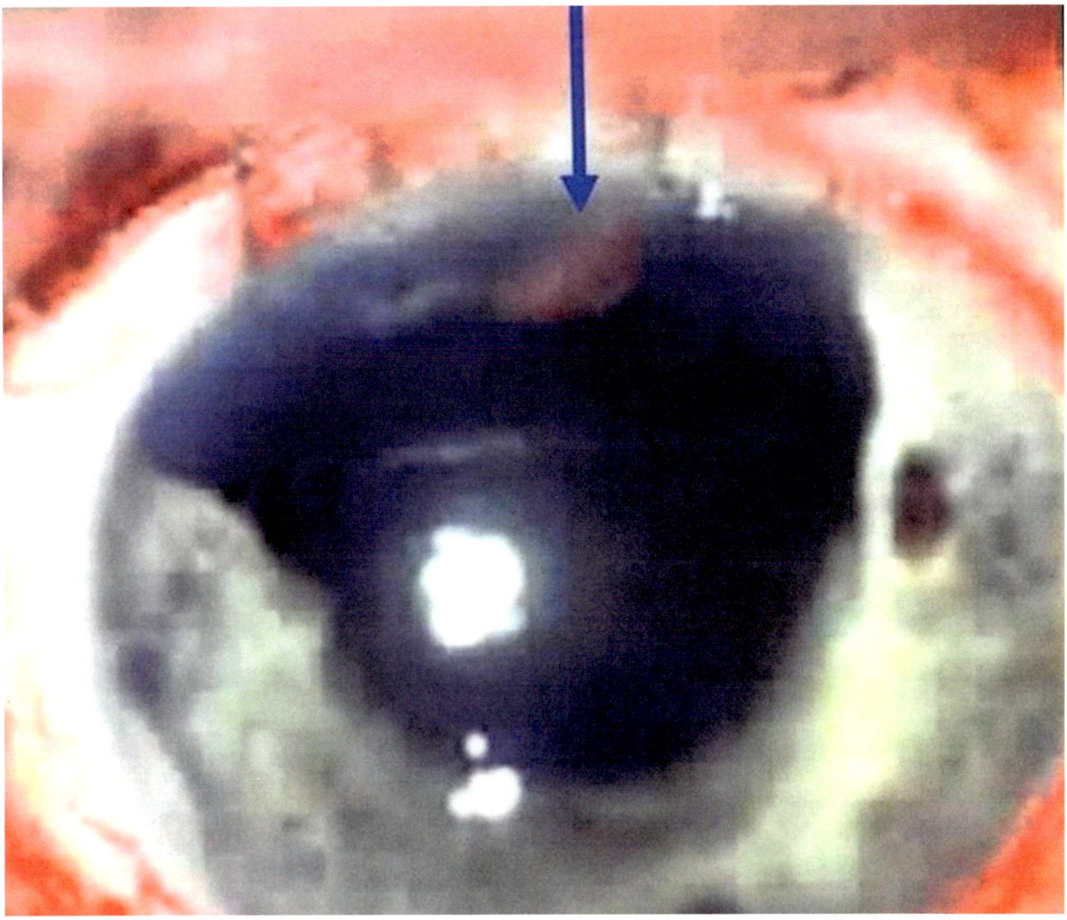

Figure 254: Superior melanotic mass in the ciliary body.

Reference:

Waheed NK, Foster CS. Masquerade Syndromes: Malignant; in: Foster CS, Vitale AT. *Diagnosis and treatment of uveitis*. Saunders. Philadelphia 2002:509-513.

Autoimmune Retinopathy

Introduction: Retinopathy in the absence of a known neoplasm with electroretinogram abnormalities has been reported. These cases may share certain clinical and immunological features of paraneoplastic retinopathies. If the patient's serum is positive for retinal autoantibodies and extensive evaluation for cancer is negative, the term autoimmune retinopathy is used. The presence of circulating autoantibodies against retinal antigens may contribute to retinal dysfunction and degeneration.

Clinical features: Patients present with sudden, or less frequently, subacute painless loss of vision, typically associated with visual field defects and photopsias. Although the retina may appear normal early on, attenuated arterioles, thinned and mottled retinal pigment epithelium, and minimally pale optic disks usually appear within several months. Vitreous cells, arteriolar sheathing, and periphlebitis suggestive of inflammation can also be seen in later stages.

Diagnosis: The diagnosis is made by the presence of unexplained visual loss with electroretinogram abnormalities and the presence of retinal autoantibodies. Evidence suggests that anti-p35 antibody is the most commonly identified antibody in the serum of patients with the disease.

Treatment: The mainstay of treatment is immunomodulatery drugs such as, systemic steroids, immunoglobulin infusion, and rituximab.

References:

1) Whitcup SM, Vistica BP, Milam AH, Nussenblatt RB, Gery I: Recoverin- associated retinopathy: a clinically and immunologically distinctive disease. *Am J Ophthalmol* 1998, 126: 230-237.
2) Mizener JB, Kimura AE, Adamus G, Thirkill CE, Goeken JA, Kardon RH. Autoimmune retinopathy in the absence of cancer. *Am J Ophthalmol* 1997, 123:607-618.
3) Peek R, Verbraak F, Coevoet HM, Kijlstra A: Muller cell-specific autoantibodies in a patient with progressive loss of vision. *Invest Ophthalmol Vis Sci* 1998, 39:1976-1979.
4) Adamus G, Sugden B, Seigal GM: Cytotoxic and apoptotic effect of anti-retinal autoantibodies of autoimmune retinopathy. *FASEB Journal* 2000, 14:A1107
5) Adamus G, Ren G, Weleber RG. Autoantibodies against retinal proteins in paraneoplastic and autoimmune retinopathy. *BMC Ophthalmol.* 2004 Jun 4;4:5.

Cancer-associated Retinopathy

Introduction: Cancer-associated retinopathy (CAR) is a rare paraneoplastic retinopathy. Cross-reacting autoantibodies against retinal antigens (recoverin and á-enolase) cause retinal dysfunction. This disease can occur in association with a number of cancers, including lung, breast, and endometrial.

History: CAR was initially described in 1976 in three patients with oat-cell carcinoma of the lungs. Thirkill and colleagues were the first to report the antigen involved in CAR, which is a 23 kD CAR retinal antigen (recoverin).

Epidemiology: There is no sex predilection for CAR. Approximately 60% of patients with small cell cancer of the lung will have CAR.

Clinical Features: Patients often present with a bilateral, painless loss of vision as a result of both rod and cone dysfunction in CAR. Visual loss may occur over a period of months or years, and visual symptoms typically precede diagnosis of the systemic malignancy. Nyctalopia, photophobia, and central scotomas are common symptoms. The fundus can appear normal early in the course of the disease. There may be however, eventual vascular sheathing, disturbances of the RPE, extensive chorioretinal atrophy, and optic disc pallor. Unfortunately, visual prognosis is poor in these patients. Presence of autoimmune hepatitis is also highly suggestive of CAR.

Pathology/Pathogenesis: Histopathologic findings reveal recoverin autoantibodies causing severe degeneration of the outer nuclear layer along with inner and outer segments of the photoreceptor layer, photoreceptor destruction, and macrophages with phagocytosed retinal pigment epithelium granules.

Diagnosis: Abnormal visual field and ERG findings are central in diagnosing patients with CAR. Color plate testing may also be useful.

Treatment: Immunosuppressive therapies, like prednisone, are the treatment of choice. Intravenous immunoglobulin, Tolpa Torf preparation, and plasmapheresis have been used with limited success.

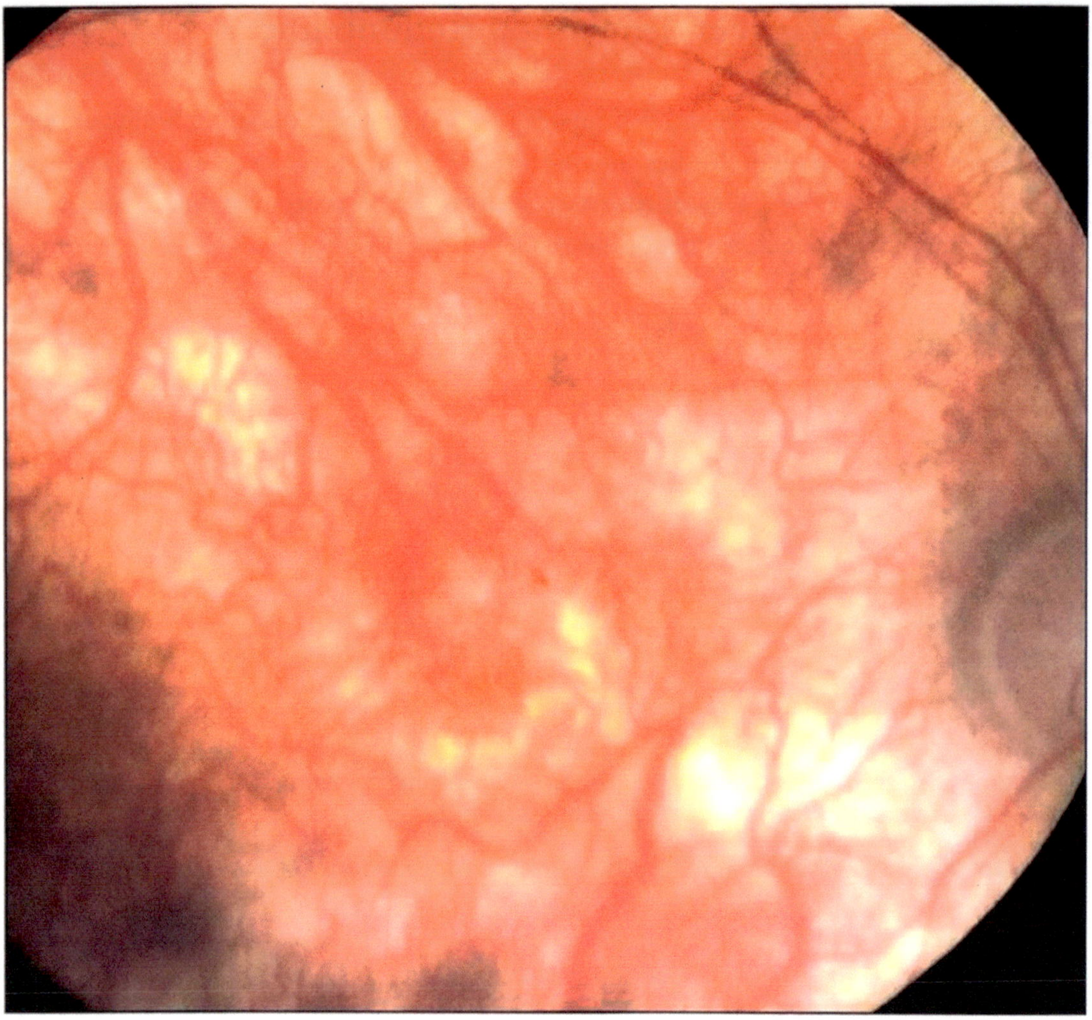

Figure 255: Cancer-associated retinopathy in a seventy-three year-old female patient. Note the extensive chorioretinal atrophy. This patient also had a remarkable history of breast cancer.

References:

1) Arnold AC, Lee AG. Systemic disease and neuro-ophthalmology: Annual update 2000. *J Neuroophthalmology*.2001: 21:46-61.
2) Whitcup SM, Vistica BP, Milam AH, Nussenblatt RB, Gary I. Recoverin-associated retinopathy: a clinical and immunologically distinctive disease. *Am J Ophthalmology*. 1998, 126:230-237.

Primary Intraocular Lymphoma

Definition: Primary intraocular lymphoma (PIOL) is a form of non-Hodgkin's lymphoma that primarily involves the retina and the vitreous. PIOL refers to a type of primary central nervous system lymphoma (PCNSL). It is a rare and lethal malignancy, which often masquerades as intraocular inflammation

History: Klingele and Hogan were the first to obtain a vitreous biopsy for positive investigation of intraocular lymphoma in 1975.

Epidemiology: The exact incidence of PIOL is unknown. It is a rare malignancy and is estimated to represent 1% of non-Hodgkins's lymphomas, 1% of intracranial tumors, and less than 1% of intraocular tumors. Reports estimate that 15-25% of patients with PCNSL will have ocular involvement. The incidence in the United States of PCNSL and therefore PIOL has tripled over the last two decades in both immunodefecient and immunocompetent patient populations. PIOL typically occurs in elderly patients, but it can affect any age. There is no racial predilection and although one eye is typically involved initially, PIOL is eventually bilateral in 80% of cases.

Pathology/Pathogenesis: The majority of intraocular-CNS lymphoma cases are of B-cell origin. Lymphoma cells are noticeable between Bruch's membrane and the retinal pigment epithelium with reactive T lymphocytes in the retina and choroid surrounding the B cells. Additionally, a thickened choroid with large gray patches of subretinal and retinal infiltration is seen.

Clinical Features: PIOL typically masquerades as a chronic posterior uveitis, with patients relating a painless decrease in their vision in the presence of floaters and in the absence of redness and pain. Hazy vitritis with clumps and sheets of vitreous cells is the most characteristic finding.

PIOL may also present with scattered retinal white lesions and yellowish subretinal or sub-retinal pigment epithelium (sub-RPE) infiltrates, which consist of deposits of malignant cells. These lesions can enlarge and coalesce or can resolve spontaneously in some cases. Lymphoma can extend through the RPE and into the retina simulating acute retinitis or infiltrate the optic nerve and mimic optic neuritis and papillitis.

PIOL masquerading as a chronic uveitis often responds well to corticosteroids initially as the majority of cells present in the vitreous are not malignant cells, but rather "reactive" lymphocytes, sensitive to steroid therapy. Eventually the vitritis becomes steroid resistant and worsens with the development of CNS symptoms. Typically this presents with personality changes as well as changes in level of consciousness as PCNSL typically involves the frontal lobe of the brain.

Diagnosis: The key to diagnosis is a high index of suspicion for any chronic posterior uveitis that is atypical or refractory to therapy, especially in middle-aged or older patients.

Imaging:. Ultrasonography provides visualization of the posterior segment while fluorescein angiography can localize areas of infiltration. The use of neuroimaging is recommended to evaluate possible CNS involvement.

Tissue Biopsy: Analysis of vitreal tissue is the cornerstone of the diagnostic workup of PIOL.

Cytology: Cytology is the gold standard for diagnosis of PIOL. Rapid preparation and gentle handling of tissues is imperative to prevent high false negative rates.

Immunohistochemistry: Cell surface markers CD19 and CD20 are pan B-cell proteins highly expressed in B-cell lymphomas. CD22 is found on early B-cells, and its presence is suggestive of B-cell lymphoma.

Cytokines: Vitreal levels of the cytokines IL-10, IL-6 and IL-12 provide ancillary testing for PIOL. Elevated IL-io is currently considered suggestive, but not diagnostic of B-cell lymphoma. IL-6 and IL-12 are elevated in inflammatory states.

Molecular Analysis: Monoclonality of a B cell population implying lymphoma can be demonstrated by polymerase chain reaction (PCR) for heavy chain immunoglobulin (IgH) gene rearrangement. PCR can also be done for translocation between chromosomes 14 and 18t (14:18).

Treatment: The current consensus on treating ocular lymphoma in the context of central nervous system disease is systemic high dose methotrexate based chemotherapy with radiation to both globes and the brain. Isolated ocular disease should be similarly treated, although radiation complications and the promise of high dose methotrexate chemotherapy regimens favor emphasis of the latter option. Recurrence of intraocular lymphoma alone should be treated with intravitreal methotrexate.

Reference

1) Choi JY, Kafkaia C, Foster CS. Primary Intraocular Lymphoma: A Review. *Seminars in Ophthalmology*, 21:125-133,2006.

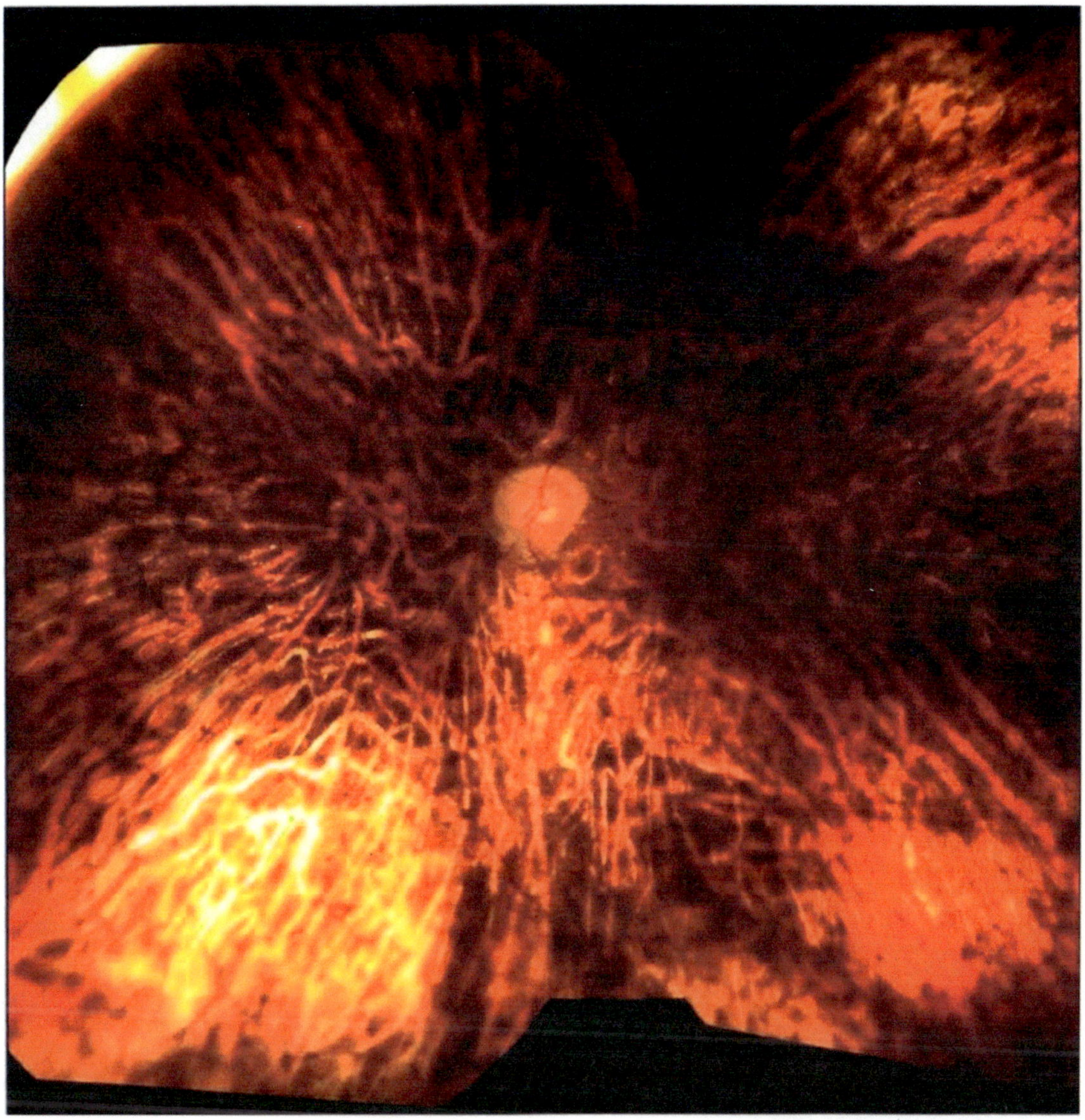

Figure 256: Diffuse retinal pigment epithelium scarring in a patient affected by intraocular lymphoma-associated posterior uveitis. Note the prominent choroidal vasculature.

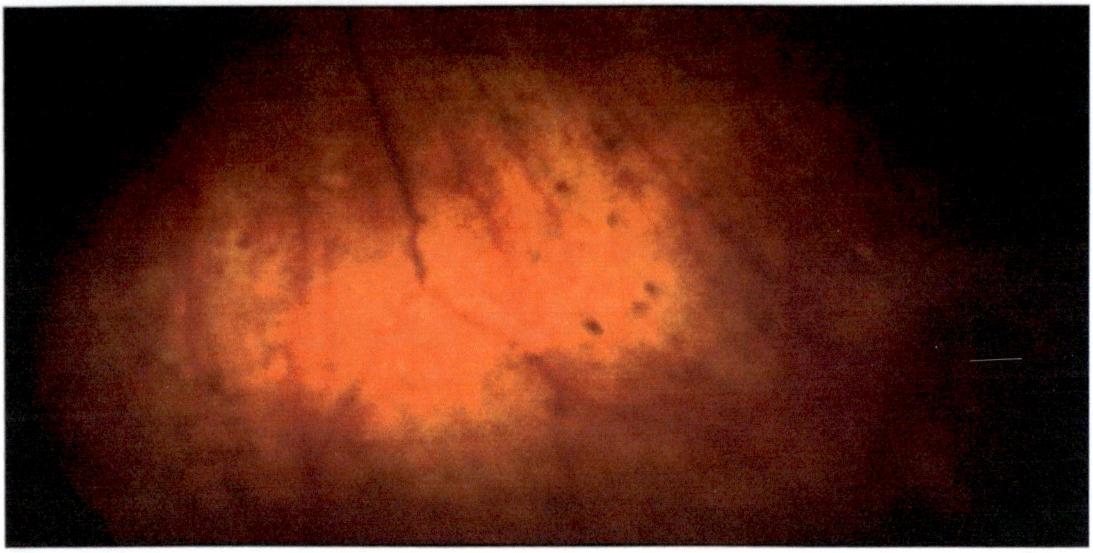

Figure 257: Inferior choroidal infiltrates and pigment clumping secondary to intraocular lymphoma.

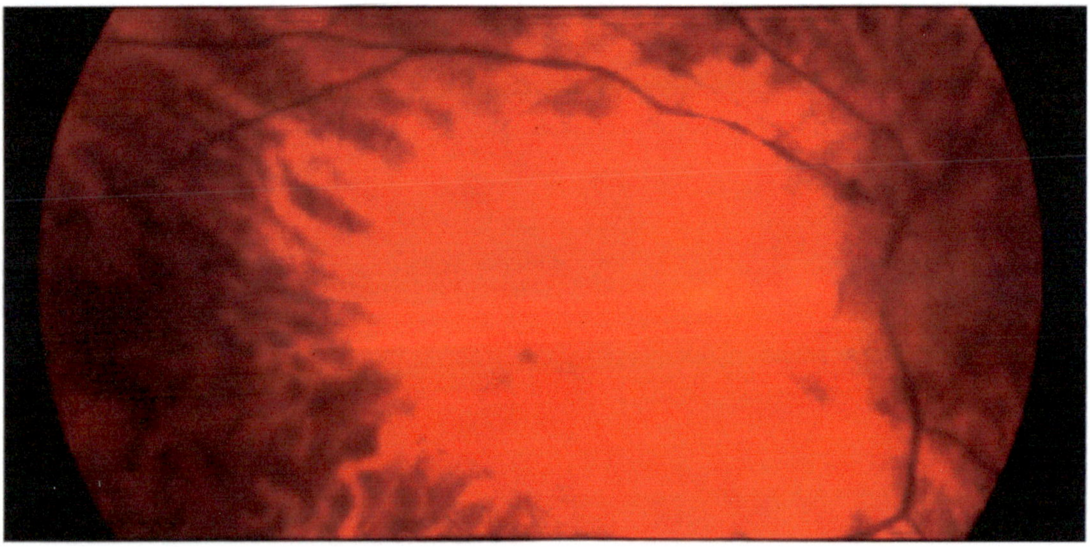

Figure 258: RPE changes and papillitis in a patient affected by primary intraocular lymphoma.

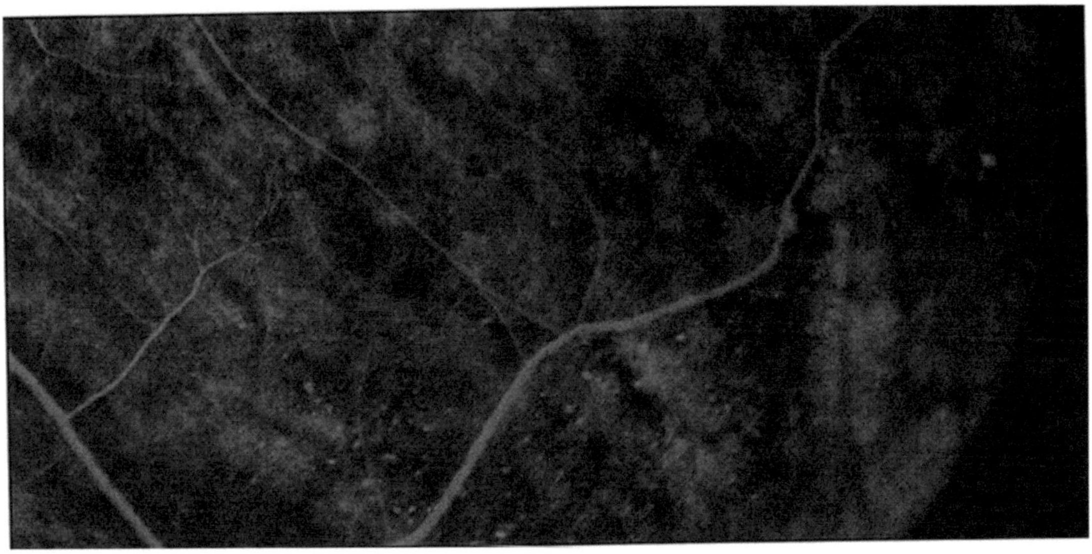

Figure 259: Layering of a sheet of leukocytes in the inferotemporal fundus of a patient with intraocular lymphoma.

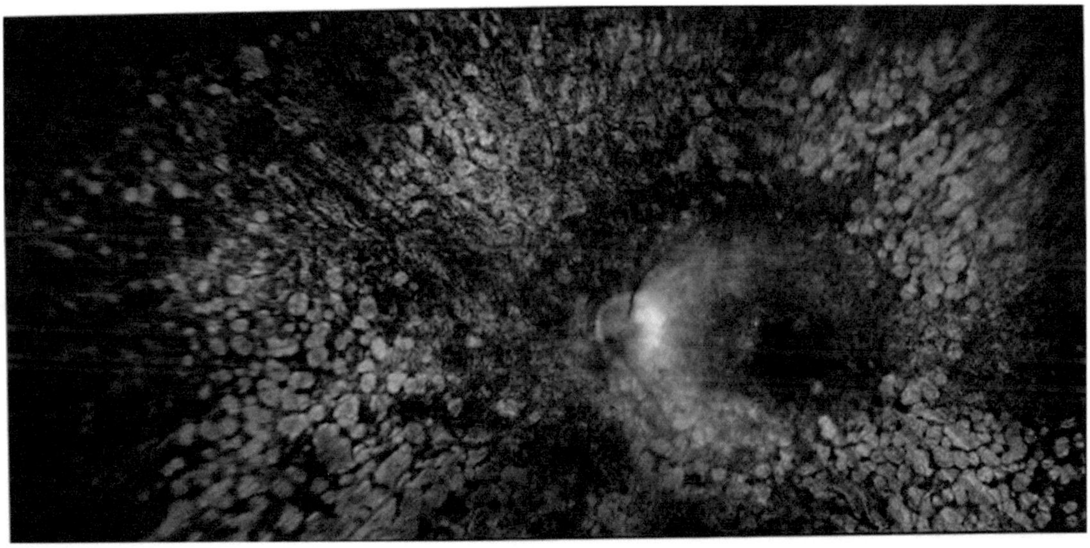

Figure 260: Extensive chorioretinal scarring due to recalcitrant inflammation seen in lymphoma posterior uveitis.

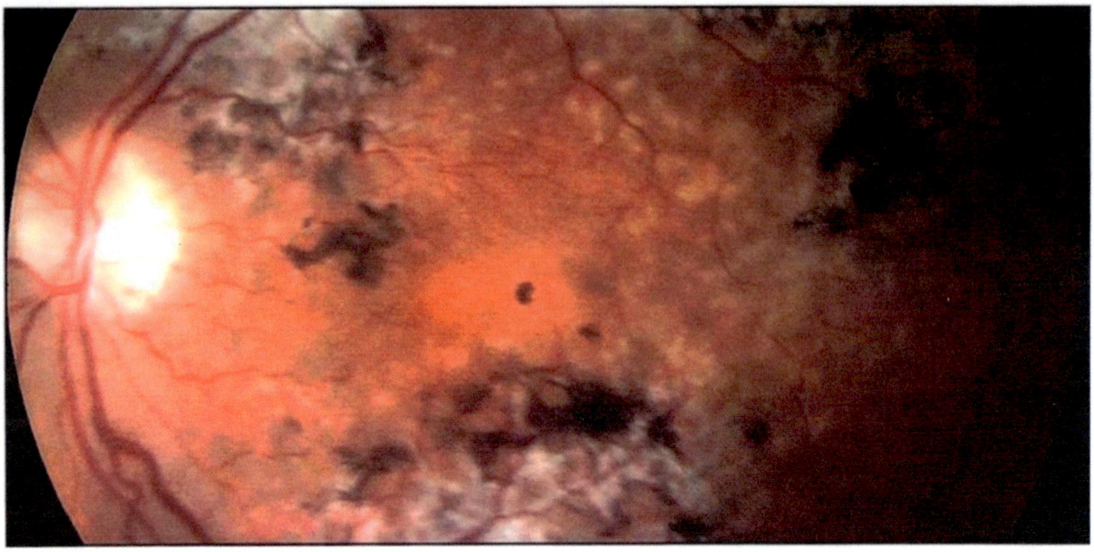

Figure 261: 76 year-old female with diffuse RPE and chorioretinal scarring and deep choroidal infiltrates as seen in intraocular lymphoma.

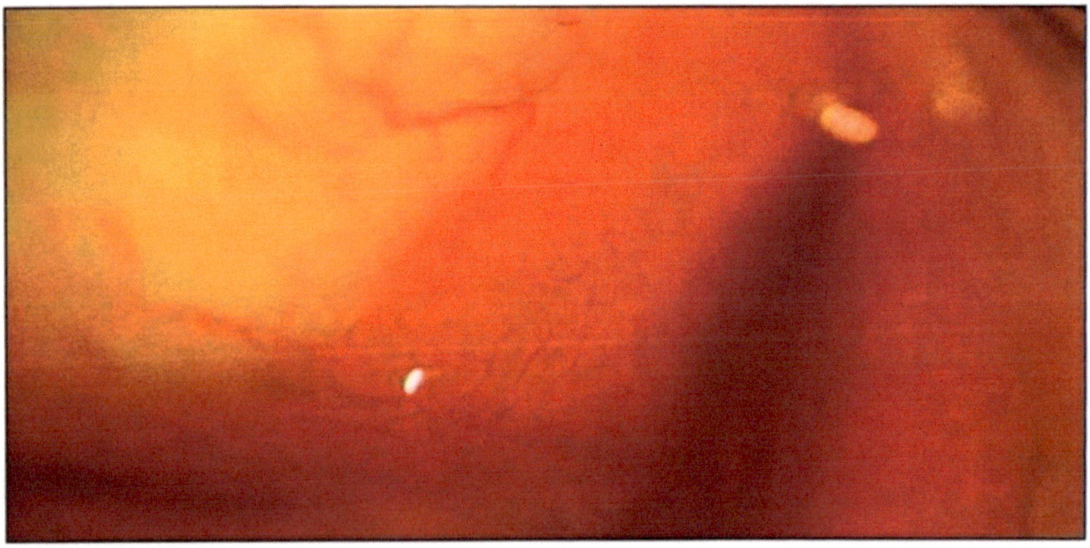

Figure 262: Salmon patch mass in temporal conjunctiva of patient afflicted by lymphoma. Note the elevation of this vascularized lesion.

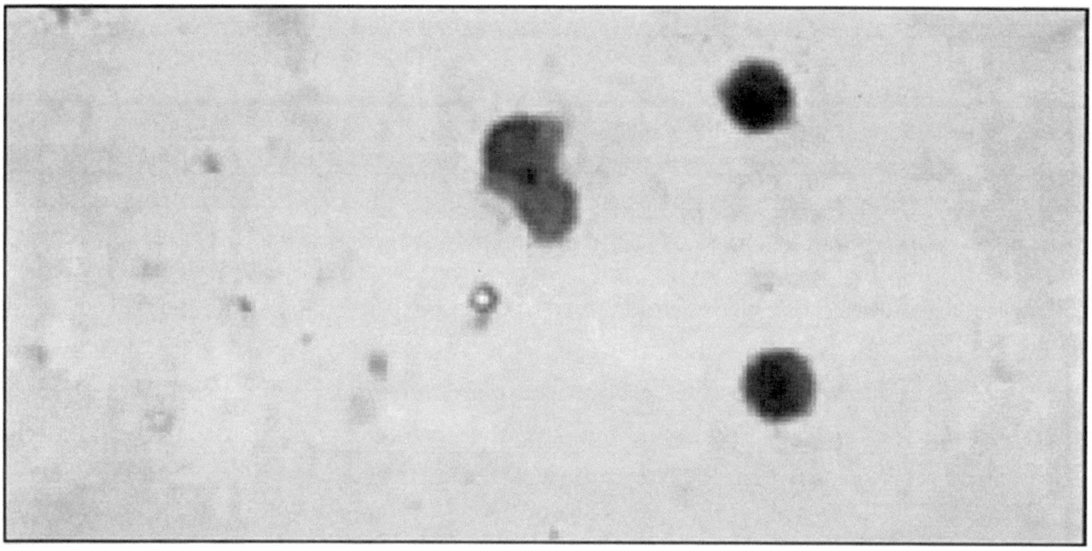

<u>Figure 263:</u> Cytologic study of the vitreous specimen garnered from a diagnostic vitrectomy reveals markedly atypical lymphoid cells in a case later proven to be intraocular lymphoma.

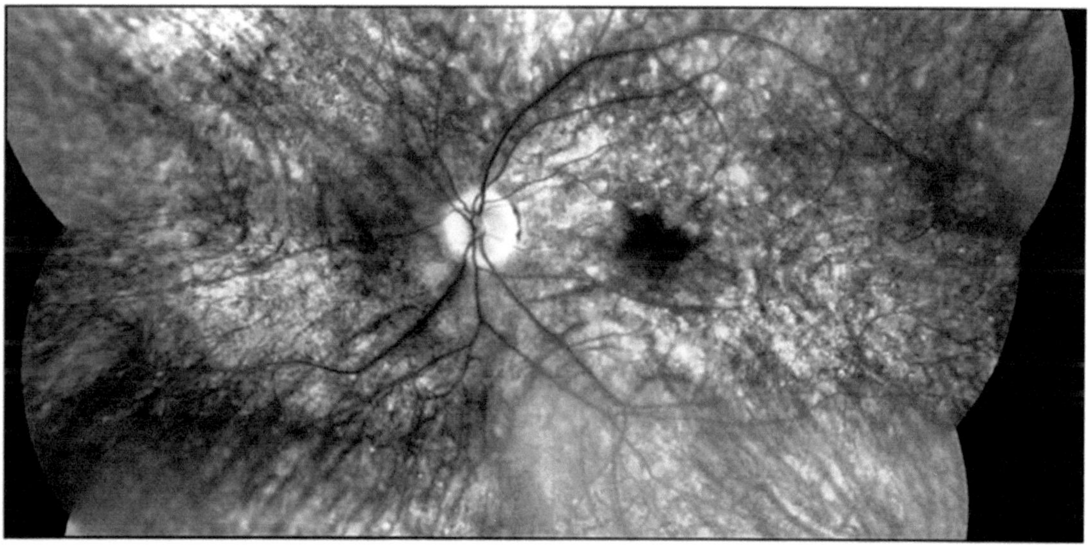

<u>Figure 264:</u> Large areas of chorioretinal atrophy, which is a typical finding of intraocular lymphoma.

Retinoblastoma

Definition: Retinoblastoma is the most common ocular tumor of childhood, and represents a malignancy arising from the photoreceptor precursor cells of the retina. This childhood malignancy can masquerade as uveitis and must be ruled out in all children presenting with signs or symptoms of intraocular inflammation.

History: The first report of retinoblastoma in medical or ophthalmic literature comes from the mid 18th century, when the case of a 3-year-old girl with bilateral ocular tumors was described. Virchow later coined the term retinal glioma until it was recognized that the tumor arose from the neuroepithelial cells of the retina. Verhoff, of the Massachusetts Eye and Ear Infirmary named the tumor Retinoblastoma. This tumor has been studied extensively as a part of molecular genetics and has been vital to our understanding of how genes cause cancer.

Epidemiology: The incidence of retinoblastoma is 1 in 20,000 children. The vast majority of these tumors present before the age of three years. 40% of cases are familial, the remainder being sporadic. Not all familial cases however, have a positive family history. Seventy percent of these tumors are unilateral,. Familial cases tend to present bilaterally.

Clinical Features: The two most common modes of presentation of retinoblastoma are leukocoria and strabismus. Less commonly, the tumor can present as intraocular inflammation. Other uncommon presentations include secondary glaucoma, proptosis and a pinealblastoma. Distant metastases usually occurs later in the disease,. Intraocular inflammation may manifest as true inflammation as a response to tumor necrosis or it may present as simulated inflammation as tumor cells enter the anterior chamber. Retinoblastoma may masquerade as any cause of granulomatous uveitis including tuberculous and syphilitic uveitis. It is essential to consider and exclude retinoblastoma in any major disease in the eye of a child which precludes a fundal view as a delay in the diagnosis of this tumor is associated with spread and associated high mortality.

Pathogenesis: The genetics of retinoblastoma have been of great interest to molecular biologists. Human cells are known to carry two copies of the retinoblastoma gene (Rb), a cancer suppressor or proto-oncogene, located on chromosome 13q14. In familial cases, children are born with one normal and one defective copy of the Rb gene. The second copy is lost through some form of somatic mutation. Loss of both copies of the allele gives rise to retinoblastoma. In sporadic cases, both normal Rb genes are lost by somatic mutation in one of the retinoblasts. Thus the mutations are present in the progeny of this retinoblast, which then forms the tumor.

Diagnosis: Retinoblastoma should be ruled out in any pediatric patient presenting with leukoria, strabismus, or uveitis . The differential diagnosis of leukoria includes persistent hyperplasic primary vitreous, posterior cataract, retrolental fibroplasia, retinoblastoma, coloboma of the choroid or optic disc and uveitis. In pediatric cases suspected of this malignancy, a family history is vital, followed by a complete eye examination. The fundal examination is usually carried out under general anesthesia, with careful documentation of the size and location of the tumor. Bone marrow aspiration and biopsy, and a lumbar puncture for cytocentrifuge examination may also be performed. Ancillary tests include CT of the orbit and head, which can rule out the presence of a pinealoblastoma, but CT scanning is of limited value in evaluating optic nerve head involvement.

Treatment: The targets for treatment in the case of retinoblastoma are the complete control of malignancy and the preservation of vision. The most commonly used treatment in patients with good prognostic factors is external beam radiation. Photocoagulation and cryotherapy are other modes of therapy. Enucleation should be considered in all eyes where there is no chance of preserving useful vision. Overall, in countries where adequate medical care facilitates early detection and treatment of this disease, the prognosis of retinoblastoma is favorable.

Reference:

Waheed NK, Foster CS. Masquerade Syndromes: Malignant; in: Foster CS, Vitale AT. *Diagnosis and treatment of uveitis*. Saunders. Philadelphia 2002:513-517.

Endophthalmitis

Introduction: Chronic postoperative endophthalmitis is characterized by recurrent episodes of low-grade inflammation, usually occurring one month after a surgical procedure, secondary to microbial invasion. Endogenous endophthalmitis is an infection due to microbes seeded to the eye from the vascular circulation, usually from an infection focus distant from the eye. These two forms of endophthalmitis can masquerade as noninfectious inflammation and uveitis.

History: Roussel and colleagues used the term chronic postoperative endophthalmitis reporting 2 cases of endophthalmitis due to Propionibacterium acnes.

Epidemiology: There are no clear statistics of the incidence of chronic postoperative endophthalmitis as cases are rare and may go undiagnosed. Endogenous endophthalmitis is uncommon, accounting for 2-8% of all endophthalmitis cases. It often occurs in immunocompromised patients such as patients with diabetes mellitus, malignancy, organ transplant, SLE, and HIV.

Clinical Features: In chronic postoperative endophthalmitis, the inflammatory episodes may occur months to years after the surgery. These usually run an indolent course and respond well to topical or periocular steroids. The inflammatory episodes typically recur when the steroid therapy is discontinued. The hallmark of the disease is a white plaque between the intraocular lens and the posterior capsule. Other features include hypopyon, iris nodules, vitritis, vascular occlusions and retinal hemorrhages, and elevated intraocular pressure.

In endogenous endophthalmitis, the patient presents with blurred vision, pain and photophobia. The vision is typically markedly decreased, to counting fingers or light perception. Other features include periorbital edema, cells, flare, hypopyon, anterior chamber fibrin, corneal edema, and elevated intraocular pressure. Vitreal condensations, such as fluff balls and pearls on a string, are associated with fungal infection.

Pathology/Pathogenesis: Organisms associated with this chronic form of postoperative infection are: P acnes, coagulase-negative Staphylococcus, Corynebacterium sp., Actinomyces, Nocardia, and Candida.

In endogenous endophthalmitis, the most common foci of infection in immunocompromised hosts are urinary tract infection, liver or gastrointestinal abscess, meningitis, cellulitis, cholecystitis and pneumonia. As for immunocompetent individuals, the infection is usually associated with endocarditis, periodontal infection, intravenous drug abuse, and indwelling intravenous catheter. Gram-positive bacteria (S aureus and streptococcal species) account for most bacterial cases and Candida is the most common cause of endogenous fungal endophthalmitis.

Diagnosis: Isolation of the microbe by Gram stain or culture of an aqueous or vitreous (ideally both) sample is essential for diagnosis.

Treatment: In chronic postoperative endophthalmitis, surgical management and total capsulectomy is more successful than treatment with intraocular antibiotics alone.

In endogenous endophthalmitis, treatment must include intravitreal antibiotics. Systemic antibiotic therapy may be used, especially when an extra-ocular focus of infection is identified.. The role of vitrectomy in endogenous endophthalmitis is not clear.

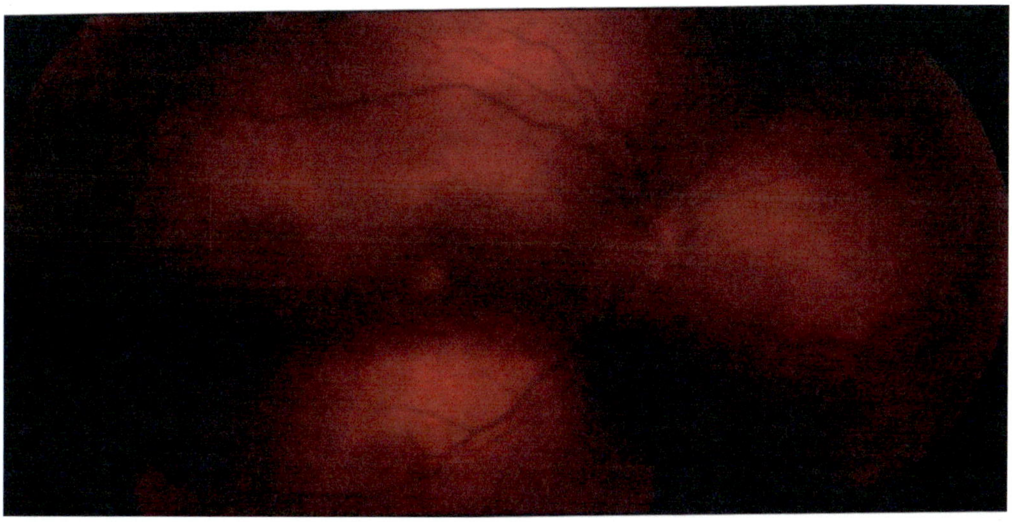

Figure 265: Superior retinal hemorrhage with juxtafoveal choroidal infiltrate in a patient with Candida albicans endophthalmitis.

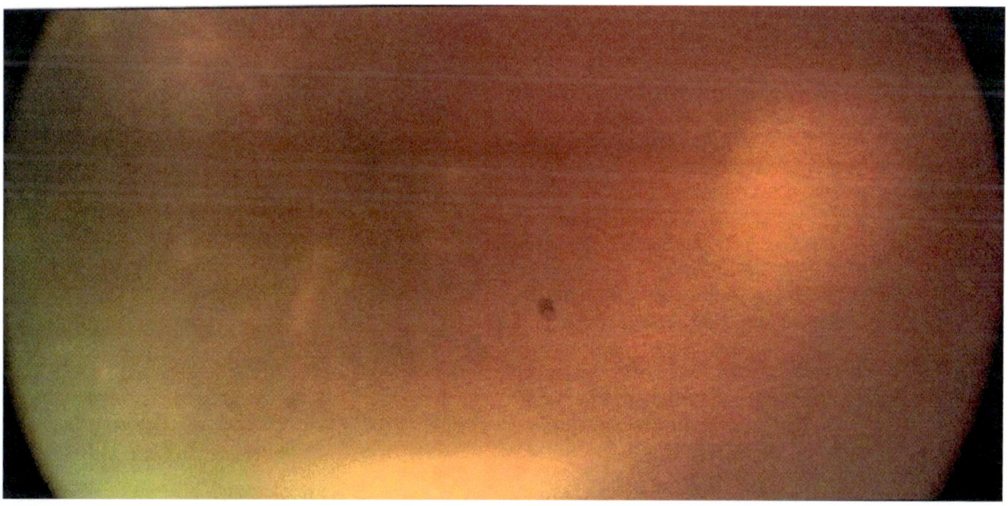

Figure 266: Retinal hypopyon secondary to S. aureus endophthalmitis. The hazy view is due to pronounced corneal edema.

Reference:

Samson CM, Foster CS. Endophthalmitis; in: Foster CS, Vitale AT. *Diagnosis and treatment of uveitis.* Saunders. Philadelphia 2002:528-536.

Intraocular Foreign Body

Definition: An intraocular foreign body (IOFB) may lodge into the anterior or posterior segment. Most IOFBs are metallic. These are usually small and sharp, and the entry site may be small and self-sealing. Various degrees of inflammation can follow a retained IOFB, with possible resulting anterior or posterior uveitis.

Epidemiology: The peak incidence of ocular injuries ranges from age 18-25 with males having a higher incidence than females.

Clinical Features: The clinical features depend on the size, nature, and location of the FB. Patients may have a transient stinging sensation and minimal pain. If the FB is large, the vision can be severely compromised due to a collapsed anterior chamber, hyphema, or vitreous hemorrhage. A corneal track or uveal pigment over sclera are usual signs of IOFB. Other signs include an iris hole, localized iris hemorrhage, iris transillumination or irregularity, lens capsule rupture, cataract, vitreous hemorrhage, and decreased intraocular pressure. Metallic foreign bodies, such as iron and copper, can cause specific toxic reactions termed siderosis and chalcosis, respectively. Other foreign bodies can be inert and become encapsulated in the eye. Uveitis secondary to an IOFB can present with pain, redness, photophobia, cells and flare, keratic precipitates, and vitreous opacities.

Pathology/Pathogenesis: The pathophysiologic mechanisms of the eye response to IOFB include mechanical, chemical/toxic, and inflammatory responses.

Diagnosis: A detailed history, including history of high risk activities, is essential for diagnosis. Careful examination for an entry wound is required. Gonioscopy should be performed to rule out an IOFB lodged in the anterior chamber angle. Dilated retinal exam with an indirect ophthalmoscope must be performed. Other tests such as plain film radiography, CT scanning, ultrasonography can be useful to detect and localize the IOFB. MM scanning is more useful in detecting vegetable, glass or plastic IOFBs, when the CT scan does not reveal a metallic FB.

Treatment: Metallic, magnetic, and vegetable matter should be removed promptly to avoid toxic reactions and endophthalmitis. Most nonorganic and nonmetallic FBs are usually inert and do not necessitate an aggressive approach. It is recommended that most IOFBs should be surgically removed by means of electromagnets or vitrectomy.

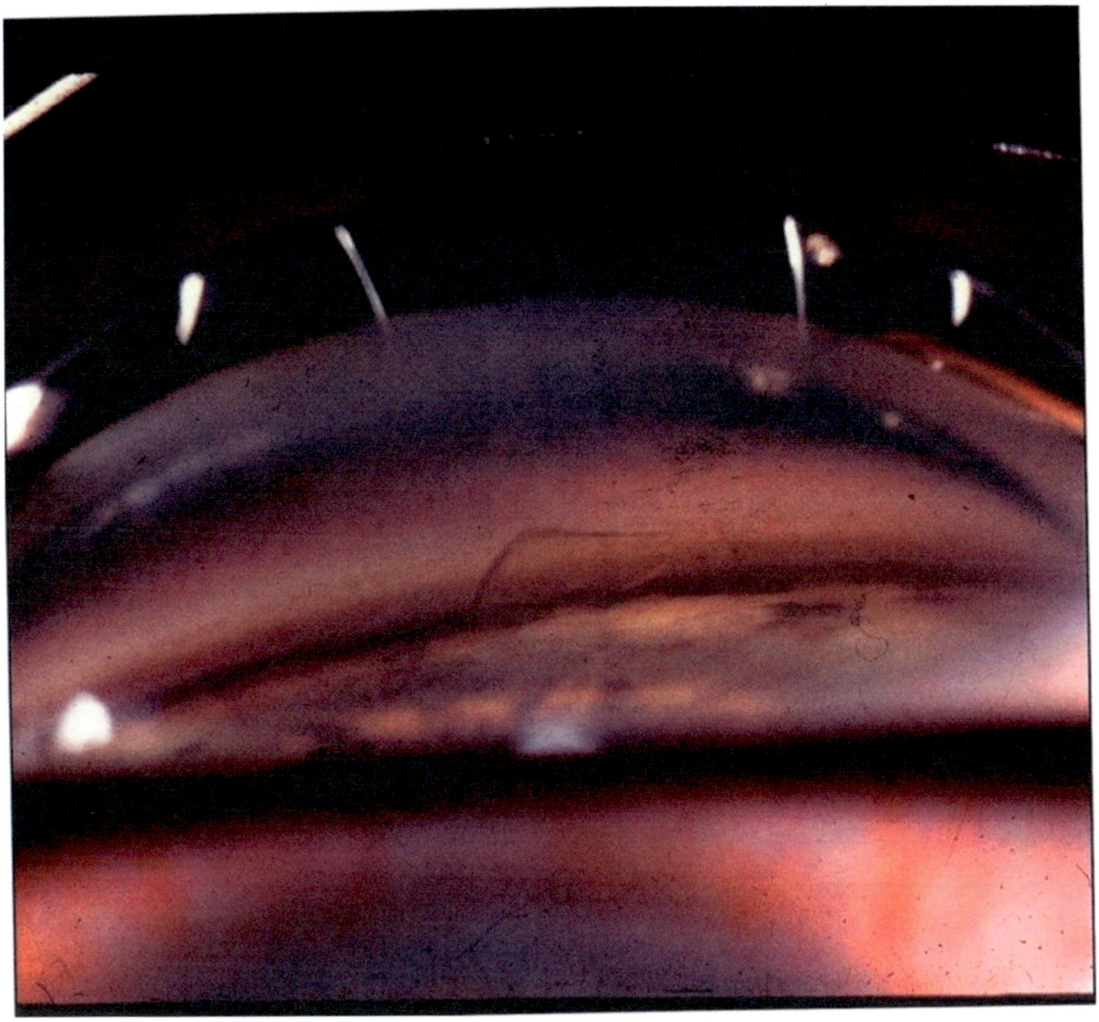

Figure 267: Residual foreign body (glass) in the angle resulting from trauma.

Reference:

Yao L, Foster CS. Intraocular Foreign Body; in: Foster CS, Vitale AT. Diagnosis and treatment of uveitis. Sauders. Philadelphia 2002:546-550.

Juvenile Xanthogranuloma

Definition: Juvenile Xanthogranuloma (JXG) is an inflammatory disorder mainly affecting the skin. It is characterized by multiple cutaneous papules. It affects infants and young children. It can occasionally affect the eye. The iris is the most commonly involved structure..

History: Adamson first reported this disease in 1905. Blank et al. then described ocular involvement in 1949.

Epidemiology: Most patients with JXG are younger than 2 years old at the time of presentation. No race or gender predilection has been described. Seventy-five percent of patients with JXG have skin manifestations only. Among patients with intraocular involvement, 85% present during the first year of life. The ocular lesions are usually unilateral, mostly regressing within months to years. JXG is rarely seen in adults.

Clinical Features:

Systemic Manifestations: The skin lesions consist of single or multiple, yellow/pink nodules up to 1 cm in diameter. They appear on the scalp, head, and neck. These commonly regress spontaneously. Extracutaneous lesions can involve the lungs, testes, spleen, gastrointestinal tract, pericardium, and bone.

Ocular Manifestations: Iris infiltration is the most common ophthalmic manifestation of JXG. This is characterized by a localized nodule or diffuse thickening of the iris stroma. The lesion can be highly vascular and may bleed spontaneously causing a hyphema and secondary glaucoma. Hyphema may manifest as the initial clinical sign of the disease. Other ocular manifestations include: salmon or yellow lymphomatous infiltration of the conjunctiva, sclera, and cornea. Lid nodules and orbital granulomas may cause proptosis. Infiltration of the optic nerve may cause obliteration of the central retinal artery and vein causing a serosanguineous retinal detachment. Chorioretinal infiltration may occur in the form of multiple subretinal lesions in the posterior pole with associated exudative retinal detachment. JXG can present with red eye, anterior chamber reaction, and may masquerade as childhood uveitis.

Pathology/Pathogenesis: The etiology is unknown. The lesions that infiltrate the iris are formed by normal histiocytes, and occasional inflammatory cells.

Diagnosis: Clinical diagnosis can be confirmed by means of skin biopsy. In cases without the skin lesions, the diagnosis may be more difficult to establish. An aqueous paracentesis with or without iris biopsy may reveal histiocytes and Touton cells confirming the diagnosis.

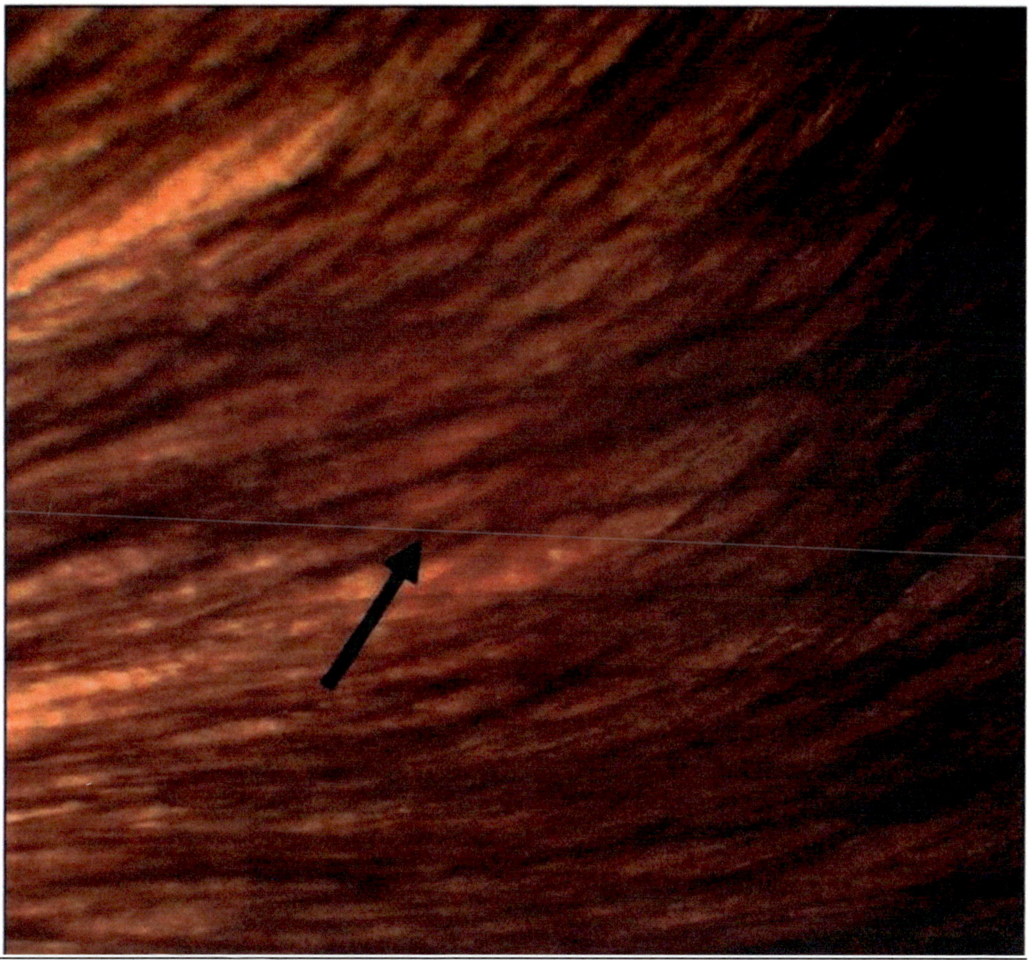

Figure 268: Juvenile xanthogranuloma-related slightly elevated papulonodule located on the scalp of an infant.

Treatment: The goal of treatment is inflammation control in the anterior chamber and the reduction of elevated intraocular pressure. Treatment options include: topical or subconjunctival steroids, and antiglaucoma therapy with acetazolamide. Systemic steroids and low-dose irradiation (300-400 cGy) can be considered in case of recurrent hyphema and glaucoma. Ocular involvement limited to the eyelid or epibulbar area does not require specific treatment.

Reference

1) Yao L, Foster CS. Juvenile Xanthogranuloma; in: Foster CS, Vitale AT. *Diagnosis and treatment of uveitis.* Saunders. Philadelphia 2002:556-558.

Pigment Dispersion Syndrome

Definition: It is characterized by a release of pigment from the epithelium of the iris or ciliary body with a deposition of pigment on intraocular structures such as the corneal endothelium, trabecular meshwork, iris, and lens. This particle dispersion can resemble anterior chamber inflammatory cells, and it can be mistaken for uveitis.

History: Von Hippel first observed the presence of pigment in the aqueous outflow in 1901. Sugar first hypothesized the possible relationship between pigment accumulation and glaucoma, and in 1949 applied the term pigmentary glaucoma.

Epidemiology: The prevalence is not known. Risk factors include: young age, male gender, myopia, and white race. The mean age of development is between 35-45 years of age. The majority of patients do not develop glaucoma.

Clinical Features: Pigment deposition on the corneal endothelium is generally in a central, vertical, spindle-shaped pattern called the Krukenberg spindle. Loss of pigment from the midperipheral pigmented epithelium of the iris results in radial transillumination defects. Gonioscopy usually shows an open angle with heavy, dark brown band of hyperpigmentation in the trabecular meshwork (TM) and inferior to Schwalbe's line (Sampaolesi line). IOP may be normal or elevated. A pigment ring on the lens can be observed at the insertion of the zonules on the posterior capsule. Iris heterochromia, due to pigment granules on the iris stroma giving it a darker appearance, can also be observed.

Pathology/Pathogenesis: Pigment granules may be released from the pigment epithelium of the iris due to contact friction. This is attributed to a backward bowing of the posterior peripheraliris against zonules that insert anteriorly on the lens surface. Released pigment is deposited in the trabecular meshwork, where small amounts can be phagocytized by the endothelial cells. Trapped pigment can cause obstruction of outflow and elevated IOP.

Diagnosis: This is a clinical diagnosis, characterized by peripheral slit like transillumination defects, increased TM pigmentation, Krukenberg's spindle, posterior concave iris, and normal or high IOP. Anterior segment ultrasound biomicroscopy can aid with a view of the peripheral iris relation to the anterior chamber and lens. RDs, lattice degeneration, retinal breaks are common findings in these patients. The optic nerve usually has a normal appearance.

Treatment: Regular examination is important in the management of these patients. IOP, optic nerve, and visual fields should be measured regularly. Medical therapy includes adrenergic antagonists and agonists. Laser trabeculoplasty and peripheral iridotomy have been shown to be effective. Filtrating surgery should be reserved for cases unresponsive to medical therapy or laser.

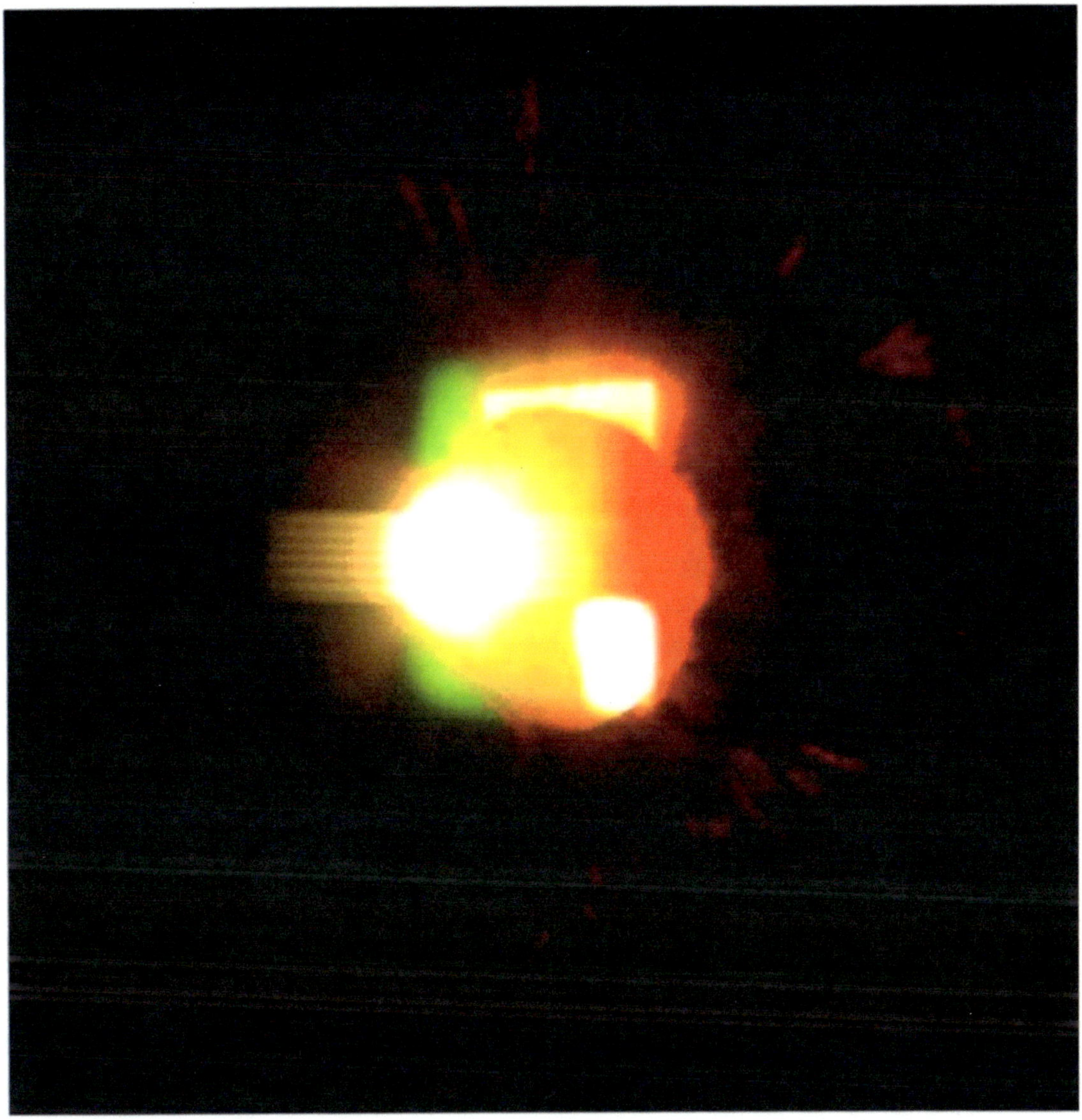

Figure 269: Loss of pigment from the midperipheral pigmented iris epithelium resulting in radial transillumination defects in pigment dispersion syndrome.

Reference:

Yao L, Foster CS. Pigment Dispersion Syndrome; in: Foster CS, Vitale AT. *Diagnosis and treatment of uveitis*. Saunders. Philadelphia 2002:550-553.

Retinitis Pigmentosa

Introduction: This is a group of hereditary retinal degenerative disease. It is characterized by progressive degeneration of retinal photoreceptors, and associated pigmented epithelial changes. Retinitis Pigmentosa (RP) can be classified as primary or secondary. Primary RP is confined to the eye and includes rod or cone degeneration and congenital onset disorders. Secondary RP is associated with single or multiple organ system diseases. RP can be inherited as autosomal dominant, autosomal recessive, or X-linked trait. Patients with RP can also have features of inflammatory disease such as pigmented vitreous cells, cystoid macular edema, and posterior subcapsular cataract, therefore this condition has been considered one of the masquerade syndromes.

History: In 1855, ponders first used the term retinitis pigmentosa to describe the disease.

Epidemiology: Worldwide, the incidence of RP is estimated to be 1 in 3500 to 4000.

Clinical Features: An Early symptom is night blindness. As it progresses, patients lose the far-peripheral field of vision, and eventually central vision can be affected. Cystoid macular edema, macular atrophy, or posterior subcapsular cataract can also affect central vision. Fundus exam findings can include small focal depigmened spots in the mid and far periphery, attenuated retinal vessels, widespread hypopigmentation, peripheral pigment migration and clumping, the characteristic bone-spicule pattern, pale optic nerve, vitreous cells or condensations.

Pathology/Pathogenesis: Histopathologic studies have shown a primary defect in the rod and cone photoreceptors, and dysfunction of retinal pigment epithelium (RPE) cells. At least 50 different mutations in rhodopsin have been found in families with autosomal dominant RP.

Diagnosis: Bilateral night blindness and progressive peripheral visual loss, starting in childhood or adolescence, with familial occurrence are the typical symptoms and history. Medical and neurological examinations are recommended in patients with RP. In patients with typical RP, depending on the severity of the disease, the electroretinogram typically shows diminished or extinguished amplitude of the a-wave and b-wave mainly in the dark-adapted state. Another typical feature is progressive visual field loss.

Treatment: Management should include periodic ocular examinations, psychological and genetic counseling, and improvement of visual function by treating refractive errors and cataracts. Peribulbar or oral steroids, as well as carbonic anhydrase inhibitors can be used for treatment of cystoid macular edema. There is no proven effective treatment to slow or halt visual loss in patients with RP.

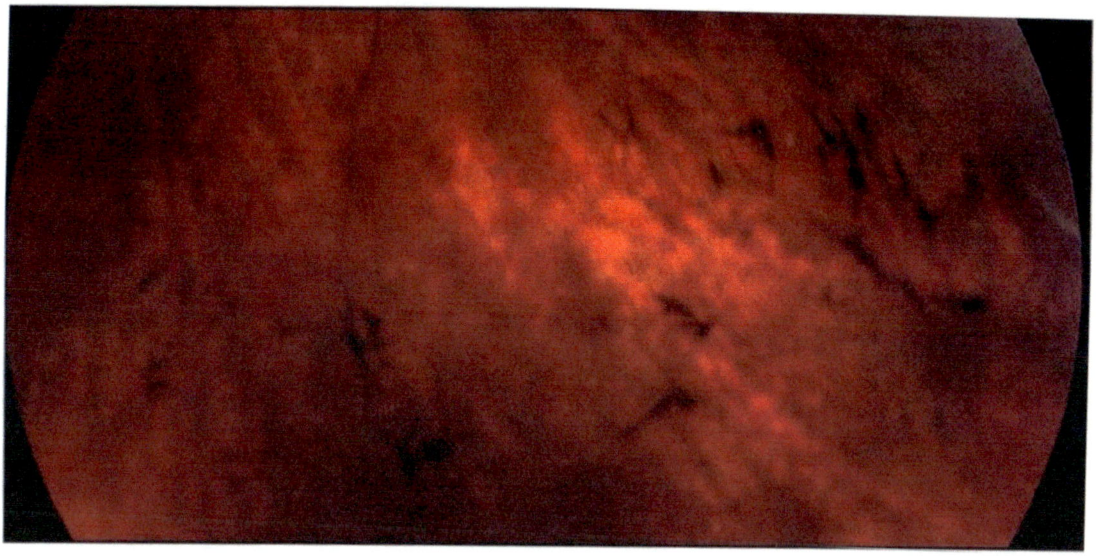

Figure 270: Inferior bone spicules in a case of atypical retinitis pigmentosa in the context of occlusive small-vessel vasculitis.

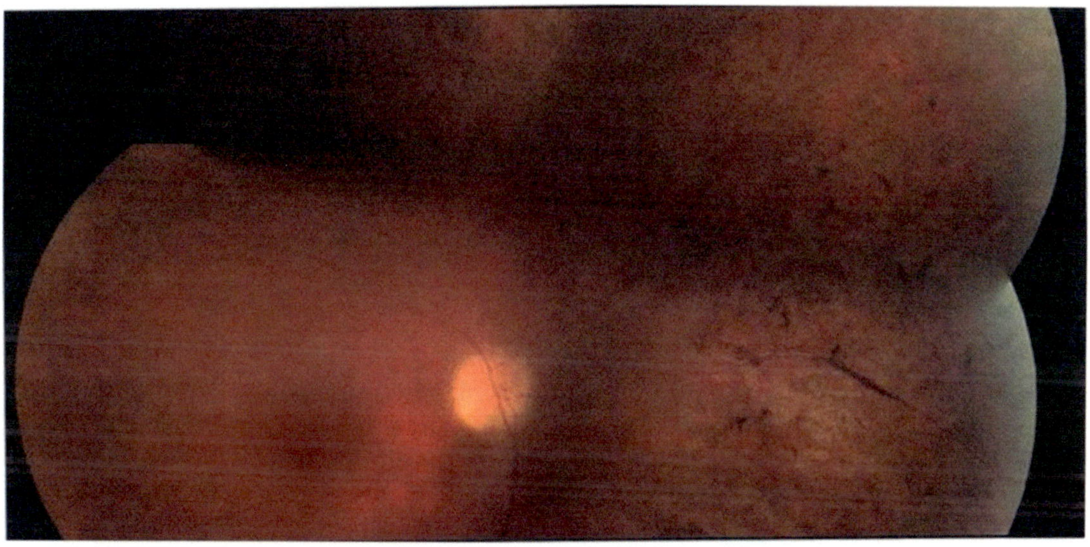

Figure 271: Atypical retinitis pigmentosa with an affected nasal and superior retina.

Reference:

Yao L, Foster CS. Pigment Dispersion Syndrome; in: Foster CS, Vitale AT. *Diagnosis and treatment of uveitis*. Saunders. Philadelphia 2002:541-546.

Rhegmatogenous Retinal Detachment

Introduction: A retinal detachment (RD) is the separation of the sensory retina from the retinal pigment epithelium (RPE), with accumulation of fluid in the space in-between. A rhegmatogenous detachment is one caused by a retinal break, tear, hole or dialyses.

History: After the invention of the direct ophthalmoscope, Coccius first observed a retinal break in 1853. In 1919, Gonin confirmed that retinal breaks cause RDs and that sealing the tear cured the detachment.

Epidemiology: The incidence of rhegmatogenous RD varies, and has been reported as 12.4 to 17.9 per 100,000 population in the United States. The mean age has been reported to be about 54 to 60 years in the US.

Clinical Features: The main symptoms include floaters, photopsias (flashes), shadows, blind areas, and blurred vision secondary to macular detachment or media clouding by pigment, vitreous hemorrhage or inflammatory debris. Relative hypotony is common in these patients. Pigment cells (`tobacco dust') and inflammatory cells in the anterior chamber and vitreous are features that can masquerade this as uveitis. Patients may also develop aqueous flare, concentric iris folds, iridodonesis, posterior synechiae, hazy vitreous, ciliary body or choroidal detachment with hypotony.

Pathology/Pathogenesis: Conditions that increase the risk of retinal breaks and rhegmatogenous RDs are: posterior vitreous detachment (PVD), lattice degeneration, myopia, cystic retinal tufts, degenerative retinoschisis, past history of cataract surgery or trauma to the eye globe.

Diagnosis: Detailed ophthalmic history, searching for predisposing conditions, and ophthalmic examination are essential to diagnose RD. On slit lamp exam, pigment debris can be seen in the anterior chamber and anterior vitreous. The ocular pressure is expected to be lower in the eye with the detachment, but it may also be elevated. On indirect ophthalmoscopy, the detached retina is usually opaque with a corrugated appearance and the subretinal fluid is clear and nonshifting. Ultrasonography is a valuable diagnostic tool in cases when the visibility is poor and the media is opaque, for example if there is vitreous hemorrhage.

Treatment: Surgical procedures include scleral buckling, vitrectomy, and internal or external subretinal fluid drainage. The retina can be pushed outward to contact choroids by application of various foreign materials such as intravitreal gas, or silicone oil. The chorioretinal adhesion may be achieved with cryotherapy, diathermy, or photocoagulation.

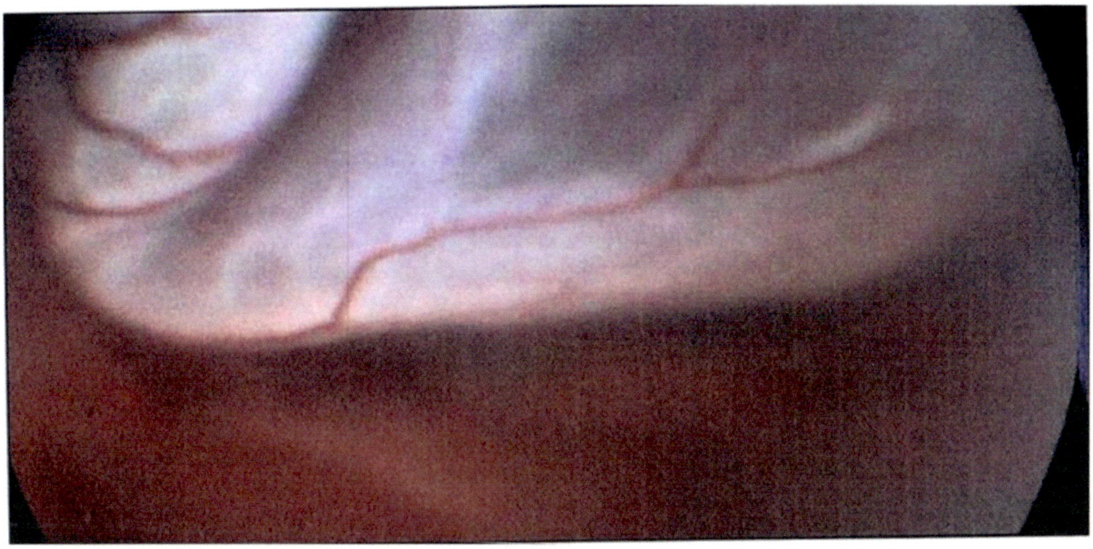

Figure 272: Masquerading rhegmatogenous retinal detachment.

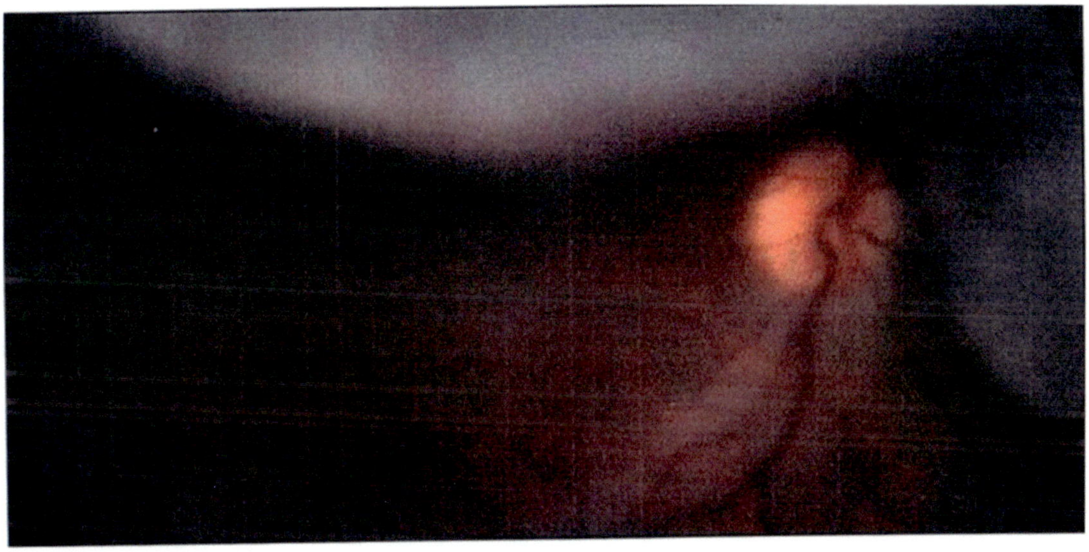

Figure 273: Retinal detachment encroaching upon the macula.

Reference

1) Yao L, Foster CS. Rhegmatogenous Retinal Detachment, in: Foster CS, Vitale AT. *Diagnosis and treatment of uveitis*. Saunders. Philadelphia 2002:537-541

Part Six:

Traumatic Uveitis

Traumatic Uveitis

Definition: Traumatic uveitis can be caused by direct or indirect mechanism. The most common causes are sports injuries, combat injuries, gun ball slingshots and ocular surgery.

Penetrating ocular trauma

The incidence of severe complications is high following penetrating trauma. Early complications include hyphema, ocular hypertension, iridocyclitis, lens dislocation or rupture, corneal and scleral laceration, endophthalmitis, choroidal rupture, and retinal detachment.

Late complications include narrow angle glaucoma, sympathetic ophthalmia, proliferative vitreoretinopathy and retinal or choroidal neovascularization. Penetrating ocular trauma is associated with chronic persistent intraocular inflammation, which often requires additional investigation to rule out other inflammatory stimulants, such as infection. The most commonly found organisms that cause endophthalmitis after penetrating trauma are the Bacillus species. Ocular trauma can also reactivate a latent herpetic infection.

Sympathetic ophthalmia is a well known complication of ocular trauma, although uncommon, it has significant morbidity. The bilateral granulomatous inflammation can occur several days to decades after the initial insult.

Nonpenetrating Ocular trauma

The main feature of ocular blunt trauma is the presence of iridocyclitis that can be associated with hyphema, miosis, ocular hypotony, ciliary flush or hemorrhage and fibrin formation in the anterior chamber. Occasionally, blunt ocular trauma may unmask a real uveitic entity. This must be suspected if the patient has a disproportionate amount of ocular inflammation following minor trauma.

Pathogenesis: morphologic reactions occur in ocular tissues. These changes include hyperemia, vasodilation, increased tissue permeability of blood vessels, disruption of the blood-ocular barrier and later a consequent cellular inflammatory response.

Treatment: Traumatic uveitis responds well to topical steroid in most patients. In severe cases, periocular or systemic steroids may be required. Supportive therapy includes cycloplegics like 1% atropine sulfate or scopolamine hydrobromide.

References:

1) Aburn N. Eye injuries in indoor cricket at Wellington Hospital: a survey January 1987 to June 1989. *N Z Med J*. 1990 Sep 26;103(898): 454-6.
2) MacEwen CJ. Sport associated eye injury: a casualty department survey. *Br J Ophthalmol.* 1987 Sep;71(9):701-5.
3) Heier JS, Enzenauer RW, Wintermeyer SF, Delaney M, LaPiana FP. Ocular injuries and diseases at a combat support hospital in support of Operations Desert Shield and Desert Storm. *Arch Ophthalmol.* 1993 Jun;111(6):795-8.
4) Bullock JD, Ballal DR, Johnson DA, Bullock RJ. Ocular and orbital trauma from water balloon slingshots. A clinical, epidemiologic, and experimental study. *Ophthalmology*. 1997 May; 104(5):878-87
5) Affeldt JC, Flynn HW Jr, Forster RK, Mandelbaum S, Clarkson JG, Jarus GD. Microbial endophthalmitis resulting from ocular trauma. *Ophthalmology*. 1987 Apr;94(4):407-13
6) Verbraeken H, Rysselaere M.Post-traumatic endophthalmitis. *Eur J Ophthalmol.* 1994 Jan-Mar;4(1):1-5
7) Seymour R, Ramsey MS. Unusually severe traumatic uveitis associated with occult ankylosing spondylitis. *Can J Ophthalmol.* 1991 Apr;26(3):156-8.
8) Rosenbaum JT, Tammaro J, Robertson JE Jr. Uveitis precipitated by nonpenetrating ocular trauma. *Am J Ophthalmol.* 1991 Oct 15;112(4): 392-5.

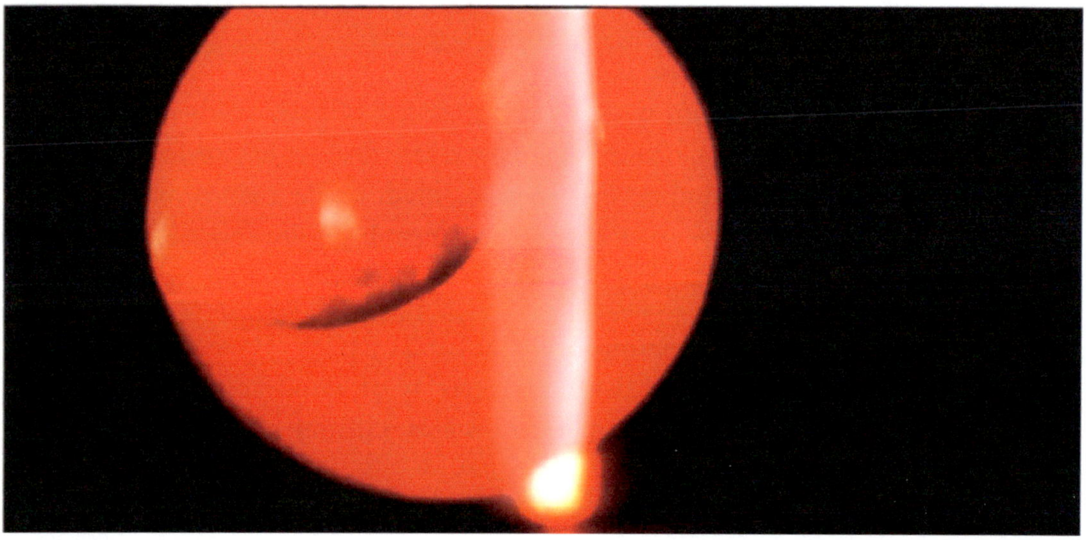

Figure 274: Transillumination view of a dislocated lens secondary to traumatic uveitis.

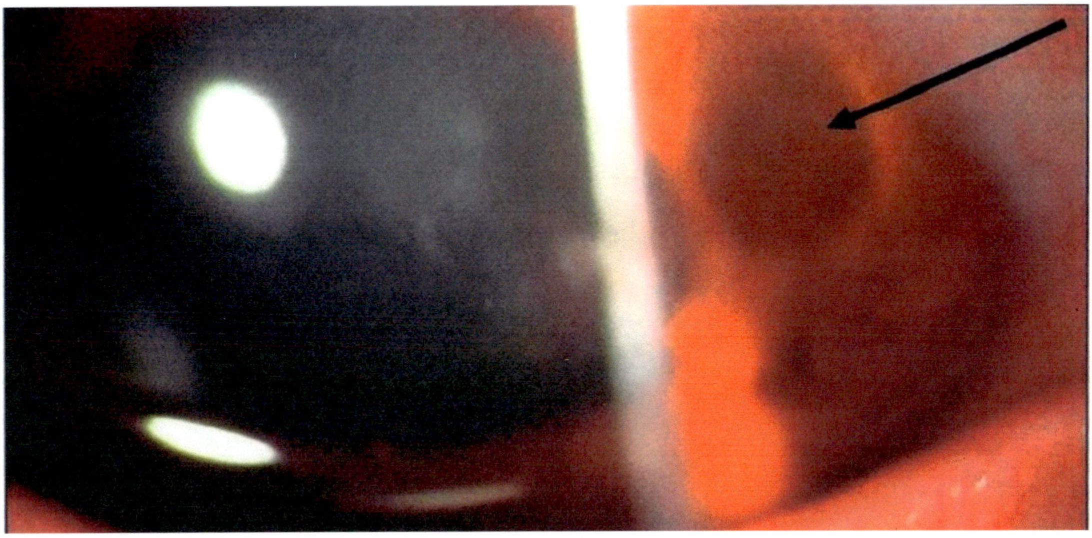

Figure 275: Nasal peripheral ulcerative keratitis secondary to traumatic uveitis.

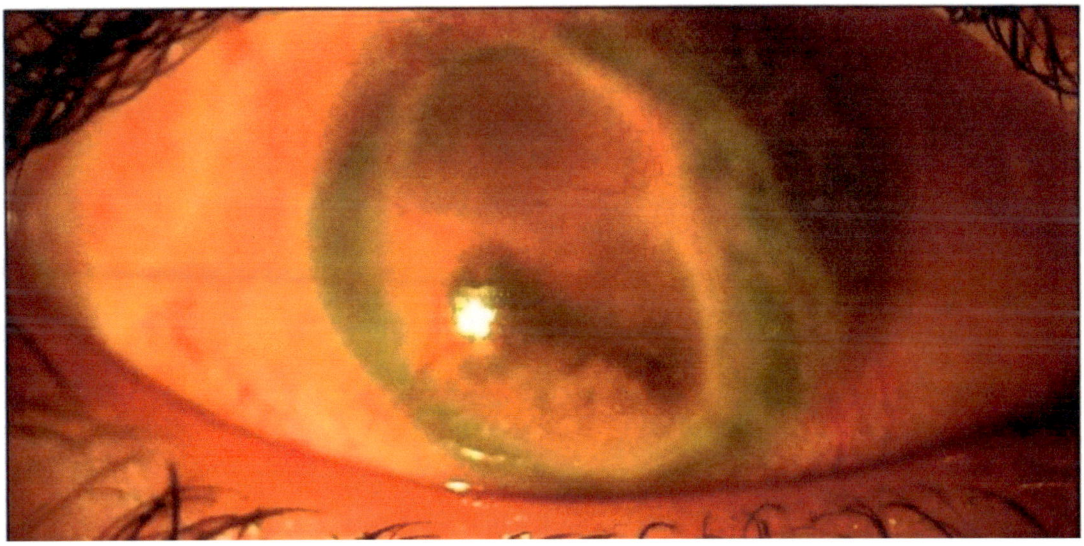

Figure 276: Secluded pupil and corneal neovascularization in a patient with traumatic uveitis.

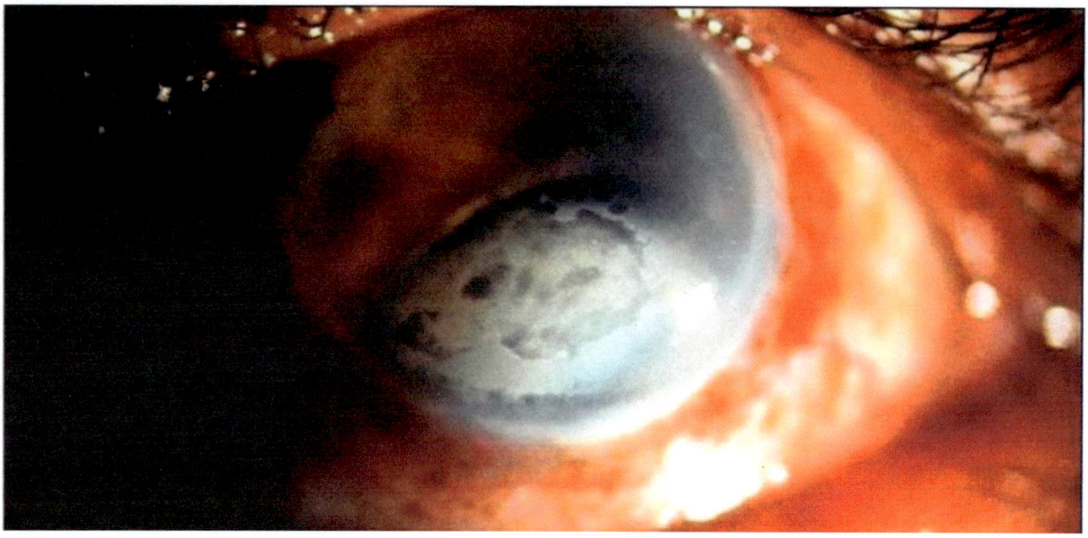

Figure 277: Traumatic uveitis with inferior and central corneal scarring.

The Ocular Immunology and Uveitis Foundation is a 501c(3), not-for-profit, tax-exempt organization. Our mission is to find cures for ocular inflammatory diseases, to correct the worldwide deficit of properly trained ocular immunologists, and to provide education and emotional support for those patients afflicted with ocular inflammatory disease.

We Believe…

* In this day and age, no patients should suffer with poor treatment for ocular inflammatory disease.

* A cure is possible for ocular inflammatory disease.

* We can correct the deficit of properly trained ocular immunologists.

* Patients should have ample support during this time of need.

www.uveitis.org

Made in the USA
Las Vegas, NV
03 November 2026

57421544R00202